APHASIOLOGY

T0383635

Volume 21   Number 6/7/8   June/July/August 2007

CONTENTS

36th Clinical Aphasiology Conference
Ghent University, Ghent, Belgium, May 29th to June 2nd, 2006

Editor

Audrey L. Holland, Regents' Professor Emerita, Department of Speech and Hearing Sciences, University of Arizona, Tucson, AZ, USA

Reviewers

Beth Armstrong
Carl Coehlo
Melissa Duff
Jean Gordon
Maya Henry
Leonard LaPointe
Laura Murray
Maggie Rogers
Barbara Shadden
Connie Tompkins
Heather Wright

Peggy Blake
Mike Dickey
Charles Ellis
Aviah Gvion
Will Hula
Nadine Martin
Sara Orjada
Katie Ross
Lew Shapiro
Kathy Youse

Heather Clark
Patrick Doyle
Naama Friedman
Julie Hengst
Richard Katz
Malcolm McNeil
Don Robin
Nina Simmons Mackie
Julie Stierwalt
Julie Wambaugh

APHASIOLOGY

SUBSCRIPTION INFORMATION

Subscription rates to Volume 21, 2007 (12 issues) are as follows:
To individuals: UK £494.00; Rest of World $817.00
To institutions: UK £1175.00; Rest of World $1940.00
A subscription to the print edition includes free access for any number of concurrent users across a local area network to the online edition, ISSN 1464-5041.
Print subscriptions are also available to individual members of the British Aphasiology Society (BAS), on application to the Society.

For a complete and up-to-date guide to Taylor & Francis's journals and books publishing programmes, visit the Taylor and Francis website: http://www.tandf.co.uk/

Aphasiology (USPS permit number 001413) is published monthly. The 2007 US Institutional subscription price is $1940.00. Periodicals Postage Paid at Jamaica, NY by US Mailing Agent Air Business Ltd, c/o Priority Airfreight NY Ltd, 147-29 182nd Street, Jamaica, NY 11413, USA. **US Postmaster**: Please send address changes to Air Business Ltd, c/o Priority Airfreight NY Ltd, 147-29 182nd Street, Jamaica, NY 11413, USA.
Dollar rates apply to subscribers in all countries except the UK and the Republic of Ireland where the pound sterling price applies. All subscriptions are payable in advance and all rates include postage. Journals are sent by air to the USA, Canada, Mexico, India, Japan and Australasia. Subscriptions are entered on an annual basis, i.e. from January to December. Payment may be made by sterling cheque, dollar cheque, international money order, National Giro, or credit card (AMEX, VISA, Mastercard).

Orders originating in the following territories should be sent direct to the local distributor.
India: Universal Subscription Agency Pvt. Ltd, 101–102 Community Centre, Malviya Nagar Extn, Post Bag No. 8, Saket, New Delhi 110017.
Japan: Kinokuniya Company Ltd, Journal Department, PO Box 55, Chitose, Tokyo 156.
USA, Canada and Mexico: Psychology Press, a member of Taylor & Francis, 325 Chestnut St, Philadelphia, PA 19106, USA
UK and other territories: Psychology Press, c/o T&F Customer Services, Informa UK Ltd, Sheepen Place, Colchester, Essex, CO3 3LP, Tel: +44 (0)20 7017 5544; Fax: +44 (0)20 7017 5198; UK.
E-mail: tf.enquiries@tfinforma.com

Typeset by H. Charlesworth & Co. Ltd., Wakefield, UK, and printed by Hobbs the Printers Ltd., Totton, Hants, UK. The online edition can be reached via the journal's website: http://www.psypress.com/aphasiology

Back issues: Taylor & Francis retains a three-year back issue stock of journals. Older volumes are held by our official stockists: Periodicals Service Company, 11 Main Street, Germantown, NY 12526, USA, to whom all orders and enquiries should be addressed. Tel: +1 518 537 4700; Fax: +1 518 537 5899; E-mail: psc@periodicals.com; URL: http://www.periodicals.com/tandf.html

APHASIOLOGY, 2007, 21 (6/7/8), 533

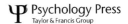

Introduction

The 36th Clinical Aphasiology Conference that spawned these Proceedings was unique. It was held in Ghent Belgium, the first CAC meeting to be held outside North America. As a result, the 2006 CAC attracted a substantial number of submissions from European researchers and clinicians, many of whom had never attended CAC before. Although I was not able to attend the meeting to see it for myself, colleagues worldwide have remarked on how exciting it was to be there and to find CAC playing on the world stage. It is also exciting to see the increased international presence in the current Proceedings. My wish is that this will be a continuing trend in the future.

This is the last Proceedings that I will be editing. Beth Armstrong will assume this role for a 3 year term starting with the 2007 CAC. I don't know whether to laugh or cry about completing my term—it takes relatively frantic effort to have one year's Proceedings ready for the next year's meeting, but with the help of a superb group of reviewers, it is obvious that it can be done. And I will miss the fun parts, the correspondence with potential authors and reviewers from whom I have learned so much, and pleasures of watching manuscripts shape up on their way to publication. I hope Beth will find, as I have, that the satisfactions outweigh the frustrations of this editing task.

The reviewers listed on the title page have toiled long and hard in the editing of these Proceedings. I have thanked them each privately, but want to thank them publicly for making my job a positive experience.

Audrey L. Holland, PhD
Professor Emerita, University of Arizona, Tuscson, AZ, USA

http://www.psypress.com/aphasiology   DOI: 10.1080/02687030701190038

APHASIOLOGY, 2007, 21 (6/7/8), 535–547

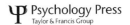

Syntactic and pragmatic aspects of determiner and pronoun production in Dutch agrammatic Broca's aphasia

Esther Ruigendijk

University of Oldenburg, Germany

Sergio Baauw

University of Utrecht, The Netherlands

Background: Agrammatic aphasic individuals produce a lower than normal number of pronouns and determiners in their spontaneous speech. Interestingly, linguistically these two types of functional categories have some properties in common. In Dutch, the language that was studied, both categories depend on case, both are marked for gender, and both carry pragmatic information. These properties relate to different levels of linguistic processing. Case is a *syntactic* property, gender is *lexically* specified for determiners, and *semantically* for pronouns (in Dutch), and the *pragmatic* function relates to the distinction between definiteness and indefiniteness; that is, whether something refers to information already introduced in the discourse or to new information respectively.

Aims: The aim of this study was therefore to find out if and how far each of these properties (case, gender, and pragmatic information) contributes to the problems agrammatic speakers have with the production of determiners and pronouns.

Methods & Procedures: We analysed spontaneous speech samples of eight Dutch-speaking agrammatic aphasic individuals with regard to the omission and production rates of determiners and pronouns, taking into account the different linguistic properties.

Outcomes & Results: The analyses revealed that the syntactic property of determiners and pronouns, *case*, contributes most to the agrammatic problems. Gender information seems to be unproblematic. Finally, our aphasic speakers omitted relatively more indefinite determiners than definite determiners. It is not completely clear yet whether this is related to a problem with indefinites. The error analysis shows that pragmatic information as such seems to be unimpaired.

Conclusions: The syntactic aspects of determiners and pronouns play an important role in the problems agrammatic speakers have with these elements. More detailed research may be needed to investigate the distinction between indefiniteness and definiteness in determiners. Our results suggest that the production of determiners and pronouns should always be treated with a focus on their syntactic property: their dependency on case-assigning categories.

Apart from the well-known impairment in verbs, verb finiteness, and complex sentences, one of the key characteristics of agrammatism in languages like English,

Address correspondence to: Esther Ruigendijk, Carl von Ossietzky Universität, Fak. III, Institut für Fremdsprachenphilologien, Ammerländer Heerstr. 114-118, 26111 Oldenburg, Germany.
E-mail: esther.ruigendijk@uni-oldenburg.de

We thank Arlette Sjerp for carrying out part of the speech analyses.

DOI: 10.1080/02687030701191911

Dutch, and German is the relatively low number of both determiners and pronouns in speech production (see, among others, de Roo, 1999; Menn & Obler, 1988; Ruigendijk, 2002). Determiners are often omitted, and significantly fewer pronouns are used by agrammatic speakers than by non-brain-damaged speakers. It is interesting that determiners and pronouns seem to be problematic at the same time in the same population, since both elements have several properties in common. First, their presence is related to the presence of categories such as verb finiteness and transitive verbs because of the *syntactic* operation of case assignment (following Chomsky, 1981; Giusti, 2002, 2006; Ouhalla, 1993). Case assignment will be discussed in more detail in the next section. Furthermore, in some languages (e.g., Dutch, German) determiners and pronouns are marked for gender. For Dutch determiners, which are studied in this paper, gender marking depends on the *lexically* specified gender of the noun that it modifies. Gender on Dutch pronouns is usually seen as a *semantic* feature, since it depends on—among other aspects—natural gender of the noun that is referred to. And finally, both types of elements have *pragmatic* properties (i.e., properties that play a role at discourse level). Indefinite determiners are used for the introduction of new entities, and definite determiners and pronouns usually refer to given or known information. Apart from these similarities, there is one important difference between determiners and pronouns, which is that pronouns can be used freestanding, whereas determiners can only be used in combination with a noun. Some of the properties of determiners and pronouns have been studied before, however, and as far as we are aware there have been no studies that examined the omission *and* production of determiners *and* pronouns in agrammatism at the same time, taking into account the similarities of these elements. Close examination of these properties may shed light on the exact nature of the agrammatic problems with determiners and pronouns.

The central question of this study is therefore if and how far each of the syntactic, lexical, semantic, and pragmatic properties contributes to the problems agrammatic speakers have with the production of determiners and pronouns.

We will first provide some linguistic background and a description of the Dutch determiner and pronoun system. After that, we will discuss previous studies that investigated aspects of determiner or pronoun production. Then we present the procedure of our spontaneous speech analysis, which we performed to find an answer to our research question. Finally, we will present and discuss our results in the light of the distinction between the syntactic, lexical-semantic, and pragmatic properties of determiners and pronouns.

LINGUISTIC BACKGROUND

Although there are clearly differences in form, function, and characteristics, determiners and pronouns share some important characteristics (case, gender, pragmatic information). These similarities led to the linguistic proposal that both determiners and pronouns[1] are the head (D) of a Determiner Phrase, a DP (Abney, 1987; see also Bernstein, 2001). This analysis is now widely accepted and has

---

[1] In fact we could speak about determiners only, since this term has also been used to include pronouns (Postal, 1966). For the sake of clarity we will use the term "determiner" to refer to an element that is used with a noun and the term "pronoun" for an element that is used freestanding.

TABLE 1
The Dutch article paradigm

	Common	Neuter	Plural
Definite	*de* man "the man" *de* vrouw "the woman"	*het* kind "the child"	*de* kinderen "the children"
Indefinite	*een* man "a man" *een* vrouw "a woman"	*een* kind "a child"	Ø kinderen "children"

the advantage that it can account for the similarities between determiners and pronouns.

In this study we focus on those determiners that can head a DP in Dutch:[2] articles, demonstratives, and possessives. In Table 1 the Dutch paradigm for one type of determiner is provided: articles. Demonstratives are another type of definite determiner, since they have to refer to an entity that has already been introduced in discourse. Demonstratives are also marked for gender and distinguish between entities that are nearby (*deze man* "this man", *dit kind* "this child") and far away (*die man* "that man", *dat kind* "that child"). Possessives also pattern with definite determiners, and are the genitive form of pronouns, which are specified for person, gender (of the antecedent[3]), and number information: *mijn* "my", *jouw* "your", *zijn* "his", *haar* "her", *ons/onze* "our", *jullie* "your", *hun* "their".

Not all nouns require a determiner in Dutch. Legitimate bare nouns are, for example, plurals like *tulpen* "tulips" or mass nouns like *water* "water", and proper names. Plurals and mass nouns may be used with or without a determiner. Used without a determiner they are indefinites, and therefore usually cannot refer back to "old information".

Dutch pronouns can be divided in several subclasses (see Haeseryn, Romijn, Geerts, de Rooij, & van den Toorn, 1997) of which we will be concerned with personal pronouns and demonstratives only. Personal pronouns are marked for gender, person, and number information, just like the possessives mentioned above. Apart from that, Dutch personal pronouns carry case and distinguish between nominative and accusative/objective, as can be seen in Table 2. The demonstrative determiners discussed above can also be used independently as pronouns, and similarly only distinguish gender and distance. Below, we briefly describe the three properties that are the focus of this study: case, gender, and pragmatic information.

---

[2] This study focuses on determiners that, at least in Dutch surface structure, are arguably in D° position. The criterion used for determining whether a determiner is in this position is the fact that it cannot co-occur with an article. Since articles are accepted to be situated in D°, the co-occurrence of an article with another determiner indicates that they occupy different positions. This is the case for numerals and (some) quantifiers, for example, *de drie vrienden* "the three friends" or *de vele boeken* "the many books", as opposed to demonstratives **de deze kamer* "the this room" or possessives **de mijn boek* "the my book".

[3] Only the first person plural possesive *ons/onze* distinguishes between common and neuter gender: *onze auto* "our car" vs *ons huis* "our house".

TABLE 2
The Dutch personal pronoun paradigm

Number	Person	Case			
		Nominative		Objective	
Singular	first	ik ("k)	"I"	mij (me)	"me"
	second	jij (je)	"you"	jou (je)	"you"
	third masculine	hij (ie)	"he"	hem ("m)	"him"
	third feminine	zij (ze)	"she"	haar (d'r)	"her"
	third neuter	het ("t)	"it"	het ("t)	"it"
Plural	first	wij (we)	"we"	ons	"us"
	second	jullie	"you"	jullie	"you"
	third	zij (ze)	"they"	hen/hun (ze)	"them"

Forms of nominative and objective pronouns in Dutch. Unaccented forms are given in brackets.

Case

Case is a linguistic notion that refers to a syntactic relationship between, for instance, a verb and its arguments. It licenses the presence of a noun phrase. According to Chomsky (1981) every visible noun phrase (NP) must have case. If a noun phrase does not have case, an utterance is ungrammatical. This holds for noun phrases in all languages. This Case Filter was adapted slightly after the introduction of the DP analysis (Abney, 1987). Ouhalla (1993) and later Giusti (2002, 2006) suggested that not NPs but DPs must have case—in other words, complete noun phrases; that is, noun phrases with a determiner or pronouns. Both determiners and pronouns are thus dependent on case and case assignment. Noun phrases (DPs) receive their case from case-assigning categories, such as verb finiteness, transitive verbs, or prepositions. Nominative case is assigned to a noun phrase in subject position by a finite verb, and accusative is assigned by the verb to its object (see Ruigendijk, 2002, for a more detailed discussion of case assignment and how this relates to agrammatic speech production). In Dutch, case is not realised morphologically on noun phrases (unlike other languages, like Russian, Finnish, or even German which has overt case marking on the DP, on the determiner, and other constituents of the DP). Dutch pronouns, however, are marked overtly for case and have a different form when they are in subject (nominative) or object position (accusative) as was shown in Table 2.

Gender

Dutch determiners and pronouns are also marked for gender. The processes by which both categories receive this feature are slightly different however. Dutch determiners only distinguish between common (masculine and feminine) and neuter, depending on the gender of the noun, which has to be learned in Dutch—that is, it is assumed to be specified lexically (Deutsch & Wijnen, 1985; Haeseryn et al., 1997). Unlike Romance languages, such as Spanish or Italian, in Dutch the word form gives no clues as to whether the noun is masculine, feminine, or neuter. Although officially masculine and feminine gender are still distinguished in Dutch grammar books and lexicons, most speakers of Dutch are unable to say whether common *de* words are masculine or feminine, with the exception of dialect speakers from southern parts of the Netherlands (see Haeseryn et al., 1997).

For pronouns, gender assignment is dependent on the natural gender of the noun that is referred to. For male humans and animals, masculine *hij* is used; for females feminine *zij*; and for objects it depends on whether the noun that is referred to is countable (in that case most of the time the masculine *hij* "he" is used) or not countable (then most of the time the neuter *het* "it" is used). In this respect Dutch is very similar to English (see van Haeringen, 1956).

Pragmatic information

The third property that determiners and pronouns share is their role on the pragmatic (also discourse) level. This level goes beyond the sentence level. An important distinction made at this *pragmatic* level is the definiteness distinction, which reflects the difference between old and new information (Heim, 1983; Kadmon, 2001). Definite forms (nouns with a definite determiner and pronouns) refer to an antecedent in the discourse (this can be a linguistic antecedent, but also, for example, something in the environment that is being pointed at), whereas indefinite forms (i.e., nouns with an indefinite determiner) introduce new information. Generally, indefinite forms cannot refer to "old" information, as is shown in [1]. In the second sentence "a boy" cannot be used to refer to the boy from the first sentence. The definite "the girl" or the pronoun "her" can refer to the girl from the first sentence.

[1] Een jongen$_j$ en een meisje$_k$ lopen op straat. *Een jongen$_j$ houdt het meisje/haar$_k$ vast.

A boy and a girl walk on the street. *A boy holds the girl/her.

PREVIOUS STUDIES ON DETERMINERS AND PRONOUNS IN AGRAMMATISM

Several studies have shown that determiners and pronouns are often omitted in agrammatism (e.g., Baauw, Roo, & Avrutin, 2002; Hofstede & Kolk, 1994; Menn & Obler, 1988; Saffran, Berndt, & Schwartz, 1989). These problems have been related to syntactic, morphological, or more general processing capacity problems. Baauw et al. (2002), for instance, examined determiner omission in Dutch agrammatism and found that more determiners are omitted in non-finite sentences than in finite sentences. The authors argued that agrammatic speakers' tendency to omit determiners and tense is due to their difficulties with the use of *syntactic* devices to structure information. Hofstede and Kolk (1994), however, assumed that the high omission rates of pronouns and determiners in spontaneous speech production were the result of a reduced *processing* capacity in combination with an adaptation by the patients of their language use to the demands of the situation. Other authors focused on morphological properties. Bates, Wulfeck, and McWhinney (1991), for example, related the problems with determiners (among other inflectional morphemes) to a selective morphological vulnerability on the basis of cross-linguistic comparisons.

Case

There are only a few studies that have investigated determiner and/or pronoun production with regard to their case features. Ruigendijk, van Zonneveld, and Bastiaanse (1999) and Ruigendijk and Bastiaanse (2002), for example, showed that the presence of determiners and pronouns in Dutch and German agrammatic production was related to the presence of case-assigning categories such as transitive verbs and verb finiteness. They therefore argued that the lack of determiners and pronouns in agrammatic production can be at least partly explained by the problems agrammatic speakers have with case-assigning categories, such as verbs and verb finiteness. The idea behind this is that when case cannot be assigned due to the absence of a case-assigning category, determiners and pronouns cannot be realised (see Ruigendijk, 2002, for a detailed account). De Bleser and others (de Bleser, Bayer, & Luzzatti, 1996; de Bleser, Burchert, & Rausch, 2005) examined the abilities of German agrammatic speakers to realise case morphology on articles. They found that although these patients did not use the morphology randomly, they had problems realising the correct article in sentences. Some of the patients applied a default strategy, using the same case most of the time (either nominative or accusative) in both subject and object position; some of the patients only had problems with case morphology in non-canonical sentences (OVS) in which they used the canonical order (SVO). Case assignment in genitive conditions and in prepositional phrases was relatively unimpaired, which led the authors to the assumption that perhaps more distant syntactic relationships (as in OVS) were more impaired than local relationships (as case assignment in PPs).

Gender

Gender information, however, does not seem to be problematic in agrammatism. De Bleser et al. (1996; 2005) did not find problems in the realisation of the article (i.e., masculine, feminine, or neuter) on a single-word task in which German agrammatic speakers had to produce the correct article for a noun. Bastiaanse, Jonkers, Ruigendijk, and van Zonneveld (2003) showed that Dutch and German agrammatic speakers did not make many gender errors in the determiners that they produced on sentence elicitation and production tasks. The same was found for pronouns in spontaneous speech (Ruigendijk, 2002).

Pragmatic information

Less clear results have been obtained on the effect of the pragmatic properties of both determiners and pronouns. Wulfeck et al. (1989) reported no errors in use of articles with respect to definiteness and the distinction between referring to old or new information in English-, German-, and Italian-speaking agrammatic individuals. However, Månsson and Ahlsén (2001) demonstrated that Swedish-speaking agrammatic patients omitted indefinite determiners more often than definite determiners on different tasks (interview, picture description, story telling). Apart from that, Månsson and Ahlsén reported omission and substitution of pronouns. The difference between definite and indefinite determiners may be related to the pragmatic properties of determiners. However, as Havik and Bastiaanse (2004) pointed out, there is also a morphological difference between the two elements in Swedish. Swedish definite determiners are bound morphemes, realised postnominally, whereas indefinite determiners are free prenominal morphemes. The different omission rates could very well be due to the difference between bound and free morphemes. Havik and Bastiaanse (2004) therefore analysed Dutch agrammatic speech production and found a non-significant effect in the opposite direction—higher omission rates for definite than indefinite determiners. However, they concluded (p. 1101) that "definiteness does not play a role in the problematic production of articles in agrammatic speakers".

All the studies discussed so far only investigated one (or two) aspects of determiners or pronouns, and most of these studies focussed on the omission pattern of determiners or pronouns. To unravel the factors that are involved in the agrammatic problems with determiners and pronouns, we replicated the earlier studies described above and in addition analysed the production rates of definite and indefinite articles *and* pronouns in Dutch agrammatic speech production, and examined whether these were produced correctly, with respect to gender and definiteness. Our goal was to acquire a more complete understanding of what exactly causes the problems with determiners and pronouns in agrammatism.

We assume that agrammatism is the result of a syntactic disorder, without discussing the exact nature of this syntactic disorder here (see Avrutin, 2006; Friedmann, 2006; Grodzinsky, 2000), since this would go beyond the scope of this study. Assuming that agrammatism is primarily the result of a syntactic disorder, and taking the earlier findings into account, we expect to find:

- a high omission and low production rate for both determiners and pronouns;
- a relation between the production of determiners and the production of case-assigning elements;
- no effect of definiteness for determiners, and no pragmatic errors for pronouns.

METHOD

We analysed the spontaneous speech production of eight Dutch individuals (four male, four female; mean age 61.1, *SD* 13.02) who were all native speakers of Dutch and diagnosed with Broca's aphasia on the basis of the Aachen Aphasia Battery (a standardised Dutch Aphasia battery; Graetz, de Bleser & Willmes, 1992). Individual data can be found in Appendix 1. The diagnosis was confirmed by their speech therapist and one of the authors (ER). The speech production of all patients was agrammatic, as indicated by problems with verb finiteness and/or a low number of verbs.

The data of the aphasic speakers were compared to those of 12 healthy individuals (6 male, 6 female; mean age 56.3, *SD* 12.86), all native speakers of Dutch. A speech sample of 300 words from each participant was transcribed and analysed following Saffran et al. (1989). This speech sample was elicited with a semi-structured interview which is part of the standard procedure within the Aachen Aphasia test and includes questions like "Can you tell me how your problems with speaking began?", "Can you tell me something about your family", or "Can you tell me something about your job/hobbies?".

First all nouns, determiners, and pronouns were counted. Proper names or fixed expressions were omitted from the data. The nouns were then scored for the presence or absence of a determiner (definite or indefinite). It was determined for all nouns whether they required the presence of a determiner. This resulted in the amount of

Nouns Requiring Determiners (NRDs) which were divided in NRDs with and without determiner. After this, noun phrases containing numerals or quantifiers were not further analysed, and are summarised under "other determiners".

For all NRDs and for all pronouns we examined whether a case-assigning category was present. As discussed above, this means a finite verb, a verb, or a preposition depending on the structural position of the NRD or pronoun. It was then decided whether determiners of the NRDs should be definite (either a definite article, a demonstrative, or a possessive) or indefinite depending on the context (see [2] with utterances of the aphasic speakers and the targets in brackets) or whether this could not be determined, to examine the omission rates of definite and indefinite determiners (represented in determiner/noun ratios).

[2] a. ... is mooi groot huis (target: .. is *een* mooi groot huis. → indefinite missing)
          ... is beautiful big house
     b. ... beslissen en eh slachthuis ja eh commissie (target: not determinable whether definite or indefinite)
          ... deciding and ah slaughterhouse yes ah committee
     c. ... hobbies, nou ja eh tuin spitten (target: ... *de* tuin spitten → definite missing)
          ...hobbies, well ah garden digging

Omission rates were calculated in the form of determiner/noun ratios, which is calculated by dividing the number of NRDs with a determiner by the total number of NRDs. This ratio was also calculated for indefinite NRDs and definite NRDs separately. Finally, for all determiners and pronouns that were realised, we examined whether they were correct with respect to case (pronouns only), gender, and pragmatic use (see [3] for examples of possible errors; note that the case error was not actually found in the data, but constructed).

[3] a. *Example of case error (constructed)*
          ... hem werkt in het ziekenhuis (acc. *hem* instead of *hij*)
          ... him works in the hospital
     b. *Example of gender error (from the data)*
          ... toen ... eh ... de ziekenhuis in H. (common *de* instead of neuter *het*)
          ... then ... ah ... the_{wrong gender} hospital in H.
     c. *Example of definiteness error (from the data)*
          ... er komt de voorstelling (definite *de* instead of indefinite *een*)[4]
          ... there comes the idea
     d. *Example of a pragmatic error (from the data)*
          The interviewer and patient talked about the place where the patient lives. He has just described the house and is about to start describing the garden, and then the interviewer asks: Is it an old farm? Answer: ja ... heeft eh .. gebouwd eh eh kijk in de haag, haag, met hier de haag ... (definite *de* instead of indefinite *een*)
          ... yes .. has ah .. build ah ah ... look in the hedge, hedge, here the hedge

---

[4] In fact this can also be seen as a syntactic error, since the use of a definite (specific) subject with the Dutch expletive "er V ..." construction is—with some exceptions of the "er is" *there is* form—illicit.

RESULTS

The spontaneous speech analysis replicated earlier results, as can be seen in Table 3 (individual data can be found in Appendix 2). Agrammatic speakers realised fewer determiners and pronouns than the controls (Mann Whitney U, determiners: $Z = -3.47$, $p = .000$; pronouns: $Z = -2.55$, $p = .01$). Their determiner/noun ratio was also significantly lower than that of the control group (Mann Whitney U: $Z = -3.74$, $p = .000$).

Case

A relationship was also observed between the realisation of a case-assigning category and the presence of a determiner in the agrammatic data: 85% of nouns with a determiner were realised in the presence of a case assigner and only 15% of nouns with determiner were realised without an available case assigner. Note that the

TABLE 3
Mean scores of the agrammatic and control groups

	Agrammatic group	Control group
# determiners – mean	15.2*	29.1
det/noun ratio	70%*	97%
# pronouns – mean	19.4*	36.8
Case		
with determiner		
+case assigner	85%	n.a.
−case assigner	15%	n.a.
without determiner		
+case assigner	43%	n.a.
−case assigner	57%	n.a.
pronouns		
+case assigner	79%	
−case assigner	21%	
% case errors		
on pronouns	0	n.a.
Gender		
% gender errors		
on determiners	10%	n.a.
% gender errors		
on pronouns	0	n.a.
Pragmatic information		
% definite determiners – mean	47.7	48.7
% indefinite determiners – mean	12.2*	28.7
% other determiners – mean	38.8	22.6
det/noun ratio definites	67%	n.a.
det/noun ratio indefinites	35%	n.a.
% pragmatic errors		
on determiners	5%	n.a.
on pronouns	0	n.a.

First the scores that show general impairment, then the case-related scores, followed by gender and pragmatic information-related data. (Det/noun ratio = determiner/noun ratio in %). The percentages of errors are based on the total number of incorrect DPs, the other errors consist of determiner omissions.   * Significantly different from score of the control group, established with Mann Whitney U test, with an alpha level of .05.

reverse does not hold: illegitimate bare noun phrases were realised approximately as often in the presence (43%) as in the absence (57%) of a case assigner. A chi-square on these four combinations ($\pm$ case assigner, $\pm$ determiner) revealed that there was a significant preference for the combination of noun phrases with a determiner with a case assigner ($\chi^2 = 11.95$, $p = .001$). For pronouns, a similar relationship was found: relatively more pronouns were with (79%) than without a case assigner (21%), and this difference is significant (Wilcoxon Signed-Rank Test, $T = 1$, $p = .031$). No errors were made with case marking on pronouns.

Gender

When determiners were realised, only a few gender (10%) errors were made (of these 10% gender errors, 7% were made by one patient who overused the non-neuter demonstrative four times for neuter nouns). No gender errors were made on pronouns.

Pragmatic information

In addition, no pragmatic errors were made with pronouns. In determiners 5% of the errors consisted of pragmatic errors. Furthermore, analyses of the omission and production rates revealed that the omission rate of the indefinite determiners (65%) was significantly higher than the omission rate of definite determiners (33%, Wilcoxon Signed-Rank Test, $T = 2$, $p = .024$) for the agrammatic speakers. They also produced relatively fewer indefinite determiners than the control group (12.2% vs 28.7% of all determiners, Mann Whitney U, $Z = -2.09$, $p = .037$), whereas the relative number of definite determiners was the same (47.7% vs 48.7%, Mann Whitney U, $Z = -0.23$, $p = .82$). Finally, there was no difference between the groups regarding the relative number of other determiners (38.8% vs 22.6%, Mann Whitney U, $Z = -1.58$, $p = .114$). This category consisted of 80% numerals and 20% quantifiers for the control group and 95% numerals and only 5% quantifiers for the agrammatic group.

CONCLUSION

As expected, and replicating earlier studies, our Dutch agrammatic patients produced (many) fewer determiners and pronouns than the healthy controls. Replicating the data of Ruigendijk et al. (1999) and Ruigendijk (2002), the presence of determiners and pronouns was found to be related to the presence of a case-assigning category. The reverse was not true: the omission of determiners was not related to the absence of a case assigner. The illegitimate bare noun phrases were realised as often with as without a case assigner. This means that sometimes even the presence of a case assigner is not enough to realise the determiner. It is not exactly clear yet how this can be explained.

As for the omission and production rates of definite and indefinite determiners, our results seem to be more in line with the Månsson and Ahlsén (2001) study than with Havik and Bastiaanse (2004), since our patients omitted more indefinite determiners than definite determiners and produced fewer indefinite determiners compared to the control group, whereas the relative number of definite determiners was the same for the agrammatic and control group. This suggests that the definiteness distinction does play a role in agrammatism. A possible explanation for the difference with the Havik and Bastiaanse results is that they did not analyse demonstrative and possessive determiners (which are definite determiners), thus ending up with a relatively low number of definite determiners (Havik, personal communication). However, this still does not explain their much lower omission rate for indefinite determiners (39%) compared to ours (65% omission). At the moment, we do not have a good explanation for these different results other than that they might reflect slight differences between patients. But note that, in our group, indefinite determiners were omitted significantly more often than definite determiners; only one of our patients (1) showed a slight difference in the opposite direction. The difference between definite and indefinite determiners may be related to preserved pragmatic abilities. Perhaps the intact pragmatic abilities can support the production of definite nouns in order to play a pragmatic role, namely marking an entity that has been introduced in discourse before, even if at the syntactic level, due to the absence of a case assigner, a bare noun phrase has to be produced. It is possible that there is an asymmetry between definite and indefinite determiners in that indefinite determiners are derived by syntax alone, and definite determiners are also motivated by pragmatics to mark the pragmatic feature.[5] Of course this explanation is still somewhat speculative. More (cross-linguistic) data are needed to find out the exact role of definiteness in agrammatism.

Summarised, these results indicate that *lexical* properties, or at least gender information of determiners, is not the cause of the agrammatic problems with these elements, which supports earlier results from de Bleser et al. (1996; 2005) and Bastiaanse et al. (2003). The same holds for the *semantic-conceptual* assignment of gender information on pronouns, which is assigned on the basis of the biological gender of the person (or animal) that is referred to. Determiners and pronouns receive gender differently, but neither process seems to affect their production performance. The claim that gender information is unimpaired in agrammatism finds additional support from studies which showed that subject–verb agreement (which requires access to the grammatical gender of the subject in various languages) is spared in agrammatic production (e.g., Friedmann, 2001; Friedmann & Grodzinsky 1997). The results do suggest that *syntactic* properties—more specifically the case assignment relationship between determiners and pronouns on the one hand and transitive verbs and verb finiteness on the other hand (cf. Ruigendijk, 2002)— play an important role. This is in line with the idea that agrammatism is primarily the result of problems with syntax (see, among others, Avrutin, 2006; and for a syntactic account of problems with determiners: de Bleser et al., 1996; de Bleser et al., 2005; Ruigendijk, 2002). Although some aspects of the data on the pragmatic properties of determiners need more research, the finding that hardly any definite determiners or pronouns are used to refer to new information and no indefinite determiners are used to refer to "old" information suggests that pragmatic knowledge is generally preserved. This replicates earlier results from Wulfeck et al. (1989). However, the difference between omission and production rates may indicate that definite determiners are less impaired than indefinite determiners. The cause of this possible difference remains for future research.

Overall, the results show that whereas syntax is impaired in these participants, leading to deficits in case-related elements such as determiners and pronouns, lexical, semantic, and pragmatic aspects are unimpaired. These results provide a clear

---

[5] We thank one of the reviewers for pointing out this interesting explanation to us.

direction for the treatment of determiners and pronouns. Both pronouns and determiners should primarily be treated with a focus on their syntactic property; that is, their dependency on case-assigning categories. This implies that an improvement of the production of these case-assigning categories should also improve the production of determiners and pronouns.

REFERENCES

Abney, S. (1987). *The English noun phrase in its sentential aspect.* PhD dissertation, MIT, Cambridge, MA.

Avrutin, S. (2006). Weak syntax. In Y. Grodzinsky & K. Amunts (Eds.), *Broca's region.* Oxford, UK: Oxford University Press.

Baauw, S., de Roo, E., & Avrutin, S. (2002). Determiner omission in language acquisition and language impairment: Syntactic and discourse factors. *Proceedings of the Annual Boston University Conference on Language Development, 26*(1), 24–35.

Bastiaanse, R., Jonkers, R., Ruigendijk, E., & van Zonneveld, R. (2003). Gender and case in agrammatic production. *Cortex, 39,* 405–417.

Bates, E., Wulfeck, B., & McWhinney, B. (1991). Cross-linguistic research in aphasia: An overview. *Brain and Language, 41,* 123–148.

Bernstein, J. (2001). The DP Hypothesis: Identifying clausal properties in the nominal domain. In M. Baltin & C. Collins (Eds.), *Handbook of contemporary syntactic theory.* Oxford, UK: Blackwell.

Chomsky, N. (1981). *Lectures on government and binding.* Dordrecht, the Netherlands: Foris Publications.

de Bleser, R., Bayer, J., & Luzzatti, C. (1996). Linguistic theory and morphosyntactic impairments in German and Italian aphasics. *Journal of Neurolinguistics, 9,* 175–185.

de Bleser, R., Burchert, F., & Rausch, P. (2005). Breakdown at the morphological level. *Stem-, Spraak- en Taalpathologie, 13,* 35–46.

de Roo, E. (1999). *Agrammatic grammar. Functional categories in agrammatic speech.* Doctoral Dissertation, Leiden, 62. Den Haag: Holland Academic Graphics.

Deutsch, W., & Wijnen, F. (1985). The article's noun and the noun's article: Explorations into the representation and access of linguistic gender in Dutch. *Linguistics, 23,* 793–810.

Friedmann, N. (2001). Agrammatism and the psychological reality of the syntactic tree. *Journal of Psycholinguistic Research, 30,* 71–90.

Friedmann, N. (2006). Speech production in Broca's agrammatic aphasia: Syntactic tree pruning. In Y. Grodzinsky & K. Amunts (Eds.), *Broca's region* (pp. 63–82). Oxford, UK: Oxford University Press.

Friedmann, N., & Grodzinsky, Y. (1997). Tense and agreement in agrammatic production: Pruning the syntactic tree. *Brain and Language, 56,* 397–425.

Giusti, G. (2002). The functional structure of noun phrases: A bare phrase structure approach. In G. Cinque (Ed.), *Functional structure in DP and IP* (pp. 54–90). Oxford, UK: Oxford University Press.

Giusti, G. (2006). On some parallels between noun phrases and clauses. In M. Frascarelli (Ed.), *Phases of interpretation.* Berlin: Mouton de Gruyter.

Graetz, P. R., de Bleser, R., & Willmes, K. (1992). *Akense Afasie Test* [Aachen aphasia test]. Lisse, the Netherlands: Swets & Zeitlinger.

Grodzinsky, Y. (2000). The neurology of syntax: Language use without Broca's area. *Behavioral and Brain Sciences, 23,* 1–71.

Haeseryn, W., Romijn, K., Geerts, G., de Rooij, J., & van den Toorn, M. C. (1997). *Algemene nederlandse spraakkunst.* Groningen/Deurne: Martinus Nijhoff uitgevers/Wolters Plantyn.

Havik, E., & Bastiaanse, R. (2004). Omission of definite and indefinite articles in the spontaneous speech of agrammatic speakers with Broca's aphasia. *Aphasiology, 18*(12), 1093–1102.

Heim, I. (1983). File change semantics and the familiarity theory of definiteness. In R. Bäuerle, C. Schwarze, & A. von Stechow (Eds.), *Meaning, use and interpretation of language.* Berlin: de Gruyter.

Hofstede, B. T. M., & Kolk, H. H. J. (1994). The effects of task variation on the production of grammatical morphology in Broca's aphasia: A multiple case study. *Brain and Language, 46,* 278–328.

Kadmon, N. (2001). *Formal pragmatics: Semantics, pragmatics, presupposition, and focus.* Oxford, UK: Blackwell.

Månsson, A-C., & Ahlsén, E. (2001). Grammatical features of aphasia in Swedish. *Journal of Neurolinguistics, 14,* 365–380.

Menn, L., & Obler, L. (1988). Findings of the cross-language aphasia study, phase I: Agrammatic narratives. *Aphasiology, 2,* 347–350.

Ouhalla, J. (1993). Functional categories, agrammatism and language acquisition. *Linguistische Berichte*, *143*, 3–36.

Postal, P. (1966). On so-called "pronouns" in English. In D. Reibel & S. Schane (Eds.), *Modern studies in English*. New York: Prentice-Hall.

Ruigendijk, E. (2002). *Case assignment in agrammatism: A cross-linguistic study* (Vol. 36). Groningen: Groninger Dissertations in Linguistics.

Ruigendijk, E., & Bastiaanse, R. (2002). Two characteristics of agrammatic speech: Omission of verbs and omission of determiners, is there a relation? *Aphasiology*, *16*(4–6), 383–395.

Ruigendijk, E., van Zonneveld, R., & Bastiaanse, R. (1999). Case assignment in agrammatism. *Journal of Speech, Language and Hearing Research*, *42*, 962–971.

Saffran, E. M., Berndt, R. S., & Schwartz, M. F. (1989). The quantitative analysis of agrammatic production: Procedure and data. *Brain and Language*, *37*, 440–479.

van Haeringen, C. B. (1956). Nederlands tussen Duits en Engels. In [unknown] (Ed.), *Algemene aspecten van de grote cultuurtalen* (pp. 27–97). Den Haag: Servire.

Wulfeck, B., Bates, E., Juarez, L., Opie, M., Friederici, A. D., & MacWhinney, B. et al. (1989). Pragmatics in aphasia: Crosslinguistic evidence. *Language and Speech*, *32*, 315–336.

APPENDIX 1

Participant information

Agrammatic speaker	Gender	Age	Aetiology	MPO
1	f	57	CVA left	5
2	f	64	CVA left	18
3	f	50	CVA left	4
4	f	58	CVA left	148
5	m	41	CVA left	30
6	m	82	CVA left (twice)	24
7	m	73	CVA left	240
8	m	68	CVA left	9

MPO = monthspost onset; f = female, m = male; CVA = cardio-vascular accident (hemisphere); Age and MPO are at the time of the interview.

APPENDIX 2

Individual scores on number of pronouns and determiners as well as on the three determiner/noun ratios

Patient	#Pronouns	#Determiners	Det/noun ratio in % *	Det/noun ratio definites in %	Det/noun ratio indefinites in %
1	22	12	91	80	100
2	53	7	47	13	0
3	21	19	78	83	20
4	9	15	72	88	0
5	25	13	73	83	0
6	11	19	89	100	70
7	12	17	72	56	25
8	2	20	54	70	10
Total	155	122	70	67	35

*This ratio can be higher than the mean of the ratios of the definites and indefinites, since for the latter ratios only cases for which we could decide whether a definite or indefinite determiner was required (on the basis of context) were counted.

APHASIOLOGY, 2007, 21 (6/7/8), 548–557

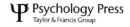

The "tree-pruning hypothesis" in bilingualism

Andrea Tissen and Sandra Weber

Zuyd University, Heerlen, The Netherlands

Marion Grande

University Hospital, RWTH Aachen University, Germany

Thomas Günther

Zuyd University, Heerlen, The Netherlands, and University Hospital, RWTH Aachen University, Germany

Background: The "tree-pruning hypothesis" (TPH) suggests that syntactic deficits in agrammatic production are highly selective: most patients have impaired tense inflection while their agreement inflection is preserved. The TPH states that the split-inflection tree is pruned at the tense node, which is why an obvious dissociation in performance exists between tense and agreement.

Aims: This study aims to determine whether the TPH applies to a bilingual individual by examining whether a dissociation in performance exists between agreement and tense inflection in the bilingual speaker's two languages: German and Luxembourgish. We expect the pattern of grammatical impairment to support the validity of the TPH in German and Luxembourgish.

Methods & Procedures: The participant examined in this study, AM, is a pre-onset balanced German–Luxembourgish speaker with Broca's aphasia and moderate agrammatism. We used a verb completion and grammatical assessment task to examine whether a dissociation in performance existed between tense and agreement in both languages.

Outcomes & Results: The results comply with the TPH. The agreement results produced by the participant were significantly better than the tense results in both German and Luxembourgish.

Conclusions: The results show a clear dissociation in each language as predicted by the TPH. This confirms that the TPH can be applied to both German and Luxembourgish.

This study investigates the tree-pruning hypothesis (TPH; Friedmann & Grodzinsky, 1997) in a bilingual individual with Broca's aphasia. Agrammatism is the leading symptom in Broca's aphasia. Traditionally, agrammatism is defined as the omission and substitution of function words and the omission of finite verbs, or the use of infinitives (Bastiaanse, Jonkers, Quak, & Put, 1996; Friedmann, 2001; Wenzlaff & Clahsen, 2004). This view states that all syntactic abilities are affected. By contrast, the tree-pruning hypothesis (TPH; Friedmann, 2001; Friedmann & Grodzinsky, 1997) predicts a more selective impairment in syntactic production. Pruning of the

---

Address correspondence to: Thomas Günther, Zuyd University, School of Speech and Language Pathology, P.O. Box 550, 6400 AN Heerlen, The Netherlands. E-mail: gunther@hszuyd.nl

---

http://www.psypress.com/aphasiology   DOI: 10.1080/02687030701191952

split-inflection tree (Pollock, 1989) results in agrammatic speakers failing to project their syntactic tree up to the higher nodes. In moderate agrammatism, the split-inflection tree is pruned between the two functional categories of agreement (AgrP) and tense (TP). This leads to an impairment of TP and all higher structures, while the AgrP and all lower parts are preserved. Evidence of this has been found in various languages; for example, in German (Wenzlaff & Clahsen, 2004), Spanish, Galician, and Catalan (Gavarró & Martinez-Ferreiro, 2004), Hebrew and Arabic (Friedmann, 2001). In Japanese, TP is considered to be localised in the lower part of the syntactic tree and so remains intact in contrast to the higher nodes (Hagiwara, 1995).

According to Chomsky's "principles and parameters theory" (1981), the grammar of each language can be attributed to a set of universal principles, some of which are fixed while others are changeable in the form of parameters. So the various grammars are represented in a single underlying structure, the split-inflection tree proposed by Pollock (1989). Language impairment may appear very differently for various reasons in bilinguals after a CVA: for example, only one or both languages may be impaired or the extent of the impairment may differ (Paradis, 2004). Use of a more neurolinguistic framework such as the "neurolinguistic theory of bilingualism" proposed by Paradis (2004) may also show that less affected language structures may possibly compensate for more affected ones. This may lead to different language impairment in each language.

By contrast, we argue that both languages should show a similar pattern of impairment in the case of a bilingual aphasic individual whose respective grammars do not differ much and who has the same pre-onset level in each language. As far as the syntactic tree for both grammars is concerned, the pruning should affect both languages: TP is impaired in both languages, while AgrP remains intact. We predict that the pattern of grammatical impairment supports the tree-pruning hypothesis in both languages. Therefore, our study aimed to examine whether language performance was better for agreement than tense, and whether this pattern could be observed in a pre-onset balanced bilingual individual with Broca's aphasia who speaks German and Luxembourgish.

OUTLINE OF GERMAN AND LUXEMBOURGISH GRAMMAR

Both languages belong to the Indo-European group of languages; Luxembourgish is also defined as a "Mosellefranconian" dialect. German used to be the official language of Luxembourg. Luxembourgish was previously used in private only and only had an oral form. It has recently been recognised as the national language, so now it has both an oral and a written form. Finite verbs encode agreement (person, number) and tense in both languages. Agreement in regular verbs is achieved by means of suffixes in German [Ge] and Luxembourgish [Lux]. These are affixed to the verb stem, which is the infinite verb form without -en. In German, the so-called agreement markers are -e, -st, -t and -en, while in Luxembourgish they are -en, -st, and -t. Irregular verbs additionally show changes in the stem morpheme in both languages.

The perfect in German and Luxembourgish is generated by means of conjugated auxiliaries *haben* [Ge] (= *to have*) and *sein* (= *to be*) combined with a participle (e.g., *ich habe **ge-**mal -t* [Ge] = *ech hun **ge-** mol -t* [Lux]). Irregular verbs are formed by the infinitive form with a change in the stem morpheme and the prefix *ge* (e.g., *ich habe **ge-** sung -en*[Ge] = *ech hun **ge-** song -en* [Lux]). Subject–verb agreement in the perfect only affects the auxiliary, while the participle remains the same. In the tense condition, the participle has the tense markers -*t* and -*ge*, and includes a possible stem change.

The past tense in regular verbs is formed by a -*t* suffix, followed by the agreement suffixes (e.g., *ich mal* -*te* [Ge]). A stem change takes place in irregular verbs (e.g., *ich ging* [Ge] = *ech goung* [Lux]).

The TPH is based on the "split-inflection-theory" (Pollock, 1989). Pollock argues that the inflection node (IP) is split into TP and AgrP, with AgrP located below TP in the syntactic tree. Others argue that languages may show differences in the split-inflection trees in both the amount and hierarchy of their functional categories (Alexiadou & Stavrakaki, 2006; Hagiwara, 1995; Milman, Dickey, & Thompson, 2004; Nanousi, Masterson, Druks, & Atkinson, 2006; Nilipour & Paradis, 1995). For Luxembourgish, there is still no evidence today for the structure of the split-inflection tree. Because Luxembourgish is defined as a Mosellefranconian dialect, which is a West Germanic language like German, we expect the Luxembourgish syntactic tree to have the same order of functional categories as found in German with AgrP below TP. Verbs are inflected by the movement of functional heads. According to the checking theory contained in the Minimalist Program (Chomsky, 1992), an inflected verb inserted in VP moves up the tree checking its inflection in Agr for person and number and in T for tense. If the derivation converges at these checkpoints, the sentence is well formed. If mismatches exist between the inflected form of the verb and the feature stored in the checkpoints, the sentence is ungrammatical. After checking the inflection, main verbs and the auxiliaries "have" and "be" move to C in the second position, in both German and Luxembourgish. In embedded clauses, the verbs stays in the final position. While the perfect is formed by conjugated auxiliaries ("have" and "be") combined with a participle, the participles also have to check their inflections at the T node. Since they are inserted in VP in final position, they may move to TP and then return to VP. As far as English is concerned, Pollock (1989), Chomsky (1991), and Rizzi (1990) suggest that AgrP and TP are lowered onto V. However, the verbs obtain their affix from the checking mechanism. If the pruned tree follows the TPH, then this mechanism is impaired in TP and all higher nodes, while AgrP and the lower part of the tree still check the inflection of the verb.

METHOD

Participant

The participant in this study (AM) was a 39-year-old male patient who had suffered a left CVA. He had Broca's aphasia and moderate agrammatism, based on the German results of the Aachen Aphasia Test (Huber, Poeck, Weniger, & Willmes, 1983). No Luxembourgish aphasia test results were available. AM also suffered from a word deafness condition that still seemed to exist at the time of testing, 20 months after his stroke. Before suffering the stroke, AM worked as a truck and bus driver. The participant was a balanced-bilingual (German–Luxembourgish) with Luxembourgish as his mother tongue. He did not learn to read and write Luxembourgish at school, but learned German in both the written and oral form. In public, he used German as the official language in all formats (writing, reading, comprehension, speaking). Luxembourgish was spoken at home only.

These data are based on a self-constructed bilingualism questionnaire based on the History of Bilingualism (part A) and the Language Background (part B) taken from *The Assessment of Bilingual Aphasia* produced by Paradis (1987).

Materials and procedures

The TPH was tested in a 2×2 factorial design, each carried out in German and Luxembourgish. Following Friedmann (2001) and Wenzlaff and Clahsen (2004), we investigated two sentence completion tasks (agreement completion and tense completion) and two grammaticality judgement tasks (agreement judgement and tense judgement). The agreement completion task presented a clause that contained a gap instead of the finite verb. The infinitive verb was placed in parentheses behind the clause (*"Er_____ eine Tasse Kaffee. (trinken)"* [Ge]; *"Hien ____ eng Taass Kaffi. (drénken")* [Lux], [*"He ____ a cup of coffee (to drink)"*]).

The participant had to enter the correctly inflected verb according to the clause-initial personal pronoun or noun. All six person and number pairings were determined by a matching procedure and were tested in German and Luxembourgish. All sentences were presented in the present tense.

In the agreement judgement task, we presented a counterbalanced set of grammatically correct and incorrect sentences. All sentences showed the same syntactic structure and all six person and number pairings, as in the agreement completion task. Incorrect sentences contained agreement violation (person and/or number). The participant had to indicate whether the verb was inflected correctly according to the clause-initial pronoun or noun. The form of the incorrectly inflected verb was matched from the remaining five person and number pairings (*"Der Hase laufen über die Wiese."* [Ge]; *"Den Hues laafen iwwert d'Wiss"* [Lux], [*"The rabbit run across the grassland."*] as an example of an incorrect item). (*"Das Kind spielt mit dem Teddybär."* [Ge]; *"D'Kand spillt mam Teddybaer."* [Lux], [*"The child plays with the Teddy."* as an example of a correct item).

The tense completion task contained two sentences, both with a clause-initial temporal adverbial. The first one included a verb already inflected; the second phrase had a gap instead of the verb. Each phrase was formed in a different tense, either present tense or perfect (or simple past), indicated by a specific temporal adverbial. The combination of auxiliary and participle in the perfect called for the participant to insert only the participle. In the present tense condition, the participant was required to alter the tense and inflect the verb correctly. (*"Gestern habe ich dir meine Telefonnummer gesagt. Heute _____ ich dir noch einmal meine Telefonnummer."* [Ge]; *"Geschter hun ech dir meng Telefonsnummer gesoot. Haut _____ ech dir meng Telefonsnummer nach eng Keier."* [Lux], [*"Yesterday I gave you my phone number. Today I _____ you my phone number again"*]).

In this example, the first sentence uses the perfect, and the second sentence uses the present tense. Both tenses were distributed approximately evenly; unfortunately there were some Luxembourgish words that are not used with the perfect. Instead, we used the simple past. We also had a nearly counterbalanced set of verb types (regular vs irregular) caused by some words with a language-specific derivation (e.g., in German a word has regular inflection, but in Luxembourgish it is irregular). Although the two sentences of a single item gave the same person and number, the whole tense completion task actually tested all six person and number pairings, determined by a matching procedure. Subject pronouns and nouns were used, as in the agreement completion task.

For the tense judgement task we presented a counterbalanced set of grammatically correct and incorrect sentences. The incorrect items only contained tense violations in person and/or number. The sentences began with a temporal adverb to indicate the required tense. The participant only had to indicate whether the verb had been derived correctly in accordance with the temporal adverb ("*Morgen waren wir in Luxemburg.*" [Ge]; "*Muer woren mir zu Letzeburg.*" [Lux], *["Tomorrow we were in Luxembourg."]* as an example of an incorrect item). ("*Jetzt bringe ich dich nach Hause.*" [Ge]; "*Elo brengen ech dech heem.*" [Lux], *["Now I'll take you back home."]* as an example of a correct item).

The distribution of tense and verb types is controlled as in the tense completion task. "*Morgen*"/"*Muer*" ("*tomorrow*") determines the future tense, "*waren*"/ "*woren*" ("*were*") is simple past. The personal pronouns were also matched in both tense tasks (tense completion and judgement).

Altogether, 160 items per language, 40 for each task, were used. This produced two dependent variables (agreement and tense) with two levels per language (completion and grammaticality judgement). The number of errors made by the participant per task provided the dependent variable. Words were judged as incorrect if an incorrect stem change took place and/or if the wrong affix or no affix was chosen. An unsolved item was always defined as incorrect. To ensure that the participant understood the tasks, we held short practice sessions at the beginning of each task. The participant was only assisted when a problem occurred due to his receptive language abilities, but never if it contained morphosyntactic aspects.

All parts were first conducted in Luxembourgish, a few days later in German. All items were presented in written and oral form, because of the participant's assumed word deafness condition. The experimenters (two native speakers) read all the test sentences out loud (including the infinitive verb forms in the completion tasks). The participant was requested to read the full sentences out loud. In the completion tasks, the participant was asked to provide the missing verb orally, while in the grammaticality judgement tasks he had to indicate whether the sentence was correct or incorrect by saying "correct" or "incorrect".

The whole session was video- and audio-taped, and the experimenters also noted down the answers. The participant could request as much time as necessary. Only the first answers were considered for further analysis.

The results of the (tense vs agreement) category were compared for each language, as were the categories within a mode (e.g., tense judgement vs agreement judgement). The results were analysed using a Pearson chi-square test ($p < .05$) to look for differences in performance between the languages and between the categories. The percentages for performance (see Table 1) were given for all 40 sentences of a task.

RESULTS

German

The participant gave significantly more correct answers in the agreement task than in the tense task, $\chi^2_{(1)} = 15.50$; $p < .001$. Performance in the agreement task was better than in the tense task in both modes. The results are shown in Table 1. The difference between agreement and tense was significant only for the sentence completion task,

TABLE 1
Correct answers (%) for agreement and tense in the modes grammaticality judgement and
sentence completion in German and Luxembourgish

Language	Task	Correct answers
German	Agreement Completion	92.5%
	Agreement Judgement	87.5%
	Tense Completion	55.0%
	Tense Judgement	72.5%
	Total	76.9%
Luxembourgish	Agreement Completion	82.5%
	Agreement Judgement	67.5%
	Tense Completion	42.5%
	Tense Judgement	75.0%
	Total	66.9%

$\chi^2_{(1)} = 14.53$; $p < .001$, and not for the grammaticality judgement task, $\chi^2_{(1)} = 2.81$; $p = .094$. In the agreement condition, the participant performed at the ceiling level. With 92.5% correct answers, the sentence completion task was somewhat better than the grammaticality judgement task (87.5%). With an overall score of 90% correct answers in the agreement task, the participant did not have any major problems completing or recognising subject-verb-agreement adequately. Performance in the tense condition was considerably poorer. With an accuracy of 55% in the completion task and 72.2% in the grammaticality judgement task, the participant only scored an overall result of 63.7% correct answers (see Table 1).

Luxembourgish

The overall comparison between the tense and agreement results shows a significantly higher accuracy in the agreement than in the tense condition, $\chi^2_{(1)} = 4.77$; $p = .029$. For the Luxembourgish part, significantly higher results for the agreement condition can only be seen in the completion tasks, $\chi^2_{(1)} = 13.65$; $p < .001$. Comparison of the judgement tasks does not reveal any significant differences in achievement, $\chi^2_{(1)} = 0.55$; $p = .459$. The accuracy in the grammaticality judgement task was higher for the tense condition (75%) than the agreement condition (67.5%). The agreement sentence completion task (82. 5%) was the best result in both categories, and is significantly higher than in the tense sentence completion task (42.5%).

Comparison of the two languages

A comparison of the number of errors in each language shows a significant difference in all four conditions: agreement completion task $\chi^2_{(1)} = 15.29$; $p < .001$, agreement judgement task $\chi^2_{(1)} = 15.06$; $p < .001$, tense completion task $\chi^2_{(1)} = 24.19$; $p < .001$, tense judgement task $\chi^2_{(1)} = 35.15$; $p < .001$. The participant performed up to 23% worse in almost every Luxembourgish task. The exception is the Luxembourgish tense grammaticality judgement task (75% correct answers), which was higher than the corresponding results for German (72.5%). The significant performance differences in the German and Luxembourgish completion tasks show that the participant generally had fewer problems with the agreement tasks than with the tense tasks. These results are illustrated in Figure 1.

DISCUSSION

Our study aimed to investigate the tree-pruning hypothesis (TPH) in a bilingual German–Luxembourgish individual with moderate agrammatism. The results of our study comply with the TPH in both languages. The pruned split-inflection tree between the two nodes of tense (TP) and agreement (AgrP) resulted in our bilingual agrammatic speaker being significantly better on agreement than on tense in the German and the Luxembourgish completion tasks. This pattern is consistent with the recent literature (Benedet, Christiansen, & Goodglass, 1998; Friedmann, 2001, 2002; Friedmann & Grodzinsky, 1997; Gavarró & Martinez-Ferreiro, 2004), whereas findings in German agrammatism are inconsistent. Burchert, Swoboda-Moll, and De Bleser (2005) only occasionally found a dissociation between tense and agreement, whereas Wenzlaff and Clahsen (2004) could confirm a dissociation between TP and AgrP. Our findings suggest that the tree-pruning hypothesis could be extended to German agrammatism too.

We found a significant difference in performance between the tense and agreement tasks, confirming the TPH in the completion tasks but not in the judgement tasks. This is consistent with the findings of Friedmann and Grodzinsky (1997) and Friedmann (2001). Results provide evidence towards an approach to a broader deficit like the "overarching agrammatism" (Grodzinsky, 2000b), with a "parallelism" of input and output. Friedmann and Grodzinsky (1997), Friedmann (2001, 2006b) argue that the deficit is a highly restricted one, which concerns disorders in production only. In contrast to a recent account, Friedmann (2006a) tries to apply the TPH for comprehension by also using passive sentences requiring TP and relative clauses requiring CP. Wenzlaff and Clahsen (2004) also found in their study that the dissociation between Tense and Agreement is not restricted to production. However, in 1997 and 2001 Friedmann and Grodzinky supposed that

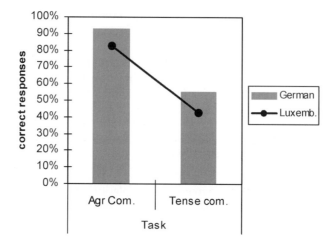

Figure 1. Correct answers to all 40 items (100%) for agreement (Agr Com.) and for tense (Tense Com.) completion in German and Luxembourgish.

the input route is either not impaired or its function is completely different from the output route. Grodzinsky (2000a) proposes that there is a comprehension disorder, but its description differs from that of the output. This assumption may explain an unexpected finding in this study: tense (75%) produced better performance than agreement (67.5%) in the Luxembourgish judgement task. However, our findings are consistent with the tree-pruning hypothesis, which originally described production only.

A comparison between both languages on the errors produced in each category showed better performance in German in three of the four tested tasks (agreement judgement, tense judgement, and agreement completion). In these cases, the participant performed up to 23% better in German than in Luxembourgish. So the German language seemed to be less impaired.

The TPH does not provide an adequate theoretical background for investigating this, because the hypothesis only explains the kind of impairment, namely a pruned syntactic tree, corroborated by a significant dissociation between tense and agreement in the production of both languages. One reason for this higher level of performance in German may relate to the modes of speaking, comprehension, writing, and reading. Our participant was a pre-onset balanced bilingual in the modes of speaking and comprehension, but not balanced in the modes of writing and reading. His performance in these two written modalities was much better in German than in Luxembourgish. This may be due to the lack of a written form of Luxembourgish during his schooldays, explaining why he did not learn to read and write Luxembourgish. Today, however, Luxembourgish has a written form, too. In fact, the participant was not as good at reading or writing Luxembourgish as he was at German. Therefore he might have had more difficulties with the test offered in written form. To reduce these possible comprehension errors, the test items were also delivered in oral form to provide him with an opportunity to compensate for the lack of Luxembourgish skills. Unfortunately, the participant also suffered from an assumed word deafness condition. So he may not have been able to rely on the oral form and had to work only on the basis of the written form. This may have affected the test results. However, since we do not know which form he preferred to work with, we cannot rule out the possibility that the missing written form of Luxembourgish may have affected the test results.

A more plausible explanation for this language imbalance results from a more neurolinguistic approach, that of the "neurolinguistic theory of bilingualism" (Paradis, 2004). Paradis claims that the language impairment in aphasia depends on the specific properties of each language. Languages can be learned formally and informally (Lebrun, 1995); depending on how a language is acquired, the deficit may be compensated (Paradis, 2004). An informal language, mostly the mother tongue, is learnt by implicit knowledge; i.e., children are not aware of the general principles underlying the language they learn. By contrast, a formal language, like a foreign language, is usually based on explicit (metalinguistic) knowledge; i.e., the speaker is conscious of the grammatical rules used. According to Paradis (2004), explicit and implicit knowledge are independent systems subserved by different cerebral mechanisms and also located in different brain areas. Therefore, a possible deficit in implicit knowledge may be compensated for by reliance on metalinguistic knowledge. Depending on whether in formal or informal language, the extent of metalinguistic knowledge use differs.

In this study, the participant's mother tongue was Luxembourgish and his second language was German. So he learned Luxembourgish informally, and his implicit knowledge was presumably very well developed. At school, Luxembourgish was neither spoken nor written. Therefore it is likely that he did not acquire an elaborate metalinguistic knowledge in Luxembourgish, which, by contrast, played an important role in the acquisition of German at school. On the other hand, his German implicit knowledge should not be as elaborate as his Luxembourgish knowledge.

A stroke is thought to affect implicit knowledge (Paradis, 2004). This impairment results in the syntactic tree being pruned between tense and agreement, which may lead to a constricted morphosyntax in German and Luxembourgish. Compensation of the impaired morphosyntax by metalinguistic knowledge is more probable in the formal language (Lebrun, 1995; Paradis, 2004), due to the better development of metalinguistic knowledge. The participant's formal language is German, so the German morphosyntactic deficit can be compensated for to a greater extent than the Luxembourgish deficit. This might explain why the German test results were much better than those for Luxembourgish.

The opportunity for compensating for the impaired implicit knowledge by means of preserved explicit knowledge may be used in treatment. Explicit knowledge must be extended so that the aphasic individual can rely mainly on the explicit language system in his or her language performance.

Conclusion

To summarise, the results of our study support the tree-pruning hypothesis in the agrammatic production of a pre-onset balanced bilingual involving the languages German and Luxembourgish. The difference in performance between German and Luxembourgish is parsimoniously explained by the "neurolinguistic theory of bilingualism".

REFERENCES

Alexiadou, A., & Stavrakaki, S. (2006). Clause structure and verb movement in Greek English speaking bilingual patient with Broca's aphasia: Evidence from adverb placement. *Brain and Language, 96*, 207–220.

Bastiaanse, R., Jonkers, R., Quak, C., & Put, M. V. (1996). The production of finite and non-finite verb forms in agrammatism. *Platform Session 1: Agrammatism, Brain and Language, 55*, 8–19.

Benedet, M. J., Christiansen, J. A., & Goodglass, H. (1998). A cross-linguistic study of grammatical morphology in Spanish- and English-speaking agrammatic patients. *Cortex, 34*, 309–336.

Burchert, F., Swoboda-Moll, M., & De Bleser, R. (2005). Tense and agreement dissociations in German agrammatic speakers: Underspecification vs. hierarchy. *Brain and Language, 94*, 188–199.

Chomsky, N. (1981). *Lectures on government and binding.* Dordrecht: Foris.

Chomsky, N. (1991). Some notes on the economy of derivation. In R. Freidin (Ed.), *Principles and parameters in comparative grammar* (pp. 417–454). Cambridge, MA: MIT Press.

Chomsky, N. (1992). A *minimalist program for linguistic theory (MIT occasional papers in linguistics).* Cambridge, MA: MIT Press.

Friedmann, N. (2001). Agrammatism and the psychological reality of the syntactic tree. *Journal of Psycholinguistic Research, 30*, 71–90.

Friedmann, N. (2002). Question production in agrammatism: The tree-pruning hypothesis. *Brain and Language, 80*, 160–187.

Friedmann, N. (2006a). Generalizations on variations in comprehension and production: A further source of variation and a possible account. *Brain and Language, 96*, 151–153.

Friedmann, N. (2006b). Speech production in Broca's agrammatic aphasia: Syntactic tree pruning. In Y. Grodzinsky & K. Amunts (Eds.), *Broca's region* (pp. 63–82). Oxford, UK: University Press.

Friedmann, N., & Grodzinsky, Y. (1997). Tense and agreement in agrammatic production: Pruning the syntactic tree. *Brain and Language, 56*, 397–425.

Gavarró, A., & Martinez-Ferreiro, S. (2004). *Tense and agreement impairment in Ibero-Romance*. [Online]. Retrieved Feb 13, 2005 from http://seneca.uab.es/ggt/Reports/GGT-04-4.pdf

Grodzinsky, Y. (2000a). The neurology of syntax: Language use without Broca's area. *Behavioral and Brain Sciences, 23*, 1–71.

Grodzinsky, Y. (2000b). Overarching agrammatism. In Y. Grodzinky, L. Shapiro, & D. Swinney (Eds.), *Language and the brain: Representation and processing – Studies presented to Edgar Zurif on his 60th birthday* (pp. 73–86). San Diego, CA: Academic Press.

Hagiwara, H. (1995). The breakdown of functional categories and the economy of derivation. *Brain and Language, 50*, 92–166.

Huber, W., Poeck, K., Weniger, D., & Willmes, K. (1983). *Der Aachener Aphasie-Test*. Göttingen: Hogrefe.

Lebrun, Y. (1995). The study of bilingual aphasia: Pitres' legacy. In M. Paradis (Ed.), *Aspects of bilingual aphasia* (pp. 11–22). Oxford, UK: Pergamon Press.

Milman, L., Dickey, M. W., & Thompson, C. K. (2004). Production of functional categories in agrammatic narratives: An item response theory analysis. *Brain and Language, 91*, 126–127.

Nanousi, V., Masterson, J., Druks, J., & Atkinson, M. (2006). Interpretable vs. uninterpretable features: Evidence from six Greek agrammatic patients. *Journal of Neurolingusics, 19*, 209–238.

Nilipour, R., & Paradis, M. (1995). Breakdown of functional categories in three Farsi–English bilingual aphasic patients. In M. Paradis (Ed.), *Aspects of bilingual aphasia* (pp. 123–138). Oxford, UK: Pergamon Press.

Paradis, M. (1987). *The assessment of bilingual aphasia*. London: Lawrence Erlbaum Associates Ltd.

Paradis, M. (2004). *A neurolinguistic theory of bilingualism*. Amsterdam: Benjamins.

Pollock, J. Y. (1989). Verb movement, universal grammar and the structure of IP. *Linguistic Inquiry, 20*, 365–424.

Rizzi, L. (1990). *Relativized minimality*. Cambridge, MA: MIT Press.

Wenzlaff, M., & Clahsen, H. (2004). Tense and agreement in german agrammatism. *Brain and Language, 89*, 57–68.

APHASIOLOGY, 2007, 21 (6/7/8), 558–569

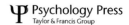

Single-word semantic judgements in semantic dementia: Do phonology and grammatical class count?

Jamie Reilly, Katy Cross, Vanessa Troiani and Murray Grossman

University of Pennsylvania, Philadelphia, PA, USA

Background: Listeners make active use of phonological regularities such as word length to facilitate higher-level syntactic and semantic processing. For example, nouns are longer than verbs, and abstract words are longer than concrete words. Patients with semantic dementia (SD) experience conceptual loss with preserved syntax and phonology. The extent to which patients with SD exploit phonological regularities to support language processing remains unclear.

Aims: We examined the ability of patients with SD (1) to perceive subtle acoustic–phonetic distinctions in English, and (2) to bootstrap their accuracy of lexical-semantic and syntactic judgements from regularities in the phonological forms of English nouns and verbs.

Methods and Procedures: Four patients with SD made minimal pair judgements (same/different) for auditorily presented stimuli selectively varied by voice, place, or manner of the initial consonant (e.g., *pa –ba*). In Experiment 2 patients made forced-choice semantic judgements (abstract or concrete) for single words varied by (1) *concreteness* (abstract or concrete); (2) *grammatical class* (noun or verb); and (3) *word length* (one- or three-syllable words).

Outcomes and Results: The most semantically impaired patients paradoxically showed the highest accuracy of minimal pair phonologic discrimination. Judgements of word concreteness were less accurate for verbs than nouns. Among verbs, accuracy was worse for concrete than abstract items (e.g., *eat* was worse than *think*). Patients were more likely to misclassify longer concrete words (e.g., *professor*) as abstract, demonstrating sensitivity to an underlying phonologically mediated semantic property in English.

Conclusions: Single-word semantic judgements were sensitive to both grammatical class and phonological properties of the words being evaluated. Theoretical and clinical implications are addressed in the context of an anatomically constrained model of SD that assumes increasing reliance on phonology as lexical-semantic knowledge degrades.

Semantic dementia (SD) is a progressive neurodegenerative disease that affects inferior, ventral, and anterolateral portions of the temporal lobe (Grossman, 2002). The early stages of SD are associated with conceptual loss and concurrent language deficits that include anomia, impaired auditory comprehension, and surface dyslexia in the context of reasonably preserved syntactic and phonological abilities. From a theoretical standpoint, selective impairment of conceptual knowledge presents an *in vivo* model for examining the interaction of semantic memory with other linguistic

Address correspondence to: Jamie Reilly PhD, Department of Neurology, 3 Gates Building, University of Pennsylvania School of Medicine, Hospital of the University of Pennsylvania, 3400 Spruce Street, Philadelphia, PA 19104-4283, USA. E-mail: reillyjj@mail.med.upenn.edu

http://www.psypress.com/aphasiology   DOI: 10.1080/02687030701191986

processes such as phonology. From a clinical perspective, the development of an aetiologically-specific language rehabilitation for SD presents a major challenge. One important step towards development of such an intervention, we argue, is to better understand how preserved functions interact with degraded knowledge. Here we examined (1) the integrity of phonetic processing in SD, and (2) sensitivity to phonological regularities that mark semantic and syntactic distinctions between English nouns and verbs.

Figure 1 illustrates a general model of the cognitive-linguistic decline associated with SD. We assume three interacting levels of processing (semantic, lexical, and phonological). Under this model, degradation of language occurs with the disease progression in an orderly manner: semantic → lexical → phonological. These cognitive changes are correlated with cortical degeneration that begins with circumscribed atrophy in the left ventral temporal lobe, progressing posteriorly and laterally, ultimately involving the temporal lobes bilaterally (see also Lambon Ralph, McClelland, Patterson, Galton, & Hodges, 2001). Performance on variables associated with different aspects of language can provide converging evidence in support of an interactive model where "top-down" semantic functioning progressively declines, and "bottom-up" contributions from phonology assume an increasingly important role in language.

One core characteristic of SD illustrated in Figure 1 is that phonological perception is spared until the latest stages of the disease. This assumption of preserved phonological processing is supported by the particular distribution of atrophy incurred in SD, which typically spares superior temporal and inferior parietal lobe structures dedicated to auditory comprehension. We predict that as lexical-semantic comprehension is compromised, patients with SD will show an increasing reliance on phonological support for language.

Research has provided evidence in favour of phonological reliance in SD in a number of ways. In immediate serial recall, patients with advanced SD have shown rapid forgetting of early list items with preservation of terminal items, a pattern that is consistent with impaired semantic comprehension in the context of preserved phonology (Martin & Saffran, 1990; Reilly, Martin & Grossman, 2005; Saffran & Martin, 1990). Another source of evidence for phonological dependence in SD is the high frequency of surface dyslexia in this population (Jefferies, Lambon Ralph, Jones, Bateman, & Patterson, 2004), a disorder wherein reading is markedly impaired for orthographically irregular words (e.g., *yacht*) with preservation of regular grapheme–phoneme correspondence (e.g., *cat*), a process that is not dependent on lexical-semantic comprehension (Coltheart, Byng, Masterson, Prior, & Riddoch, 1983)

Phonological effects have been investigated in serial recall and reading in SD. However, few studies have examined the integrity of subtle acoustic perceptual distinctions such as voice onset time (i.e., phonemic categorical perception), and place and manner of articulation. In one such study, patients with severe semantic impairment showed a normal shift in phonemic categorical perception ($b \rightarrow p$) as voice onset time was truncated in 10-ms increments from +120ms (always perceived by healthy listeners as /b/) to −120ms (always perceived as /p/) (Kwok, Reilly, & Grossman, 2006). In addition, participants with advanced SD successfully discriminated pairs of pure tones varied by frequencies of 0Hz, 25Hz, or 200Hz, demonstrating preserved auditory perception of nonlinguistic stimuli.

One aspect of phonology that has not been investigated in SD is pattern induction, or the ability to recognise and exploit phonological regularities in

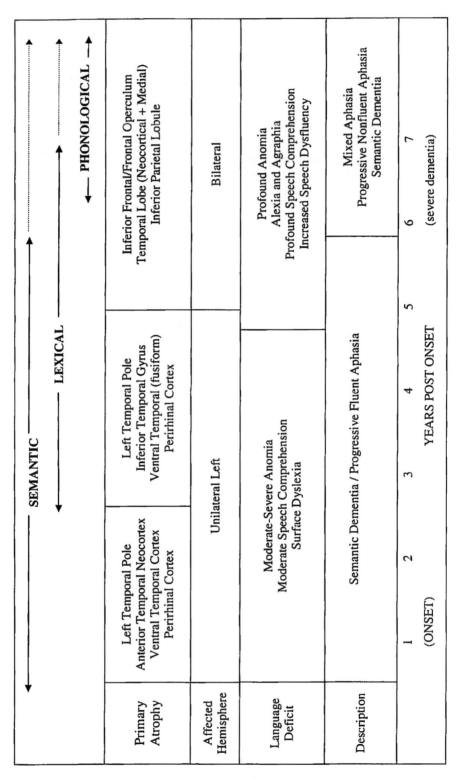

Figure 1. A model of the erosion of semantic–lexical–phonological support in semantic dementia.

language. Healthy listeners use statistical probabilities such as word length, phonotactic probability, and neighbourhood density to assign syntactic roles, parse word boundaries, and resolve semantic ambiguities (Saffran, Aslin, & Newport, 1996). Stress patterns tend to mark English nouns and verbs differently, and verbs tend to be shorter than nouns across many natural languages (Kelly, 2004; Langenmayr, Gozutok, & Gust, 2001). Similarly, phonological and morphological markers distinguish English abstract and concrete words. Concrete nouns tend to be shorter, more phonologically dense, and of higher cumulative phonotactic probability (Reilly & Kean, 2007). It is unclear whether patients with SD can make reliable decisions about phonology, and if so, whether they can use phonological patterns to bootstrap judgements of semantic and syntactic properties of words. One reason to investigate this issue is to determine whether reliable access to phonology can facilitate language processing in SD.

DISTINCTIVENESS OF CONCRETENESS AND GRAMMATICAL CLASS

Different neurological substrates support fine-grained semantic processing and storage distinctions between abstract and concrete words (e.g., *truth* versus *dog*). This distinction is evident in functional-imaging investigations among healthy adults that have shown inferior and lateral ventral temporal lobe activation for concrete words relative to abstract words (Binder, Westbury, McKiernan, Possing, & Medler, 2006) and in naming deficits encountered in patients with circumscribed brain damage. In deep dyslexia, for example, abstract words are sometimes strikingly impaired relative to concrete words. In contrast, patients with damage to ventral visual association cortex have shown the opposite trend, with a naming deficit for concrete words relative to abstract (Bird, Lambon Ralph, Patterson, & Hodges, 2000; Breedin, Saffran, & Coslett, 1994; Yi, Moore, & Grossman, 2007). One explanation we favour for this *reverse concreteness effect* is that damage to visual association cortex disproportionately disrupts highly salient visual features that underlie concrete word representation, whereas abstract words are less visually and more verbally mediated (see also Paivio, 1985).

In addition to concrete–abstract word differences, neuropsychological and imaging findings also support an anterior–posterior distinction between verbs and nouns, with greater recruitment of the left inferior frontal gyrus and premotor cortex for action verbs relative to nouns (Friederici, Opitz, & von Cramon, 2000). Studies of verb processing in dementia are rare. However, one recent investigation showed marked impairment in word-to-definition matching for verbs relative to nouns in semantic dementia (Yi et al., 2007). The same patients showed a robust reverse concreteness effect, with impaired matching of action verbs (e.g., *eat*) relative to abstract verbs (e.g., *think*).

In summary, some core differences exist between nouns and verbs and abstract and concrete concepts. Furthermore, phonological form is predictive of both distinctions. The extent to which patients with SD rely on phonologically mediated semantic and grammatical regularities to support their language processing is unknown. Here we examined two hypotheses germane to this issue: (1) that phonological perception is preserved in SD, and (2) that patients with SD exploit phonological regularities such as word length in making probabilistic judgements of words varied by their semantic and grammatical properties.

EXPERIMENT 1: MINIMAL PAIR JUDGEMENTS

Method

Participants. Participants included four male, monolingual English speakers with no comorbid psychiatric illness (e.g., major depression) or history of cerebrovascular disease. Table 1 summarises relevant demographic and neuropsychological data for the following patients: RZ, JF, JR, and LL (average age = 70.5). Patients are all currently retired and living at home with spouses who assist with daily activities and communication. These patients represent a range of anomia from mild (RZ) to severe (JR), with speech characterised as fluent with the exception of word-finding pauses.

Diagnoses were derived from a combination of imaging, neuropsychological, and linguistic testing in accord with a modification of published criteria for SD (Grossman & Ash, 2004; Neary et al., 1998). Table 1 lists patients ranked by severity of semantic and naming impairment via z-scores of their Pyramids and Palm Trees test performance (words and pictures; Howard & Patterson, 1992) compared with 18 age-matched healthy controls (mean age = 70.3, $\sigma = 8.0$), and by severity of naming impairment gauged by Boston Naming Test score (Goodglass & Kaplan, 1983) compared with 25 age-matched healthy controls (mean age = 66.76; $\sigma = 9.8$). Each patient's z-score for naming and semantic categorisation was calculated based on the mean and standard deviation of the control group [(Observed Patient Score − Mean Score of Controls)/Standard Deviation of Controls].

Figure 2 represents an illustrative voxel-based morphometric (VBM) image of patient LL, demonstrating areas of significant grey matter atrophy ($p < .01$ corrected) compared with a local brain template of age-matched controls ($N = 12$).

TABLE 1
Patient demographic, naming, and neuropsychological data

ID	Age	Ed	Months post	MMSE	Animal fluency	BNT (of 15) Raw	BNT (of 15) Z-score	PPT (words) Raw	PPT (words) Z-score	PPT (pictures) Raw	PPT (pictures) Z-score
RZ*	76	12	72	25	18	15	0.63	50	−0.48	52	1.02
JF	63	12	60	21	4	9	−3.84	45	−5.72	40	−7.42
JR	80	16	60	6	2	3	−8.30	n/a	n/a	41	−6.71
LG	50	16	30	29	7	10	−3.10	42	−8.15	42	−6.01
LL	63	16	96	21	0	2	−9.06	37	−9.05	30	−14.44
SB	69	14	n/a	22	2	4	−7.56	24	−25.40	n/a	n/a

Age and Education are reported in years; n/a = Testresult not available; *Months post* = Months post onset of initial complaint; *MMSE* = MiniMental State Examination (Folstein, Folstein, & McHugh, 1975); *BNT* = BostonNaming Test Score for a subset of 15 low, medium, and high frequency (Goodglass & Kaplan, 1983); *PPT* = Pyramids & Palm Trees test (Howard & Patterson, 1992); *Animal Fluency* = Animals named in 60 seconds. Each patient's associated z-score is with reference to an age-matched control group (control means: BNT = 14.72; PPT words = 50.6; PPT pictures = 50.5).

*RZ is a newly diagnosed SD patient. Although his semantic deficit is not evident on the BNT or PP tests, it is evident on MMSE and a different lexical categorisation task. When shown six vegetables, three fruits, and three tools, in both picture and word format, and asked "Is this a vegetable?", RZ classified all the fruits as vegetables (9/12 correct; control mean correct is 11.6 for words and 10.9 for pictures).

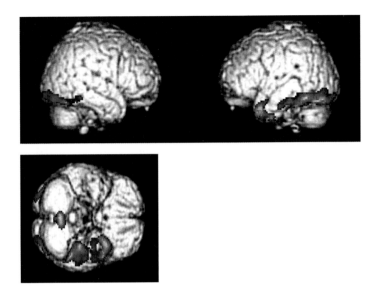

Figure 2. Voxel-based morphometric images (lateral and ventral) of Patient LL. Areas of higher intensity red to yellow indicate voxels with atrophy significant at $p < .01$ (corrected).

LL's distribution of atrophy, typical of moderate SD, encompassed the left anterior temporal lobe and the entirety of the left inferior temporal neocortex. Grey matter atrophy extended posterior to temporo-occipital cortex and ventrally through the left fusiform gyrus. Superior temporal and inferior parietal structures critical for auditory perception (e.g., primary auditory cortex and Wernicke's area) and inferior frontal areas implicated in grammatical processing were spared.

Experimental procedure. We constructed 48 pairs of consonant + vowel(CV) stimuli, varying the initial consonant and holding the vowel constant (e.g., /pa/, /ma/, /na/). Of these minimal pairs, half were identical (e.g., *ma – ma*), whereas the remaining pairs differed selectively by only voice, place, or manner of articulation. That is, eight pairs of items differed only by the presence of voicing in the initial consonant (e.g., *pa – ba*), eight pairs differed by manner of articulation (e.g., *da – na*), and the remaining eight pairs differed by place of articulation (e.g., *ga – na*). Stimuli were recorded by a female speaker in a sound booth using a Marantz PMD 670 digital audio recorder (DAT). Individual wavefiles were matched to an identical volume (50dB) using the Praat waveform editor (Boersma & Weenink, 1996). Wavefiles were recorded in stereo (dual-channel) format using a 16-bit, 44100-Hz sampling rate, and then filtered for noise. Two independent judges confirmed intelligibility of these stimuli through 100% accurate repetition. Wavefiles were presented via Sennheiser stereo headphones that completely covered the ear.

Testing was completed in the patients' homes using a Dell Inspiron laptop computer while an examiner simultaneously heard stimuli via a headphone splitter. E-Prime presented auditory stimuli in randomly ordered pairs with a 1000-ms interstimulus interval. Participants were instructed to listen while viewing an unchanging monitor display that asked *"Are these the same?"*. YES and NO were signalled by a keypress of either "M" (colour-coded green) or "Z" (colour-coded red). Participants first completed a familiarisation sequence to a criterion of 75% correct where they made same/different judgements for eight pairs of CVC stimuli.

Results

Patients performed more accurately in their minimal pair phonetic discrimination as a function of greater semantic impairment. This is confirmed by the negative correlation between minimal pair discrimination accuracy and each of the modalities of the Pyramids and Palm Trees tests, *Pearson* $r = -.75$, $p = .03$ (Howard & Patterson, 1992) (see Table 1 for z-scores on each measure). Milder patients showed phonetic discrimination not significantly different from chance, whereas more severe patients discriminated minimal pairs with higher accuracy (JF = 54%; RZ = 62%; JR = 73%; LL = 90%).

Discussion

Patients showed a paradoxical trend in their discrimination accuracy for minimal pairs. Individuals with milder semantic impairment performed less accurately in their phonetic judgements than patients with more severe semantic impairment. One possible explanation is that residual lexical-semantic knowledge in milder patients may degrade their performance for minimal pairs constructed with sparse phonology (e.g., *ga*, *ta*, *ma*). CV stimuli often form legal words (e.g., *ma*, *pa*). Furthermore, many real words can be created through the addition, omission, or substitution of a single phoneme to the bigram /#a/. This property, known as phonological neighbourhood density, produces wordlikeness or lexicality effects that may influence the accuracy of minimal pair phonologic discrimination (Gathercole, 1995; Luce & Pisoni, 1998). Aphasic adults show similar effects of lexical interference with an advantage in judgements of rhyming for pseudowords over real words (Kalinyak-Fliszar, Kohen, & Martin, 2006). SD patients with more advanced lexical-semantic degradation would theoretically not experience top-down lexical interference. These findings can therefore be interpreted in two ways: (1) patients with SD show poor phonetic perception, or (2) patients with milder SD show lexical interference effects for stimuli with high wordlikeness. We argue that the observed results support a lexical interference effect similar to that encountered in word and nonword rhyme judgements in aphasia (Kalinyak-Fliszar et al., 2006). This interference hypothesis is supported by these patients' performance on other paradigms that require intact phonological perception, such as auditory lexical decision wherein the individuals who performed at chance levels in their minimal pair discrimination here showed higher accuracy in judging nouns from plausible pseudowords (RZ = 84%; JF = 75%) (Reilly, Grossman, & McCawley, 2006). In contrast, the patients with the highest accuracy of minimal pair discrimination performed more poorly in making auditory lexical decisions (JR = 71%; LL = 71%). Thus, subtle deficits observed in acoustic perception in this patient sample may reflect lexical density effects for the patients with milder semantic impairment. Taken together, the current results interpreted in the context of preserved single-word repetition and auditory lexical decision abilities support grossly preserved phonological processing in this sample. However, a larger sample size and age-matched control group is necessary to assert this hypothesis with greater confidence.

EXPERIMENT 2: SINGLE-WORD CONCRETENESS JUDGEMENTS

We examined sensitivity to phonological regularities that mark English abstract and concrete verbs and nouns, hypothesising that phonological form will influence accuracy of single-word judgements as a function of grammatical class (noun/verb) and concreteness (abstract/concrete). We tested this hypothesis via forced choice semantic judgements for verbs and nouns varied by length and concreteness. This experiment employed a 2 (noun/verb) × 2 (abstract/concrete) × 2 (short/long word length) within-subjects design. The dependent measure was accuracy of single-word concreteness judgements compared with adult norms from the Cambridge Psycholinguistic database (Coltheart, 1981).

Method

Participants. Four male patients completed this experiment (JF, SB., LG, and RZ). Table 1 summarises relevant neuropsychological and demographic data. This sample includes two of the patients who completed Experiment 1 (RZ and JF) and two newly diagnosed SD patients (SB and LG). The two most semantically impaired patients from Experiment 1 (JR and LL) were excluded after multiple unsuccessful attempts at completing this experiment.

Materials. Stimuli included nouns ($n = 40$) and verbs ($n = 40$) matched for word concreteness using norms from the MRC Psycholinguistic database (Coltheart, 1981). Mean concreteness values on a 100–700-point scale were 376.33 and 429.18 for verbs and nouns respectively, $t(64) = 1.90$, $p = .06$. Concrete versus abstract stimuli collapsed across grammatical class had average concreteness ratings of 316 ($\sigma = 36.65$) and 486 ($\sigma = 91.73$), with higher values associated with stronger word concreteness (e.g., *truth* → *beach*) (Coltheart, 1981). These concreteness values were obtained from participants who were younger than the present SD sample. However, word concreteness has proven to be a stable construct with little known age-related variance across mature subjects within a single language (Barca, Burani, & Arduino, 2002; Kerr & Johnson, 1991).

Within each grammaticality and concreteness condition, half of the stimuli were three syllables in length, the remainder monosyllabic. Therefore, this factorial design employed eight cells with 10 stimuli per cell. Illustrative examples are as follows:

Abstract, 1 − syllable, Verb = *think*   Abstract, 3 − syllable, Noun = *attitude*

Concrete, 1 − syllable, Verb = *bake*   Concrete, 3 − syllable, Noun = *policeman*

Written frequencies of nouns and verbs were matched (Noun $\mu = 37.08$ per million, $\sigma = 4.0$; Verb $\mu = 39.50$ per million, $\sigma = 5.7$) $p > .05$ (Kučera & Francis, 1982). Stimuli were digitised as wavefiles using the identical audio sampling procedure, digital audio recording equipment, and female speaker described in Experiment 1. E-Prime software presented stimuli and logged responses using a Dell Inspiron laptop computer.

Experimental procedure. Participants were tested at a laptop computer equipped with stereo headphones, and were informed that they would hear words. Their task was to answer the following question about each new word: "*Can you see, hear, or touch this?*" Participants signalled YES or NO by pressing either M or Z (colour-coded green and red). Prior to the experimental trial, participants completed a familiarisation sequence where they made concreteness decisions with feedback for five items (e.g., *rope, hat*). There was no time restriction for this task.

Data analyses. Accuracies were scored in relation to the MRC Psycholinguistic database norms (Coltheart, 1981). For example, a response of "NO" to "*Can you can see, hear, or touch this?*" was scored as correct for abstract stimuli based on the grouping described above. Based on these accuracy scores, a proportion correct was calculated for each patient's performance within each cell in the design. Contrasts were conducted on proportions using three within-subjects factors: (1) concreteness (abstract/concrete); (2) word length (short/long); and (3) grammatical class (noun/verb). An item analysis was also performed by calculating an average accuracy score for each stimulus item collapsed across patients.

Results

Subject analyses. Group analyses conducted via a repeated measures within-subjects ANOVA revealed a significant two-way interaction between concreteness and word length, $F(1, 3) = 49.00$, $p < .001$.

One-syllable words were identified with similar accuracies regardless of whether they were abstract (58%) or concrete (55%). However, patients showed a stronger influence of phonology among three-syllable words, tending to misclassify longer concrete words (e.g., *professor, decorate*) as *abstract*. Accuracy for three-syllable abstract words was 66%, whereas accuracy for three-syllable concrete words was 46%. In addition to a phonological–semantic interaction, there was also a significant two-way interaction between word class and concreteness. Abstract verbs were identified with superior accuracy to concrete verbs (65% versus 36%); concrete and abstract nouns showed similar accuracies of identification (65% versus 59%) $F(1, 3) = 10.5$, $p = .05$.

Item analyses. Patients were impaired for verbs (36%) relative to nouns (65%) $t(38) = 4.42$, $p < .01$. However, this main effect occurred in the presence of a number of two-way interactions between word length, word class, and concreteness. First, there was a significant word length by concreteness interaction among response accuracies, $F(1, 72) = 4.16$, $p = .05$. This interaction was such that for three-syllable words, accuracy was significantly higher for abstract (66%) over concrete items (46%) $t(32.5) = 2.89$, $p = .01$. In contrast, one-syllable words showed similar accuracies regardless of their concreteness (58% abstract; 55% concrete) $p > .05$. Thus, the word length manipulation had a negative impact on judgement accuracies for concrete stimuli (e.g., *apartment* misclassified as abstract).

The second observed interaction was between concreteness and word class, $F(1, 72) = 16.64$, $p = .01$. Patients performed significantly more poorly for concrete verbs (36%) over abstract verbs (65%), tending to misclassify concrete verbs as *abstract*, $t(38) = 5.04$, $p < .001$. Within nouns, this effect was not as apparent, as similar item agreement was elicited between abstract (59%) and concrete nouns (65%).

Discussion

These interactions suggest that lexical-semantic judgements are sensitive to the phonologic properties of words in SD. Patients were impaired for verbs relative to nouns. In addition, patients showed a reversal of the typical concreteness effect, with a disadvantage in identifying concrete over abstract verbs. These response patterns replicate the findings of Yi et al. (2007) who reported similar noun–verb discrepancies in a different paradigm (i.e., word-to-definition matching) where patients with SD showed disadvantages for verbs, and within verbs were less accurate for concrete than abstract items. The authors accounted for these effects via a distributed hierarchical model of semantic memory in which nouns share many overlapping visually salient semantic features across exemplars (e.g., tails, legs, snouts of ANIMALS), whereas verbs lack this level of redundancy. Therefore, in the face of degraded feature knowledge, shared features can compensate in part for degraded knowledge of a specific exemplar for nouns (e.g., *labrador retriever*) (Gonnerman, Andersen, Devlin, Kempler, & Seidenberg, 1997). By comparison, the poorly structured hierarchical organisation of the verb semantic network limits the potential for shared features, resulting in greater difficulty for verbs than nouns.

In addition to grammatical class, listeners here showed an influence of word length in their judgement accuracies. Longer words were more likely to be classified as *abstract*, regardless of their actual semantic properties. This pattern is consistent with the phonological regularity in English abstract words, which are on average longer, more derivationally complex, and share fewer similar-sounding neighbours (Reilly & Kean, 2007). Thus, phonological manipulations also affected semantic judgement accuracy. We argue that these findings provide preliminary support for the active use of statistical regularities in language to aid in making higher-level semantic distinctions.

GENERAL DISCUSSION

A temporally dynamic behavioural model is valuable towards tailoring interventions to strengths at different stages of the disease. Here we have argued for an interactive model of SD that assumes increasing dependence on phonology and phonological regularities within language as dementia severity worsens. Patients with SD have shown contributions of intact phonology through repetition, immediate serial recall, and in patterns of reading associated with surface dyslexia (Jefferies et al., 2004; Knott, Patterson, & Hodges, 1997; Reilly et al., 2005). Patients with highly degraded semantic comprehension in the current study paradoxically showed the highest accuracy of judging subtle phonetic cues in minimal pair stimuli. Further evidence for an augmented role of phonology in language processing was apparent in the moderating effects of word length when making single-word semantic judgements. That is, longer words were often erroneously misclassified as *abstract*. This phonological bootstrapping effect plays a significant role in normal speech perception, where word length and syllable stress permit the rapid assignment of syntactic and thematic roles during online sentence processing. Similar cues may also facilitate semantic processing, as revealed through corpus analyses of speeded naming latencies and age of acquisition where healthy adults showed strong interaction effects between word length and imageability (Reilly & Kean, 2007).

Listeners with intact lexical-semantic knowledge appear to seamlessly overcome phonological and prosodic irregularities in speech. For example, *canoe* and *guitar* have lexical stress patterns more typical of verbs. Although listeners comprehend these nouns, they also show longer latencies to name and identify them compared to words with prototypical stress (e.g., *doctor* and *lawyer*). Therefore, subtle phonological effects in healthy listeners may incur more serious processing errors in patients with semantic impairment.

The progressive course of SD typically spares superior temporal and inferior parietal structures critical for phonological storage and phonetic perception. Consequently, patients with SD experience clinically preserved phonological perception until the late stages of the disease. Phonology is a residual strength in SD that should be capitalised upon in the selection of target stimuli. Patients here showed evidence of using phonological regularities to solve semantic problems in their single-word judgements. Thus, careful attention to both the phonological and semantic attributes of a therapeutic set may be warranted. Patients with SD may have the greatest success in relearning a small, closed set of words with careful attention to an optimal fit between phonological form, grammatical class, and meaning.

REFERENCES

Barca, L., Burani, C., & Arduino, L. S. (2002). Word naming times and psycholinguistic norms for Italian nouns. *Behavior Research Methods, Instruments, & Computers, 34*(3), 424–434.

Bird, H., Lambon Ralph, M. A., Patterson, K., & Hodges, J. R. (2000). The rise and fall of frequency and imageability: Noun and verb production in semantic dementia. *Brain and Language, 73*, 17–49.

Binder, J. R., Westbury, C. F., McKiernan, K. A., Possing, E. T., & Medler, D. A. (2006). Distinct brain regions for processing concrete and abstract concepts. *Journal of Cognitive Neuroscience, 17*(6), 905–917.

Boersma, P., & Weenink, D. (1996). *Praat, a system for doing phonetics by computer. Version 3.4. Report 132*. Institute of Phonetic Sciences of the University of Amsterdam.

Breedin, S., Saffran, E. M., & Coslett, H. (1994). Reversal of the concreteness effect in a patient with semantic dementia. *Cognitive Neuropsychology, 11*, 617–660.

Coltheart, M. (1981). The MRC psycholinguistic database. *Quarterly Journal of Experimental Psychology, 33*A, 497–505.

Coltheart, M., Byng, S., Masterson, J., Prior, M., & Riddoch, M. J. (1983). Surface dyslexia. *Quarterly Journal of Experimental Psychology, 35*A, 469–495.

Folstein, M. F., Folstein, S. E., & McHugh, P. R. (1975). Mini-Mental State: A practical method for grading the state of patients for the clinician. *Journal of Psychiatric Research, 12*, 189–198.

Friederici, A., Opitz, B., & von Cramon, D. Y. (2000). Segregating semantic and syntactic aspects of processing in the human brain: An fMRI investigation of different word types. *Cerebral Cortex, 10*, 698–705.

Gathercole, S. E. (1995). Is nonword repetition a test of phonological memory or long-term knowledge? It all depends on the nonwords. *Memory & Cognition, 23*(1), 83–94.

Goodglass, H., & Kaplan, E. (1983). *The assessment of aphasia and related disorders* (2nd ed.). Philadelphia, PA: Lea & Febiger.

Gonnerman, L. M., Andersen, E. S., Devlin, J. T., Kempler, D., & Seidenberg, M. S. (1997). Double dissociation of semantic categories in Alzheimer's disease. *Brain and Language, 57*, 254–279.

Grossman, M. (2002). Frontotemporal dementia: A review. *Journal of the International Neuropsychological Society, 8*, 566–583.

Grossman, M., & Ash, S. (2004). Primary progressive aphasia: A review. *Neurocase, 10*(1), 3–18.

Howard, D., & Patterson, K. (1992). *The Pyramids and Palm Trees Test: A test of semantic access from words and pictures*. Bury St. Edmonds, UK: Thames Valley Test Company.

Jefferies, E., Lambon Ralph, M. A., Jones, R., Bateman, D., & Patterson, K. (2004). Surface dyslexia in semantic dementia: A comparison of the influence of consistency and regularity. *Neurocase, 10*(4), 290–299.

Kalinyak-Fliszar, M., Kohen, F., & Martin, N. (2006). Effects of lexicality and short-term memory span on performance of rhyming judgement tasks: Evidence from aphasia. *Brain and Language, 99*, 178–179.

Kelly, M. H. (2004). Word onset patterns and lexical stress in English. *Journal of Memory and Language, 50*, 231–244.

Kerr, N. H., & Johnson, T. H. (1991). Word norms for blind and sighted subjects: Familiarity, concreteness, meaningfulness, imageability, imagery modality, and word associations. *Behavior Research Methods, Instruments & Computers, 23*(4), 461–485.

Knott, R. A., Patterson, K. E., & Hodges, J. R. (1997). Lexical and semantic binding effects in short-term memory: Evidence from semantic dementia. *Cognitive Neuropsychology, 14*(8), 1165–1216.

Kucera, H., & Francis, W. N. (1982). *Computational analysis of present-day American English*. Providence, RI: Brown University Press.

Kwok, S., Reilly, J., & Grossman, M. (2006). Acoustic-phonetic processing in semantic dementia. *Brain and Language, 99*, 145–146.

Lambon Ralph, M. A., McClelland, J. L., Patterson, K., Galton, C. J., & Hodges, J. R. (2001). No right to speak? The relationship between object naming and semantic impairment: Neuropsychological evidence and a computational model. *Journal of Cognitive Neuroscience, 13*, 341–356.

Langenmayr, A., Gozutok, M., & Gust, J. (2001). Remembering more nouns than verbs in lists of foreign language words as an indicator of syntactic phonetic symbolism. *Perceptual and Motor Skills, 93*, 843–850.

Luce, P. A., & Pisoni, D. B. (1998). Recognising spoken words: The neighbourhood activation model. *Ear and Hearing, 19*, 1–36.

Martin, N., & Saffran, E. M. (1990). Repetition and verbal STM in transcortical sensory aphasia: A case study. *Brain and Language, 39*, 254–288.

Neary, D., Snowden, J. S., Gustafson, L., Passant, U., Stuss, D., Black, S. et al. (1998). Frontotemporal lobar degeneration: A consensus on clinical diagnostic criteria. *Neurology, 51*, 1546–1554.

Paivio, A. (1985). *Mental representations: A dual coding approach*. New York: Oxford University Press.

Reilly, J., Grossman, M., & McCawley, G. (2006). Concreteness effects in the lexical processing of semantic dementia. *Brain and Language, 99*, 218–219.

Reilly, J., & Kean, J. (2007). Formal distinctiveness of high- and low-imageability nouns: Analyses and theoretical implications. *Cognitive Science, 31*, 1–12.

Reilly, J., Martin, N., & Grossman, M. (2005). Verbal learning in semantic dementia: Is repetition priming a useful strategy? *Aphasiology, 19*(3/4/5), 329–339.

Saffran, J. R., Aslin, R. N., & Newport, E. L. (1996). Statistical learning in 8-month old infants. *Science, 274*, 1926–1928.

Saffran, E. M., & Martin, N. (1990). Lexical involvement in short-term memory. In G. Vallar & T. Shallice (Eds.), *Neuropsychological impairments of short-term memory*. New York: Cambridge University Press.

Yi., H., Moore, P., & Grossman, M. (2007). Reversal of the concreteness effect for verbs in semantic dementia. *Cognitive Neuropsychology, 21*(1), 1–19.

APHASIOLOGY, 2007, 21 (6/7/8), 570–586

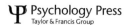
Psychology Press
Taylor & Francis Group

As far as individuals with conduction aphasia understood these sentences were ungrammatical: Garden path in conduction aphasia

Naama Friedmann

Tel Aviv University, Israel

Aviah Gvion

Tel Aviv University, and Reuth Medical Center, Tel Aviv, Israel

Background: Recent studies have indicated that working memory is not a unitary resource and that different types of working memory are used for different types of linguistic processing: syntactic, semantic, and phonological. Phonological working memory was found to support the comprehension of sentences that require re-access to the word-form of a word that appeared earlier in the sentence.

Aims: This study explored the relation between phonological working memory and sentence comprehension by testing the comprehension of garden path sentences in individuals with conduction aphasia who have very limited phonological working memory. Our prediction was that if phonological working memory limitation hampers word-form reactivation, only the comprehension of garden paths that require word-form reactivation will be impaired, whereas garden paths that require only structural reanalysis will be better preserved.

Methods & Procedures: Five individuals with conduction aphasia and 15 matched controls participated in working memory tests and a garden path comprehension test. The phonological working memory assessment included a battery of 10 tests, which showed that four of the individuals, who had input conduction aphasia, had very limited phonological working memory, and one individual, with output conduction aphasia, had unimpaired working memory. The comprehension study included 60 garden path sentences of three types: structural garden paths, which require only structural reanalysis, lexical garden paths, which require lexical re-access in addition to structural reanalysis, and optional-complement garden paths, which require re-access to the lexical-syntactic frame of the verb in addition to the structural reanalysis.

Outcomes & Results: The main result was that the individuals with input conduction aphasia showed different degrees of impairment in different types of garden path sentences. The lexical garden paths were exceptionally hard for them, with a mere 10% correct, and significantly more difficult than the structural garden paths. The individual with output conduction aphasia whose working memory was intact comprehended the lexical garden paths similarly to the normal controls.

Conclusions: These findings indicate that phonological working memory impairment only affects the comprehension of sentences that require phonological, word-form

Address correspondence to: Dr Naama Friedmann, Language and Brain Lab, School of Education, Tel Aviv University, Tel Aviv 69978, Israel. E-mail: naamafr@post.tau.ac.il

The research was supported by a research grant from the National Institute for Psychobiology in Israel (Friedmann 2004-5-2b), and by the Joint German–Israeli Research Program grant (Friedmann GR-01791). We thank Irena Botwinik-Rotem, Tali Siloni, and Michal Biran for discussions of this study.

http://www.psypress.com/aphasiology   DOI: 10.1080/02687030701192000

re-access. The type of sentence and the type of processing it requires should be taken into account when trying to predict the effect of working memory limitation on a patient's ability to understand sentences. Whereas individuals with input conduction aphasia can understand complex syntactic structures well, they have considerable difficulties understanding sentences that also require re-access to a word-form.

"Because the little boy hid the ice-cream that his brother wanted to eat melted." This sentence is a garden path sentence. As readers or listeners move from one word to the next, they encounter the verb *hid*, which can be intransitive or followed by a direct object. Some readers/listeners strongly expect a direct object after the verb, so their initial interpretation of *the ice-cream* is as the object of the verb *hid.* As the sentence proceeds they are surprised to encounter the verb *melted*, suggesting that they have initially mis-analysed the sentence and therefore have been "led down the garden-path". This mis-analysis requires the parser to reanalyse the sentence.

Garden path sentences, then, clearly require processing over and above other types of sentences. But is this processing related to phonological working memory, or is it memory resources of a different kind? The current research sought to answer this question via the examination of garden path comprehension in a group of individuals with conduction aphasia who have very limited phonological working memory.

Phonological working memory (pWM) is a specialised short-term memory for the retention of phonological information. The relation between pWM and sentence comprehension has been intensely discussed, debated, and examined in various populations with pWM limitation: individuals with aphasia (Friedmann & Gvion, 2003; Martin, 1987; Martin & Feher, 1990; Martin & He, 2004; Martin & Romani, 1994; Martin, Shelton, & Yafee, 1994; Romani & Martin, 1999; Smith & Geva, 2000, for a review; Waters, Caplan, & Hildebrandt, 1991; Wright & Shisler, 2005), young typically developing children (Willis & Gathercole, 2001), individuals with developmental short-term memory limitation (Hanten & Martin, 2001), and elderly people (DeDe, Caplan, Kemtes, & Waters, 2004; Zurif, Swinney, Prather, Wingfield, & Brownell, 1995).

In recent years a growing body of data has accumulated, showing that pWM is related to sentence comprehension only for sentences (and tasks) that crucially rely on lexical-phonological processing. Many studies that assessed the effect of syntactic complexity on individuals with limited pWM capacity—using the comprehension of passives, object relative clauses, garden-path sentences, reflexives, and judgement of subject–verb agreement in various distances—found no impairment in comprehension or in grammaticality judgement (Butterworth, Campbell, & Howard, 1986; Butterworth, Shallice, & Watson, 1990; see Caplan & Waters, 1999 for a review; Friedmann & Gvion, 2003; Friedmann & Shapiro, 2003; Hanten & Martin, 2000, 2001; Martin & Feher, 1990; Martin, Inglis, & Kuminiak, 2004; Martin & Romani, 1994; Waters & Caplan, 1996; Waters et al., 1991; Willis & Gathercole, 2001).

Other studies showed that tasks that require phonological processing are difficult for individuals with limited phonological memory. These studies, which tested phonological processing by means of verbatim repetition, found that verbatim repetition was impaired for long sentences. Importantly, the comprehension of these sentences was found to be preserved, as reflected in the paraphrases, which maintained the meaning of the sentences. These findings were reported for individuals with aphasia (Martin et al., 1994), young typically developing children with low spans (compared to children with high spans, Willis & Gathercole, 2001), and children with acquired phonological memory deficit (Hanten & Martin, 2000).

In an earlier study (Friedmann & Gvion, 2003) we examined sentence comprehension in individuals with conduction aphasia who had very limited spans. We compared the comprehension of relative clauses, which require syntactic-semantic reactivation, and the comprehension of sentences with ambiguous words, which require lexical-phonological reactivation. In both sentence types, interpretation required reactivation of an earlier constituent in the sentence. In relative clauses it was the antecedent that had to be re-accessed, and in the sentences with ambiguous words the re-access of the ambiguous lexical item was required in order to reanalyse the sentence. In both sentence types we used the same manipulation—loading pWM by increasing the number of words (and syllables) between a word and the position of its reactivation.

Syntactic-semantic reactivation was studied using subject and object relative clauses. Relative clauses include a moved constituent (antecedent), which needs to be reactivated at its original position (the gap position) in order for the sentence to be interpreted (Nicol & Swinney, 1989; Swinney, Ford, Frauenfelder, & Bresnan, 1988; Swinney, Zurif, & Nicol 1989; Zurif et al., 1995). Love and Swinney (1996) have shown that this reactivation is "deeply" semantic (and guided by syntax), rather than phonological, in nature. In order to test whether the comprehension of these sentences is affected by limited pWM we manipulated the gap-antecedent distance by adding 2, 5, 7, or 9 words between the moved constituent and the position of its reactivation (for example, in the sentence *This is the woman with the brown pants and the white shirt that the girl hugs* ←, there are 12 words between the *woman* and its reactivation, marked by an arrow). The results showed that individuals with conduction aphasia who had very limited spans comprehended subject and object relatives well and were *unaffected* by the distance between the antecedent and the gap. We concluded that when semantic-syntactic reactivation is required, phonological working memory limitation does not impair comprehension.

Phonological reactivation was studied in the same participants by using sentences with ambiguous words, positioned in a context strongly biased towards one of the meanings. The sentences were designed to be disambiguated with the alternative meaning and in a way that required reanalysis (for example: "The PEN that the man received from his wife when he retired was packed with woolly sheep", see the rationale, description of stimuli, and experimental design in Friedmann & Gvion, 2003; Gvion & Friedmann, 2007). Note in this example that it appears the meaning of *pen* will be a "writing implement" but it becomes obvious later in the sentence that the meaning should be "a corral". Unlike relative clauses, the reactivation required in these sentences at the disambiguation position had to be phonological in nature, and re-access to only its meaning would not suffice. Here is why: as Swinney (1979) and Onifer and Swinney (1981) discovered, immediately after an ambiguous word is heard, all its meanings are activated. As the sentence unfolds, only the meaning that seems relevant for the biasing context remains active, and the other meanings decay (see also Love & Swinney, 1996; Swinney, Prather, & Love, 2000). Going back to the sentences we used: when, at a later point in the sentence, it turns out that the meaning that remained active is not the one relevant for the sentence, the other meaning has already decayed. Accessing meaning only would hence yield the irrelevant meaning, and thus cannot be used to understand the sentence. Reanalysis requires the reactivation of the *phonological word form* of the original ambiguous word, in order to re-access all possible meanings and choose the contextually correct meaning.

In this experiment, too, the distance between the word and its reactivation was manipulated for short (2–3 words) and long (7–9 words) distances. The prediction was that if phonological working memory is needed to support re-access to the word-form, then the individuals with conduction aphasia with the limited spans will fail to comprehend these sentences when the disambiguation position is too far; namely, after the correct meaning has already decayed. The results indeed showed that the patients performed significantly better and well above chance on the short distance sentences, but performed very poorly and significantly worse than matched controls on the long distance disambiguation sentences. Thus, these results clearly suggest that not all types of sentences are impaired when pWM is impaired; only sentences that require phonological reactivation (or phonological maintenance) are affected.

Other studies also suggest the existence of *semantic* WM which can be selectively damaged (Martin & Romani, 1994; Martin et al., 1994). In the case studies that Martin and her colleagues describe, retention of semantic information throughout the sentence was disturbed whereas comprehension of various syntactic structures was unimpaired (Martin, 2003; Martin & Romani, 1994; Romani & Martin, 1999), and the verbatim repetition was preserved or at least much better than semantic ability (Hanten & Martin, 2000; Willis & Gathercole, 2001).

Taken together, the data from these studies strongly suggest a domain-specific working memory (WM) system in which each type of WM supports a different type of linguistic processing. According to this view, different WM types support syntax, semantics, and phonology (Friedmann & Gvion, 2003; Gvion & Friedmann, 2007; Haarmann, Davelaar & Usher, 2003; Hanten & Martin, 2000; Martin & He, 2004; Martin & Romani, 1994; Martin et al., 1994; Romani & Martin, 1999). Each such WM type is responsible for the retention and the reactivation of the relevant type of linguistic material, and each type of memory addresses the sentence differently: content-addressable retrieval for syntactic-semantic processing versus search-based mechanism for phonological processing (McElree, 2000).

How is phonological WM related to the comprehension of garden path (GP) sentences? The two studies so far that asked this question yielded contradicting results. MacDonald, Just, and Carpenter (1992) studied the performance of high- and low-span participants in comprehending GP and non-GP sentences. The participants with low spans made more comprehension errors than the participants with high spans in the GPs, although their reading times were shorter. MacDonald and her colleagues concluded that the comprehension of garden paths is related to working memory. The account they offered was that the participants with high spans maintain two possible syntactic representations at the same time, a competence that enables them to process GPs better, at the cost of longer reading times. The participants with low spans maintain only the more plausible representation and as a result fail comprehending the GP. However, a later study by Waters and Caplan (1996) compared the performance of participants with high, medium, and low spans in various sentence types including GP sentences and found no significant correlation between pWM spans and the acceptability judgement of GP sentences. One possible source for this inconsistency of results may be the different requirements of the tasks, as MacDonald et al. (1992) tested comprehension, whereas Waters and Caplan (1996) used acceptability judgement.

In light of the results from these past studies indicating the existence of different WM types that are required in different types of sentences, a different source for the mixed results regarding the relation between GP and pWM arises. If indeed only sentences that require phonological reactivation are impaired when phonological working memory is limited, whereas sentences, even complex ones, that require only syntactic-semantic processing are unimpaired, then the reason for the mixed results might be the mixed types of garden path sentences presented in these experiments. It might be that there are different subtypes of GPs, which require different types of processing, thus taxing different types of WM.

The main characteristic of GPs is that they require structural reanalysis (cf. Pritchett, 1992, and articles in Fodor & Ferreira, 1998). These sentences include a temporary syntactic ambiguity that is initially analysed in one way, but as the sentence continues to unfold has to be reanalysed and be assigned a different structure. Importantly for our discussion, whereas structural reanalysis is always required in a GP, and in fact defines it as such, sometimes additional reanalysis is required: Some sentences involve reanalysis of a lexical item.

Garden variety of garden paths

One type of garden path requires only structural reanalysis. For example, in the sentence *"Edgar met his former student and his collaborator left the room"*, the parser initially identifies *his collaborator* as the object of *met*, and then, when it reaches *left*, a structural reanalysis takes place and *his collaborator* is put in the subject position of the coordinated clause. No word changes its meaning in this sentence, and a purely structural reanalysis is required. We term this type of GP *structural GP*.

The other type of GP, *lexical GP*, requires lexical re-access and reanalysis in addition to the structural reanalysis. One example of this type of GP are sentences that include a word that is ambiguous between a noun and a verb reading, as in the sentence *The building blocks the sun faded were red* (taken from Milne, 1980).[1] In such a sentence not only does the parser need to change the structure of the sentence and reanalyse the word *blocks* as part of the NP *the building blocks* rather than as the main verb, it also needs to re-access the word-form of the lexical item *blocks* in order to reactivate all the meanings and choose a different meaning from the one that was initially chosen. Another type of garden path that might also require re-access to the lexical entry is garden paths that are built around an ambiguous verb: a verb that is associated with two thematic frames, each describing a different event. For example, the verb *hid* in *While the little boy hid his lollipop disappeared* is initially analysed with a complement and has the meaning of hiding something, and then, when it is reanalysed to having no complement, it changes its meaning to the boy himself hides. In such a case too, re-access to the lexical entry of the verb is required because its thematic grid and its meaning changed.

One open question (which we try to answer empirically in the current study) is whether lexical re-access is also required in order to change thematic frame of the verb even when the core meaning of the verb (the event denoted by the verb) does not change. In a garden path sentence such as *When the vegetarian decided to eat a pizza was delivered to her roommate*, which we term *optional-complement GP*, the analysis

---

[1] A memorial GP: When the man who invented this garden path climbed Mount Everest betrayed him.

changes from a verb that takes a complement to a verb that does not, without changing the meaning of the verb *eat*. It might be that in this type of GP too, the lexical entry of the verb should be re-accessed in order to retrieve all complementation options and choose a different one from the one initially chosen.

Shapiro and his colleagues (Shapiro, Gordon, Hack, & Killackey, 1993; Shapiro, Zurif, & Grimshaw, 1987) discovered that when a verb is heard, all its complementation options (argument structure frames) are initially activated, as indicated by the longer access time to verbs with more argument structure frames. Swinney and his colleagues (Love & Swinney, 1996; Onifer & Swinney, 1981; Swinney, 1979) demonstrated that when an ambiguous word is encountered, all its meanings are initially activated, but then only the relevant meaning remains active, and the rest of the meanings decay. If we unite the outcomes of these two lines of research, we might expect that when a verb with multiple argument structure frames is encountered, all its frames are activated, but then only one frame remains, and the others decay. If so, we would expect GPs that require reanalysis of the argument structure of the verb to require lexical re-access, to allow for the reactivation of all thematic frames and the choice of the correct frame. Hence, we would expect optional-complement GPs to behave like lexical-structural GPs.

One study we conducted with healthy individuals already indicates that structural and lexical GPs indeed interact differently with phonological working memory. Margalit, Friedmann, and Gvion (2005) tested the comprehension of structural and lexical GPs in 40 Hebrew-speaking individuals aged 25–40 without language impairment. The main result was that whereas structural GPs did not interact with word span and digit span, the comprehension of lexical GPs was significantly correlated with both word span ($r = .41$, $p < .01$) and digit span ($r = .34$, $p < .05$).

In the current study we wish to further examine the processing of different types of GP by assessing GP comprehension in individuals with conduction aphasia who have a pWM limitation. In light of the results from our previous experiments, we expect garden path sentences that require lexical-phonological reactivation to be related to pWM, whereas GPs that involve only structural reanalysis are not expected to be affected by pWM limitation.

METHOD

In order to examine the relationship between limited phonological working memory and the comprehension of the various types of garden path sentences, we administered a set of tasks that measured the participants' phonological working memory, and a garden path comprehension experiment.

Participants

The participants, YF, NT, KS, and ST, were four Hebrew-speaking individuals with input conduction aphasia (repetition conduction aphasia) following ischaemic strokes, with or without impairment in the output component. They were three men and one woman; two of them were right-handed and two left-handed. They were identified with conduction aphasia using the Hebrew version of the Western Aphasia Battery (WAB, Kertesz, 1982; Hebrew version by Soroker, 1997). Their mean age was 55.8 ($SD = 14.2$ years, range: 39–73). All had at least 12 years of education and had pre-morbidly full control of Hebrew. They were tested 4–6 months post their stroke ($M = 5$ months, $SD = 1.2$). Inclusive criteria for participation in the study were impaired repetition of sentences and nonwords and limited phonological working memory in recall and recognition spans (see section on WM measures below). Three of the patients also had deficits in phonological output lexicon or in the phonological output buffer as shown in their phonological paraphasias (substitutions, transpositions, or deletions of segments) in spontaneous speech, repetition, and naming.

Another participant with a crucially different profile of conduction aphasia was DK, a 52-year-old right-handed man with 17 years of education, who had output (reproduction) conduction aphasia as a result of an ischaemic stroke with preserved phonological working memory (see next section).

We also tested a matched control group that included 15 age-matched individuals without language impairment (mean age 54, $SD = 10.4$ years; range: 38–73). They were 5 men and 10 women, all with at least 12 years of education.

Phonological working memory assessment

The phonological WM of the participants with input conduction aphasia was measured by an extensive phonological working memory battery (FriGvi: Friedmann & Gvion, 2002). The battery included 10 tests: 5 were recall span tests, and 5 were recognition tests. The recall span tests included five sequences on each level, and each level included increasingly large sets of items. The words were read at a one per second rate. Span was defined as the maximum level at which at least three sequences per level were fully recalled; an additional half point was given for success in two out of five sequences. The five recall span tests included a *basic word span* test, with semantically unrelated sequences of 2-syllable words; *long word span* with 4-syllable words; *phonologically similar word span* with word sequences that were phonologically similar, sharing all but a single phoneme; *nonword span* that included 2-syllable nonwords; and *digit span*. The five recognition tests included listening span, word span, probe test, and digit- and word-matching tests. The *listening span* was a Hebrew version of the listening span task (Caspari, Parkinson, LaPointe, & Katz, 1998; Daneman & Carpenter, 1980; Tompkins, Bloise, Timko, & Baumgaertner, 1994), adapted for individuals with aphasia. The test was composed of five levels (two to six simple 3–4-word sentences per set) each containing five sets. Final target words were 1–2-syllable nouns. The participants made true/false judgements to each sentence in increasingly large sets of unrelated sentences, and then recognised the final word in each sentence. Recognition of the final words was assessed by pointing to the words in a set of $2n + 1$ presented words; the *word recognition span* included the words from the listening span and required the same type of recognition. In the *probe test* the participant heard a sequence of eight 2-syllable words and then another list of eight words for which s/he was requested to judge whether each word appeared in the first list. Half of the words in the second list appeared in the first list, the other half were semantic or phonological distractors. The *matching digit span* test was taken from PALPA 13 (Kay, Lesser, & Coltheart, 1992; Hebrew version by Gil & Edelstein, 2001), the participants heard two sequences containing the same digits and were required to judge whether the order of the items is the same. The *matching word span* was similar to the matching digit span task, but included two-syllable

TABLE 1
Spans of the participants with conduction aphasia in each of the recall and recognition tests, and normal mean and standard deviation for each test.

Participant	Word span	Long word span	Similar word span	Non-word span	Digit span	Listening span	Recognition word span	Probe test %match	Matching word span	Matching number span
ST	4*	3.5*	2.5*	2*	5.5*	2.5*	4*	69*	4*	4*
YF	3*	1.5*	2*	2*	2*	5*	4*	51*	3*	7
NT	2*	1.5*	2*	1*	3*	4*	3*	56*	3*	3*
KS	4*	3.0*	3*	1*	3*	5.5	5*	74*	3*	3*
Norms	5.33	4.32	4.29	3.35	6.96	5.79	5.78	84.83	6.13	6.65
(SD)	(0.75)	(0.63)	(0.63)	(0.49)	(1.14)	(0.43)	(0.36)	(8.12)	(1.01)	(0.63)
DK (output)	4.5	3.5	2.5	2	6	6	6	87	7	7

* Significantly below the norm, $p < .01$.

words instead of digits. (See Friedmann & Gvion, 2003, and Gvion & Friedmann, 2007, for detailed description of the tests in this battery and for norms taken from 60–146 healthy individuals in various age groups.)

The performance of the individuals with input conduction aphasia on the pWM tasks was poor—as seen in Table 1—and significantly poorer than that of a large group of healthy controls in at least 8 out of the 10 tasks, using Crawford and Howell's (1998) t-test for the comparison of an individual to a control group, $p < .01$. All the matched participants who were included in the study were within the normal range on all WM tasks in the battery.

With respect to DK, the individual with output conduction aphasia, because he had an output deficit DK showed poorer than normal performance on the tests that involved overt output, the recall tests, but in the recognition tests where no speech output was required, his spans were normal.

The comprehension of different types of GP sentences

The main research question of this test was whether there is a difference between the comprehension of GPs that require only syntactic reanalysis and GPs that also require lexical reanalysis. A secondary aim of the study was to examine whether GPs that require reanalysis of verbs with optional complements behave like syntactic or lexical GPs. In order to do this we also included such optional-complement GP sentences.

Materials

A total of 60 GPs were presented: 20 structural, 20 lexical, and 20 optional-complement GPs.[2]

The structural GPs included either a coordinated object that became reanalysed as the subject of a coordinated phrase (Example 1; the sentences in

---

[2] Two of the participants heard 24 structural GPs.

the examples below include the Hebrew transliterated sentences, followed by a literal translation and then free translation) or sentences with a phrase that was initially interpreted as a complement and then was reanalysed as an adjunct when the real complement was encountered. This second type included either an embedded clause that was interpreted initially as the sentential complement of the verb, but then was reanalysed as a relative clause (for example: *The boy told the groom that the bride left to run after her*), and sentences in which a prepositional phrase was initially taken to be the complement of the verb and then reanalysed as an adjunct (*The journalist was interested in my opinion only in his editor's opinion*).

The lexical GPs included six sentences with a noun–verb or verb–adjective ambiguity (Example 2), and 14 sentences with a verb with two possible argument structures, each carrying a different meaning of the verb (Example 3).

In the optional-complement GPs we used verbs like *knit* that take optional complements. These verbs can appear either without a complement (*The grandmother knitted*), or with one (*The grandmother knitted a sweater*). Unlike the lexical-thematic GPs in Example 3, here the omission or addition of the optional complement did not change the core meaning of the verb (Example 4).

1a. Ruthi kona le-itim sifrei omanut ve-itonei nashim hi lo kona af-pa'am.
    Ruthi buys sometimes books-of art and-journals women she not buys ever.
    "Ruthi sometimes buys art books and women's magazines she never buys."
  b. Yuval tamid kone sfarim atikim ve-itonim civoniyim ve-xadashim shel ofna ve-icuv
    hu lo kone af-pa'am.
    Yuval always buys books antique and-journals colorful and-new of fashion and-
    design he not buys ever.
    "Yuval always buys antique books and new glossy fashion and design magazines he never buys."
  2. xevrat haitek mexapeset menahel proyektim u-mazkira she-ha-saxar gavoha
    Firm hi-tech searches manager projects and-secretary/reminds that-the-salary high
    "A hi-tech firm searches for a project manager and mentions [ambiguous with a secretary] that the salary is high."
  3. biglal she-ha-saparit hexlika searot shel lakoxa hitpazru le-xol ever
    Because that-the-hairdresser straightened/slipped hair of client scattered to-all sides
    "Because the hairdresser slipped [the transitive means straightened] a client's hair scattered all over."
  4. be-zman she-hatabax bishel marak nishpax al ha-ricpa
    While that-the-chef cooked soup spilled-over on the-floor
    "While the chef cooked soup spilled onto the floor."

Earlier studies of GP in unimpaired individuals indicated a length effect in the comprehension of GPs. Ferreira and Henderson (1991, see also Christianson, Hollingworth, Halliwell, & Ferreira, 2001) demonstrated that the distance between the head of the temporarily ambiguous phrase and the point where the parser detects a processing error (the error signal position) affects comprehension. GPs with short head–error signal distance were found easier to process than the ones with longer distances. We therefore controlled for the distance between the point of temporal ambiguity and the point of reanalysis, with half of the sentences of each type including short distance (1–3 words, see example 1a), and half including a longer distance of 5–9 words (see example 1b).

The 60 sentences were divided into three sets of 20 sentences, each set presented in a different session. The sets were constructed so that short and long sentences that shared the same ambiguous word or the same syntactic ambiguity were never introduced in the same set. Each set included the three types of GPs (7, 7, and 6 of each type), half long and half short. The order of the sessions was randomised among participants.

Procedure

Each sentence was presented auditorily only once, in a monotonous (flat) intonation that did not disclose the meaning of the sentence. The participant was requested to paraphrase it as accurately as possible. In cases of difficulties in oral paraphrasing, hand gestures were accepted as well.

Coding of responses. The responses were transcribed and recorded during the sessions and were separately analysed by four judges. Reliability exceeded 95%, and the few disagreements that arose were resolved by consensus. The participants' paraphrases were analysed according to the following criteria: the response was coded as correct if the paraphrase indicated that a correct reanalysis was done and the participant interpreted the ambiguous phrase correctly. Deletion or substitution of information outside the relevant phrase were not counted as incorrect. Initial erroneous responses that were followed by self-corrections were counted as correct. Responses that indicated a failure to interpret the ambiguous phrase, or responses in which the participants said that a sentence was odd and they could not paraphrase it, were counted as incorrect. Partial responses or responses that were not clear enough to indicate the interpretation were excluded from analysis (i.e., the sentence was removed from the total number of sentences).

RESULTS

The results for each of the participants with input conduction aphasia and the matched controls are presented in Figure 1. The principal finding was that the phonological working memory limitation mainly impaired the comprehension of GPs that required lexical reanalysis (in addition to structural reanalysis), whereas the GPs that required only structural reanalysis were much better preserved.

Input conduction aphasia

Our main research question was whether, when phonological working memory is impaired, there is a difference between the comprehension of GPs that require only syntactic reanalysis and GPs that also require lexical reanalysis. In a two-way ANOVA with a repeated measure on sentence type, a main effect was found for sentence type (structural, lexical), $F(1, 17) = 66.05$, $p < .0001$, $\eta_{p^2} = 0.80$ as well as a main effect for the group (control, conduction), $F(1, 17) = 31.74$, $p < .0001$, $\eta_{p^2} = 0.65$. Importantly, there was a significant interaction between group and sentence type, $F(1, 17) = 17.64$, $p < .001$, $\eta_{p^2} = 0.51$. With respect to the matched controls, although they comprehended both types of GPs, with a mean performance of 84% ($SD = 10$) in the structural GPs and a mean of 69% ($SD = 20$) in the lexical GPs, lexical GPs were significantly harder for them than structural GPs, $t(14) = 4.22$,

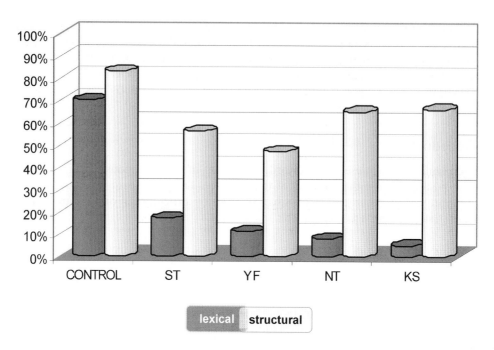

Figure 1. Comprehension of structural GPs and lexical-structural GPs.

$p < .001$, $d = 2.25$. The lexical GPs were harder for both groups, possibly because they require two types of reanalysis. Importantly however, the difference between the structural and the lexical GPs was significantly larger for the conduction aphasia group. The individuals with conduction aphasia understood 50 out of 84 structural GPs, and only 8 out of 77 lexical GPs, a difference that was highly significant both using chi-square, $\chi^2 = 42.1$, $p < .0001$, and using paired t-test, $t(3) = 7.45$, $p = .005$, $d = 8.60$. This difference between structural and lexical GPs also held when we compared the comprehension of the aphasia group for only the short structural vs lexical GPs, $t(3) = 5.25$, $p = .01$, $d = 6.06$, and when we compared only the long structural vs lexical GPs, $t(3) = 14.37$, $p < .001$, $d = 16.60$.

The individual data, presented in Table 2, show that whereas two of the individuals with conduction aphasia did not differ from the control group in their comprehension of structural GPs, and two did (using Crawford-Howell t-test for the

TABLE 2
Percentage correct in the two types of GP

Participant	Structural GP	Lexical-structural GP	χ^2
ST	56.5	17.6	$\chi^2 = 6.2$, $p = .01$
YF	47.1	11.8	$\chi^2 = 5.1$, $p = .02$
NT	65.0	8.3	$\chi^2 = 16.7$, $p < .001$
KS	66.7	5.3	$\chi^2 = 15.6$, $p < .001$
Average (SD)	58.8 (9.0)	10.8 (5.3)	
Control participants	84 (10.4)	69 (20.1)	

comparison of an individual to a control group, $p < .05$), all four participants were significantly poorer than the control group in the comprehension of the lexical GPs, $p < .03$. Each participant with conduction aphsia understood structural GPs significantly better than lexical GPs, as seen in Table 2.

No difference was found between lexical GPs in which the ambiguity stemmed from a noun–verb ambiguous word (2/24 correct responses) and lexical-thematic GPs in which the ambiguity was related to a verb that was associated with two thematic frames, each with a different meaning (6/53), $\chi^2 = 0.16$, $p = .69$, insinuating the similarity in lexical access to these two types of lexical ambiguity.

An indication that at least some of the GPs they failed to understand were actually taken as ungrammatical was that each of the individuals with conduction aphasia repeatedly commented that the sentences they failed to paraphrase seemed odd or ungrammatical (ST made this comment 13 times, YF 14 times, NT 10 times, and KS 10 times).

With respect to the effect of the distance between the point of temporary ambiguity and the point of reanalysis, similarly to earlier studies the longer GPs were harder than the shorter ones for the control participants. Their comprehension of short-distance GPs was significantly better than the long ones in both structural GPs, $t(14) = 5.37$, $p < .001$, $d = 2.87$, and lexical GPs, $t(14) = 2.88$, $p = .01$, $d = 1.54$. However, the individuals with conduction aphasia did not show this difference. The long structural GPs did not differ significantly from the short structural GPs, $t(3) = 1.41$, $p = .12$ (although approaching significance, also in χ^2 analysis, $p = .08$); nor did the long lexical GPs differ from the short lexical GPs, $t(3) = 0.96$, $p = .20$ ($p = .17$ in χ^2). An individual analysis using χ^2 yielded no significant difference between the short and the long GPs for any of the individuals with conduction aphasia.

Do optional complements require lexical re-access? Another research question pertained to verbs that take optional complements. In the garden paths that included these verbs, the initial analysis assigned a complement to the verb, and following the reanalysis the verb did not have a complement. Our question was whether this type of reanalysis requires only structural reanalysis or also lexical re-access to the verb. Now that we know that the individuals with conduction aphasia have considerably more difficulty in the comprehension of GPs that require lexical re-access, we can answer this question by testing whether the comprehension of the optional-complement GPs patterns with the lexical GPs or with the structural GPs. This analysis showed that the optional-complement GPs in the conduction aphasia group patterned with the lexical GP rather than with the structural ones. The structural GPs were not only significantly better than the lexical GPs, they were also significantly better than the optional-complement GPs, $t(3) = 16.73$, $p < .001$, $d = 19.31$. Importantly, no significant difference was found between the comprehension of optional-complement GPs and lexical GPs, $t(3) = 2.51$, $p = .09$. For the control participants too, the optional-complement and the lexical GPs did not differ, $t(14) = 1.80$, $p = .09$. It seems, then, that for the input conduction aphasia participants, the optional-complement GPs were as hard as the lexical GPs, and much harder than the structural GPs, indicating that a similar lexical re-access has to take place in the optional-complement GPs as well.

Output conduction aphasia with preserved WM

The final analysis related to the way DK, the participant with output conduction aphasia who had preserved phonological memory, understood the various types of GPs. Given his intact pWM he is expected, despite his conduction aphasia, to be able to understand lexical GPs. The comparison of DK's performance to that of the input conduction participants revealed that his performance on the lexical-thematic GPs was significantly better than each of the individuals with input conduction aphasia, $p < .05$, significantly better than the group, $\chi^2 = 15.58$, $p < .0001$, and not different from the control participants, $t(14) = 0.9$, $p = .38$. His performance on the structural GPs was slightly worse than that of the group with input conduction aphasia, $\chi^2 = 4.11$, $p = .04$ (on individual comparisons his performance on the structural GPs was only significantly poorer than NT's performance and not significantly different from the others). The comparison of DK's performance to that of the control participants using Crawford-Howell t-test showed that there was no difference between his performance and that of the matched control group on the lexical and optional-complement GPs ($p > .38$), but his performance was poorer on the structural GPs, $p < .01$.

DISCUSSION

The aim of the current study was to explore the relation between phonological working memory and sentence comprehension by testing the comprehension of garden path sentences in individuals with conduction aphasia who have very limited pWM. Previous studies strongly indicate that the WM system is domain specific, with each type of WM supporting a different type of linguistic processing: syntactic, semantic, and phonological. Consequently, an impairment in one type of WM impairs the comprehension of sentences that require the relevant type of processing. Thus, pWM limitation only impairs the comprehension of sentences that require phonological (word-form) processing. And indeed, our earlier studies with individuals with conduction aphasia who had phonological WM impairment indicated that whereas their comprehension of syntactically complex sentences may have been unimpaired, the comprehension of sentences that require maintenance or phonological re-access to an earlier lexical item was severely compromised.

Continuing this line of thought, similar reasoning can be applied to the comprehension of garden path sentences in populations with limited pWM by classifying GPs according to the type of processing they require. Whereas the defining characteristic of a GP sentence is that it requires a syntactic reanalysis, the current study tested the conjecture that GPs can be classified on the basis of whether or not they also require lexical (word-form) reanalysis. We suggested a classification of garden path sentences into those that require only structural reanalysis and those that also require lexical word-form re-access. Our prediction was that if phonological WM limitation hampers the comprehension of sentences that require lexical reactivation, only garden paths that require lexical re-access should be impaired, whereas the comprehension of garden path sentences that require only structural reanalysis will be better preserved.

The main result was that the lexical GPs were exceptionally hard for the individuals with conduction aphasia, and significantly more difficult than the structural GPs. Whereas the structural GPs yielded 59% correct responses, the lexical GPs were only 10% correct, indicating that the pWM limitation indeed affected mainly the comprehension of GP sentences that required lexical re-access, over and above the structural reanalysis. These results are also important because (with the exception of our earlier work: Friedmann & Gvion, 2003; Gvion & Friedmann, 2007) the effect of impaired phonological WM on sentence processing was only tested by means of verbatim repetition, but not in comprehension. The current study thus supports the earlier findings from an additional angle—that of a comprehension task.

Another research question related to whether or not the reanalysis of the verb's complement structure also requires lexical re-access. We tested GPs in which a verb was initially analysed as having a complement, and later reanalysed as standing alone, without a complement. The results indicated that the individuals with conduction aphasia in this study had similar difficulty in optional-complement GPs as with the GPs with lexical ambiguity, suggesting that the thematic reanalysis also required lexical re-access. This points to an interesting similarity between lexical access to ambiguous words and lexical access to verbs that have multiple options of complementation. As we have already noted, Swinney and his colleagues found that upon encountering an ambiguous word, exhaustive lexical access takes place, which retrieves all possible meanings of this word. Shapiro and his colleagues (Shapiro et al., 1993, 1987) discovered a phenomenon similar in nature with respect to verbs with multiple complementation options. They showed that when a verb is heard, all its complement options (argument structure frames) are activated, as indicated by the longer access time to verbs with more argument structure options. The current results support this view and indicate that a change of the thematic frame pertaining to an optional complement is on a par with a change in the chosen meaning of ambiguous words. Both require re-access to the lexical entry.[3]

Another result of the current study related to the effect of the distance between the temporary ambiguity and its resolution. As previous studies of GP processing have already reported (Christianson et al., 2001; Ferreira & Henderson, 1991), the longer the ambiguous region, the less likely is it that the sentences will be fully reanalysed. The current study replicated this result for the control group, who had significantly more difficulties in the comprehension of long- compared to short-distance GPs. The individuals with conduction aphasia did not show this difference, possibly because the short GPs already exceeded their capacity.

One important conclusion of this study relates to the distinction between two subtypes of conduction aphasia. In marked contrast to the poor comprehension that the individuals with input conduction aphasia showed in lexical GPs, DK, the individual with output conduction aphasia who had preserved phonological memory, understood these GPs well, and not differently from the control group.

Finally, these findings shed light on the extent of comprehension impairment we should expect from patients with limited pWM in everyday situations. The data accumulated so far, together with the current findings, are encouraging. It seems that only in very specific sentences that require phonological re-access do individuals with

---

[3] These results might also contribute to a linguistic debate regarding the representation of optional complements. They suggest that it is not the case that verbs with optional complements have a single thematic frame, which can be filled either with an overt NP or with an empty category, but rather that these constitute two different frames.

limited pWM have comprehension difficulties. However, how often do we encounter a lexical GP? How many times are we required to re-access ambiguous words that are positioned in a context strongly biasing towards one of the meanings, which gets disambiguated at a later point in the sentence towards the other meaning? How often are we required to repeat long sentences verbatim? Luckily, not often. Thus, in general we should not expect sentence comprehension difficulties as a result of phonological WM limitation. In most of the sentences and passages that we hear or read, semantic and syntactic encoding suffice for comprehension, and this should probably be the main guideline with which therapists should approach these patients (encode the meaning, do not try to remember the words!).

Thus, the current study sheds some new light on the nature of conduction aphasia, the processing of garden path sentences, and the relation between working memory and sentence comprehension.

REFERENCES

Butterworth, B., Campbell, R., & Howard, D. (1986). The uses of short-term memory: A case study. *Quarterly Journal of Experimental Psychology A, 38*, 705–737.

Butterworth, B., Shallice, T., & Watson, F. (1990). Short-term retention without short-term memory. In G. Vallar & T. Shallice (Eds.), *The neuropsychological impairments of short-term memory* (pp. 187–241). Cambridge, UK: Cambridge University Press.

Caplan, D., & Waters, G. S. (1999). Verbal working memory and sentence comprehension. *Behavioral and Brain Sciences, 22*, 77–126.

Caspari, I., Parkinson, S. R., LaPointe, L. L., & Katz, R. C. (1998). Working memory and aphasia. *Brain and Cognition, 37*, 205–223.

Christianson, K., Hollingworth, A., Halliwell, J. F., & Ferreira, F. (2001). Thematic roles assigned along the garden path linger. *Cognitive Psychology, 42*, 368–407.

Crawford, J. R., & Howell, D. C. (1998). Comparing an individual's test score against norms derived from small samples. *The Clinical Neuropsychologist, 12*, 482–486.

Daneman, M., & Carpenter, P. (1980). Individual differences in working memory and reading. *Journal of Verbal Learning and Verbal Behavior, 19*, 450–466.

DeDe, G., Caplan, D., Kemtes, K., & Waters, G. (2004). The relationship between age, verbal working memory, and language comprehension. *Psychology and Aging, 19*, 601–616.

Ferreira, F., & Henderson, J. M. (1991). Recovery from misanalyses of garden-path sentences. *Journal of Memory and Language, 30*, 725–745.

Fodor, J. D., & Ferreira, F. (1998). *Reanalysis in sentence processing.* Dordrecht: Kluwer.

Friedmann, N., & Gvion, A. (2002). *FriGvi: Friedmann Gvion battery for assessment of phonological working memory.* Tel Aviv University, Israel.

Friedmann, N., & Gvion, A. (2003). Sentence comprehension and working memory limitation in aphasia: A dissociation between semantic-syntactic and phonological reactivation. *Brain and Language, 86*, 23–39.

Friedmann, N., & Shapiro, L. P. (2003). Agrammatic comprehension of simple active sentences with moved constituents: Hebrew OSV and OVS structures. *Journal of Speech Language and Hearing Research, 46*, 288–297.

Gil, M., & Edelstein, C. (2001). *Hebrew version of the PALPA.* Ra'anana, Israel: Loewenstein Hospital Rehabilitation Center.

Gvion, A., & Friedmann, N. (2007). *Sentence comprehension and working memory limitation in conduction aphasia: The role of type of processing.* Manuscript submitted for publication.

Haarmann, H. J., Davelaan, E. J., & Usher, M. (2003). Individual differences in semantic short-term memory capacity and reading comprehension. *Journal of Memory and Language, 48*, 320–345.

Hanten, G., & Martin, R. C. (2000). Contributions of phonological and semantic short-term memory to sentence processing: Evidence from two cases of closed head injury in children. *Journal of Memory and Language, 43*, 335–361.

Hanten, G., & Martin, R. C. (2001). A developmental phonological short-term memory deficit: A case study. *Brain and Cognition, 45*, 164–188.

Kay, J., Lesser, R., & Coltheart, M. (1992). *PALPA: Psycholinguistic Assessments of Language Processing in Aphasia*. Hove, UK: Lawrence Erlbaum Associates Ltd.

Kertesz, A. (1982). *Western aphasia battery*. Orlando, FL: Grune & Stratton.

Love, T., & Swinney, D. (1996). Co-reference processing and levels of analysis in object-relative constructions: Demonstration of antecedent reactivation with the cross-modal priming paradigm. *Journal of Psycholinguistics Research, 25*, 5–24.

MacDonald, M. C., Just, M. A., & Carpenter, P. A. (1992). Working memory constraints on the processing of syntactic ambiguity. *Cognitive Psychology, 24*, 56–98.

Margalit, S., Friedmann, N., & Gvion, A. (2005). Components of verbal working memory and their relation to the comprehension of garden path sentences and sentences with lexical ambiguity. *Language, Brain, and Development, 4*, 33–35.

Martin, R. C. (1987). Articulatory and phonological deficits in short-term memory and their relation to syntactic processing. *Brain and Language, 32*, 159–192.

Martin, R. C. (2003). Language processing: Functional organization and neuroanatomical basis. *Annual Review of Psychology, 54*, 55–89.

Martin, R. C., & Feher, E. (1990). The consequences of reduced memory span for the comprehension of semantic versus syntactic information. *Brain and Language, 38*, 1–20.

Martin, R. C., & He, T. (2004). Semantic short-term memory and its role in sentence processing: A replication. *Brain and Language, 89*, 76–82.

Martin, R. C., Inglis, A. L., & Kuminiak, F. (2004). Complex sentence comprehension in a patient with a semantic short-term memory deficit. *Brain and Language, 91*, 122–123.

Martin, R. C., & Romani, C. (1994). Verbal working memory and sentence comprehension: A multiple-components view. *Neuropsychology, 8*, 506–523.

Martin, R. C., Shelton, J. R., & Yafee, L. S. (1994). Language processing and working memory: Neuropsychological evidence for separate phonological and semantic capacities. *Journal of Memory and Language, 33*, 83–111.

McElree, B. (2000). Sentence comprehension is mediated by content-addressable memory structures. *Journal of Psycholinguistic Research, 29*, 111–123.

Milne, R. (1980, August). *Parsing against lexical ambiguity*. Proceedings of the COLING-80 Conference: The 8th International Conference on Computational Linguistics, Tokyo.

Nicol, J., & Swinney, D. (1989). The role of structure in coreference assignment during sentence comprehension. *Journal of Psycholinguistic Research, 18*, 5–19.

Onifer, W., & Swinney, D. (1981). Accessing lexical ambiguities during sentence comprehension: Effects of frequency of meaning and contextual bias. *Memory and Cognition, 9*, 225–236.

Pritchett, B. L. (1992). *Grammatical competence and parsing performance*. Chicago: University of Chicago Press.

Romani, C., & Martin, R. (1999). A deficit in the short-term retention of lexical-semantic information: Forgetting words but remembering a story. *Journal of Experimental Psychology: General, 128*, 56–77.

Shapiro, L. P., Gordon, B., Hack, N., & Killackey, J. (1993). Verb-argument structure processing in complex sentences in Broca's and Wernicke's aphasia. *Brain and Language, 45*, 423–447.

Shapiro, L. P., Zurif, E., & Grimshaw, J. (1987). Sentence processing and the mental representation of verbs. *Cognition, 27*, 219–246.

Smith, E. E., & Geva, A. (2000). Verbal working memory and its connections to language processing. In Y. Grodzinsky, L. P. Shapiro, & D. Swinney (Eds.), *Language and the brain: Representation and processing* (pp. 123–141). San Diego, CA: Academic Press.

Soroker, N. (1997). *Hebrew western aphasia battery*. Ra'anana, Israel: Loewenstein Hospital Rehabilitation Center.

Swinney, D. (1979). Lexical access during sentence comprehension: (Re)consideration of context effects. *Journal of Verbal Learning and Verbal Behavior, 18*, 645–660.

Swinney, D., Ford, M., Frauenfelder, U., & Bresnan, J. (1988). *On the temporal course of gap-filling and antecedent assignment during sentence comprehension*. Unpublished manuscript.

Swinney, D., Prather, P., & Love, T. (2000). The time-course of lexical access and the role of context: Converging evidence from normal and aphasic processing. In Y. Grodzinsky, L. P. Shapiro, &

D. Swinney (Eds.), *Language and the brain: Representation and processing* (pp. 273–292). New York: Academic Press.

Swinney, D., Zurif, E., & Nicol, J. (1989). The effects of focal brain damage on sentence processing: An examination of the neurological organization of a mental module. *Journal of Cognitive Neuroscience, 1*, 25–37.

Tompkins, C. A., Bloise, C. G. R., Timko, M. L., & Baumgaertner, A. (1994). Working memory and inference revision in brain damaged and normally aging adults. *Journal of Speech and Hearing Research, 37*, 896–912.

Waters, G., & Caplan, D. (1996). Processing resource capacity and the comprehension of garden path sentences. *Memory and Cognition, 24*, 342–355.

Waters, G., Caplan, D., & Hildebrandt, N. (1991). On the structure of verbal short-term memory and its functional role in sentence comprehension: Evidence from neuropsychology. *Cognitive Neuropsychology, 8*, 81–126.

Willis, C. S., & Gathercole, S. E. (2001). Phonological short-term memory contributions to sentence processing in young children. *Memory, 9*, 349–363.

Wright, H. H., & Shisler, R. J. (2005). Working memory in aphasia: Theory, measures, and clinical implications. *American Journal of Speech-Language Pathology, 14*, 107–118.

Zurif, E., Swinney, D., Prather, P., Wingfield, A., & Brownell, H. (1995). The allocation of memory resources during sentence comprehension: Evidence from the elderly. *Journal of Psycholinguistic Research, 24*, 165–182.

APHASIOLOGY, 2007, 21 (6/7/8), 587–603

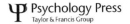

Treatment of input and output phonology in aphasia: A single case study

Sabine Corsten and Markus Mende

RWTH Aachen University, Germany

Jürgen Cholewa

College of Education, Heidelberg, Germany

Walter Huber

RWTH Aachen University, Germany

Background: Based on models of speech perception and production, different stages in phonological processing can be distinguished: phonetic, sublexical, and lexical levels of decoding and encoding respectively. In theory they can be selectively impaired. To address the specific level of phonological processing disruption we developed training material that entailed practice demands for each level of processing.

Aims: This paper aims to demonstrate the utility of this material-based approach by presenting the results of PS, a 52-year-old man with chronic conduction aphasia who showed both decoding and encoding difficulties at sublexical levels.

Methods & Procedures: The main component of the treatment programme was practice of minimal phonemic contrasts. The training material consisted of monosyllabic stimuli that were systematically varied for certain linguistic criteria, such as phonemic contrast position (onset/coda), lexicality (words/pseudowords), and phonetic complexity (increasing/unspecific sonority). The impact of these factors was studied in an alternating-treatments design employing control tests to assess baseline, outcome, and maintenance. The treatment lasted for 6 weeks during which phonological processing was practised under six treatment conditions. All exercises were computer assisted, and each session consisted of three main tasks: discrimination, identification, and reproduction.

Outcomes & Results: As predicted, the participant showed improvement during therapy when practising those items that called specifically for sublexical phonological processing.

Conclusions: This study demonstrates that an impairment-specific and material-based therapy approach is promising for the treatment of impaired sublexical phonological processing. Furthermore, the results suggest common mechanisms of input and output phonology.

Address correspondence to: Walter Huber PhD, Section of Neurolinguistics, Department of Neurology, RWTH Aachen University, Pauwelsstrasse 30, D-52074 Aachen, Germany. E-mail: huber@neuroling.rwth-aachen.de

The current work is supported by a grant of the German Research Foundation (DFG *HU 292/7-2*). We thank Klaus Willmes for statistical advice and the two anonymous reviewers for helping us to improve the manuscript and to clarify many issues.

http://www.psypress.com/aphasiology   DOI: 10.1080/02687030701192034

The aim of the study was to evaluate a theory-driven computer-based treatment programme for disorders of phonological decoding and encoding in aphasia. Even though phonological decoding and encoding can be selectively impaired, these deficits very often appear to be in an associated way in aphasic subjects (Martin & Saffran, 2002). Allport (1984) described associated impairments of input and output phonology for conduction aphasia. In a review, Ravizza (2001) discussed such an association in apraxia of speech. This suggests that the treatment programme should focus on both differences and similarities in decoding and encoding as specified in recent theories of single word processing. Common to most models of word processing is the distinction between three levels of phonological decoding and encoding each (as illustrated in Figure 1): a phonetic level, a sublexical level, and a

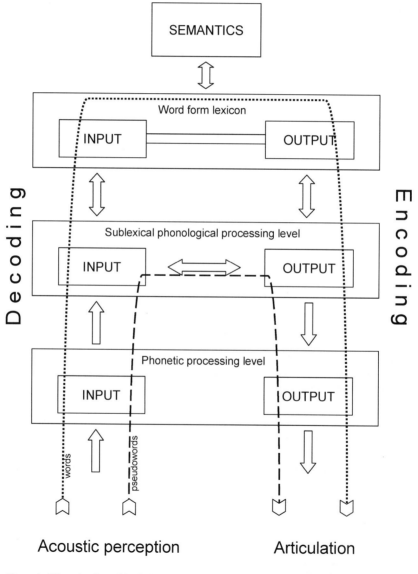

Figure 1. Three-level model of phonological processing: Word and pseudoword repetition.

lexical level (see Martin & Saffran, 2002). This distinction is a common feature of otherwise rather distinct models of *speech perception* (e.g., cohort model, Marslen-Wilson, Moss, & van Halen, 1996; interactive TRACE-model, McClelland & Elman, 1986; SHORTLIST-model, Norris, 1994) and of *speech production* (e.g., sequential model, Levelt, 2001; Levelt, Roelofs, & Meyer, 1999; connectionist model, Abel, Huber, & Dell, 2004; Dell, 1986; Dell, Schwartz, Martin, Saffran, & Gagnon, 1997; Hanley, Dell, Kay, & Baron, 2004).

All models of phonological decoding postulate a level at which the speech signal is detected as language and at which temporal and spectral analysis takes place. This is called the *acoustic-phonetic analysis processing stage* (e.g., Cutler & Clifton, 1999). Participants with a deficit at this level cannot reliably judge two spoken items (words or pseudowords) as the same or different (Gow & Caplan, 1996). Discrimination ability is influenced by phonetic similarity (Newman & Dell, 1978). At the next stage, the decoded speech sound information is transformed into a *sublexical* representation containing syllabic, phonemic, or even featural units (for a discussion, see Slowiaczek, McQueen, Soltana, & Lynch, 2000). Participants with impairments of sublexical phonological decoding show difficulties in the identification of pseudowords, for example in spoken word to written word matching tasks with phonologically related distractors. Rhyme judgements are also performed at least in part on this level (Martin & Saffran, 2002) as this task requires segmentation into onset and coda constituents of the stimuli. Therefore, in case of a sublexical disorder, rhyme judgements are also affected, especially for pseudowords.

During auditory word recognition the process of lexical activation can be characterised as incremental, and the word-initial position is important in activating the word forms (Connine, Titone, Deelman, & Blasko, 1997). At the lexical level, parallel graded activation of multiple candidate words takes place. Competition of phonologically similar word forms is one important process at this level independent of the underlying lexicon model (cf. Dell & Gordon, 2003; Marslen-Wilson et al., 1996). Deficits on the lexical phonological stage lead to difficulties in lexical decision tasks. Participants are not able to judge a spoken item as a word or a pseudoword (legal neologisms).

During encoding, the first step is word retrieval from the mental lexicon. In Levelt's model this is a two-step procedure. First a lemma is selected which carries semantic and grammatical information; second, the corresponding word form, i.e., an abstract phonological code, is activated. Word form retrieval is explained in terms of access to lexical addresses, which are organised according to phonemes in initial word position (cf. review in Brown, 1991; see also Nickels & Howard, 2000). Further, the structure of the word form lexicon is organised according to phonological similarity or neighbourhood (Vitevitch, 2002). In case of impairment, it is assumed that formal paraphasias (word forms confusion) are influenced by phonological neighbourhood effects (Best, 1996; Blanken, 1990; but see discussion of a post-lexical explanation in Nickels & Howard, 2000). Therefore, phonological similarity and more specifically phonological onset should be focussed on during treatment.

The second step of phonological encoding is sublexical transformation of words into phonemes and syllables. According to Levelt and colleagues (1999), for each lexical entry the abstract phonological code is spelled out as an ordered set of phonological segments. Simultaneously, the metrical shape is generated.

Reproduction of pseudowords requires post-lexical encoding as well. Their encoding can be purely sublexical, i.e., no previous lexical processing takes place (see Figure 1). In aphasia, segmental phonological errors like substitutions are a common symptom. Repeated attempts to correct such segmental errors can be seen (e.g., Joanette, Keller, & Lecours, 1980), resulting in sequences of phonemic approximations (conduite d'approche). A disorder on this level is typically attributed to reproduction conduction aphasia (see, e.g., Caplan, Vanier, & Baker, 1986; Kohn, 1992). Furthermore, increase of errors in coda position is reported in the literature (Wilshire & McCarthy, 1996). Given these findings, treatment of sublexical impairment should include words and pseudowords with specific contrasts in the coda position.

At the third step, phonetic encoding, the segmental composition is transformed into an articulatory program which guides the process of articulation. An impairment at this level leads to typical symptoms of apraxia of speech such as articulatory groping and phonetic distortions (Ziegler, 2002). The error pattern is influenced along with other parameters, by syllabic complexity (Odell, McNeil, Rosenbek, & Hunter, 1990). The functional relation between input and output components of phonological processing needs special consideration (see for a review Schiller & Meyer, 2003). Neurolinguistic evidence is presented for the existence of either a single phonological system (e.g., Allport, 1984; Caramazza, Berndt, & Basili, 1983), functionally connected phonological input and output networks (Miceli, Gainotti, Caltagirone, & Masullo, 1980), or two separate functionally independent phonological input and output processors (Dell et al., 1997; Nickels & Howard, 1995; Romani, 1992; Shallice, Rumiati, & Zadini, 2000). These theoretical differences might result from lack of adequate and systematic assessment in this area (Martin, Schwartz, & Kohen, 2006). Recently Martin et al. (2006) found evidence for associated processing between two separate phonological systems (see also Martin & Saffran, 2002).

In summary, phonological impairments can emerge at different stages in speech perception and production, which might be specifically addressed when treatment is deficit oriented. In our approach, we targeted the different processing stages by manipulating the stimuli to be practised. For the treatment of phonetic encoding impairments, varying phonetic complexity of the stimuli appears to be important. Sonority for instance is a potential complexity measure. As individuals with phonetic deficits are not in the focus of this paper, the impact of phonetic complexity as measured by varying degrees of sonority will not be discussed here in greater detail (but see Corsten, Mende, Cholewa, & Huber, 2005).

Treatment with pseudowords should focus on the sublexical level of processing in decoding as well as in encoding. Pseudowords require segmental processing of phonemes rather than relying on lexical and/or semantic information. Full sublexical segmentation and sequencing for each stimulus is triggered by training pseudowords in a minimal pair context with the contrast position in coda as opposed to onset. Coda contrasts are expected to be more difficult as full segmentation is mandatory. Using an earlier version of the phonological encoding training programme, we were able to demonstrate both the pseudoword and the coda effect in a participant with reproduction conduction aphasia (Corsten, Mende, Cholewa, & Huber, 2004).

At the lexical level, phonological similarity between words should be sensitive to impairment of word form activation. This should specifically hold for contrasts in the onset position, as onsets are assumed to be the guiding principle of word form retrieval.

In the present study, we report a participant, PS, with a combined sublexical phonological decoding and phonological encoding deficit. It was hypothesised that PS should benefit most from processing pseudowords with minimal contrasts in the coda position.

METHOD

Participant

PS, a 52-year-old right-handed German engineer, suffered a left-hemisphere CVA in the posterior MCA territory 11 months prior to treatment. The lesion included Wernicke's area and extended into the inferior parietal lobe. Before the experimental treatment, PS received multimodal language activation therapy for 1–2 sessions per week. During the study, PS was admitted as an inpatient to the Aachen Aphasia Ward for intensive training of his aphasic disturbances (for a description of the general treatment regimen see Huber, Springer, & Willmes, 1993). The standard treatment focused on communicative skill training and role playing for everyday life situations. This treatment took place once a day. In addition PS received two sessions daily of experimentally controlled phonological training. No other treatment of his phonological disorder took place besides the experimental therapy.

The Aachen Aphasia Test (AAT, Huber, Poeck, Weniger, & Willmes, 1983) was used to assess PS's spontaneous language. His spontaneous speech was fluent with many phonemic paraphasias, frequent sequences of phonemic approximations (conduites d'approche) and word-finding difficulties. There were no signs of either apractic or dysarthric errors. Imitation of bucco-facial movements was flawless. His digit span forward was 3 items, measured by the German version of the Wechsler Memory Scale – revised (WMS-R, Härting et al., 2000). On the AAT subtests, repetition was severely impaired (35th percentile) in contrast to substantially higher performance in all other tests (72nd percentile for written language, 85th for naming, 68th for comprehension, 65th for the Token Test) (Huber et al., 1983). His AAT profile was typical for conduction aphasia.

In order to determine PS's phonological encoding impairment more specifically, we administered a German oral naming test (Wortproduktionsprüfung: Blanken, Döppler, & Schlenck, 1999) which included 60 pictures of objects that varied in word frequency (range 0–1603 of the CELEX database; Baayen, Piepenbrock, & Gulikers, 1995), word length (one-syllable, two-syllable, and three-syllable items, 20 each), and phonological complexity (based on number of single consonants and consonant clusters). On this test, 75% of PS's errors consisted of segmental phonemic paraphasias and sequences of phonemic approximations, which we concluded were due to sublexical encoding impairments.

Additionally, a significant length effect was found; three-syllable words were significantly more difficult than one-syllable words (Fisher's exact test, two-tailed, $p < .001$). This is in agreement with a deficit at the sublexical stage (Caplan et al., 1986; Wilshire & McCarthy, 1996). No effects of either frequency or complexity were found, thus excluding the presence of severe deficits on either the lexical or the phonetic level of encoding. In summary, the results from the oral naming test supported the diagnosis of conduction aphasia.

Treatment control tests

We developed several control tests to delineate PS's phonological impairment in greater detail and to plan the deficit-oriented treatment. These control tests were also used for monitoring progress during treatment. Only uninflected nouns and pseudowords that were not part of the treatment material were used as stimuli. The control tests required both receptive and expressive processing.

As shown in Table 1 (baseline performance), PS's auditory discrimination capacity of monosyllabic pseudowords (same/different judgements) was slightly impaired. Sublexical phonological identification was examined by means of monosyllabic pseudowords using a spoken-to-written item-matching format having four written items with one target item (e.g., *sunsch*) and three phonologically related distractors (e.g., *sunf, sunch, suns*). PS matched only 41% of the items correctly, which shows a profound disorder in sublexical phonological decoding in addition to his sublexical phonological encoding impairment. Reading aloud was nearly unimpaired, precluding dyslexia. In contrast, PS demonstrated only mild difficulties in rhyme judgement tasks involving words and pseudowords respectively. Difficulties in rhyme judgements appear to have been compensated for by acoustic-phonetic analysis, which was well preserved in PS.[1]

The expressive control tests required repetition and reading aloud of monosyllabic items in separate tasks. All responses were tape-recorded (Sony DTC 690 DAT-Recorder) and phonological performance was scored on a 5-point scale (see Appendix A). PS demonstrated a clear phonological impairment in repetition, which was significantly more severe than in reading aloud (see baseline performance in Table 1). This held true for words as well as for pseudowords (Wilcoxon exact signed-ranks test, two-tailed, $p < .001$ each). Given the significant dissociation between severely impaired repetition and only slightly impaired oral reading, we either had to assume that the deficit in phonological decoding was predominant, or that phonological encoding was also impaired but was compensated for in reading aloud due to the additional graphemic information and/or the lower short-term memory demands. The assumption of an additional encoding deficit was supported by PS's oral naming, which contained a substantial number of sublexical phonological encoding errors.

The issue of associated sublexical encoding and decoding impairments will be further pursued during the discussion of the training. The different conditions of treatment covered both receptive and expressive processing at the three levels of processing. Thereby, specific deficits were expected to result in specific treatment effects.

In summary, we assumed that PS had a combined sublexical phonological impairment in both decoding and encoding. We expected PS would benefit most from training of pseudowords contrasted at the coda position, as this condition focuses most on sublexical segmentation and sequencing of phonemes. We also

---

[1] As an alternative to rhyme tasks we studied lexical decisions tasks (real words versus legal and illegal neologisms) in the development of the treatment programme. It turned out that even patients with global aphasia performed correctly at well above chance. Possibly this is due to activation of meaning rather than phonological word form alone. Therefore we disregarded lexical decision.

TABLE 1
Control test (C) performances

Test	n	Mean baseline $(C1+C2)$	C3	C4	C5	C6	C7 (Follow-up)	Trend[1] (outcome)	C7 vs C6[2] (maintenance)
Input									
Auditory discrimination pseudowords	48	83.33	77.08	77.08	87.5	85.42	94.79	.058	.182
Identification pseudowords	48	41.15	29.17	43.75	45.83	44.79	51.04	.136	.566
Rhyme judgement words	48	85.42	83.33	87.5	93.75	91.67	66.67	.016	.004
Rhyme judgement pseudowords	48	85.42	78.13	87.5	81.25	89.58	56.25	.056	.000
Output									
Repetition words	48	64.06	64.58	73.44	81.25	84.9	77.6	.000	.080
Repetition pseudowords	48	38.54	33.85	48.44	31.25	52.08	52.08	.012	.916
Reading aloud words	48	91.15	97.4	93.75	90.63	95.31	95.31	.17	.880
Reading aloud pseudowords	48	87.42	72.92	91.15	84.38	85.94	85.42	.12	.815

Phonological scores in %, p values for outcome and maintenance effects. Baseline performances are given as means of each test because there were no significant differences between the single baseline performances. [1]Page rank test for monotone trends. [2]Wilcoxon exact signed-ranks test, two-tailed.

expected that practice should generalise to the untreated items of the control tests. Finally, we expected improvement in the identification and repetition of pseudo-words, with generalisation to untreated words.

Treatment material

We used a minimal phonemic contrast practice for treatment. The training material consisted of monosyllabic uninflected German nouns and pseudowords combined in item sets of four. Individual items or sequences of two to four items always were practised in the context of the full item set of four.

The six conditions of training material are shown in Table 2. Each condition consisted of 48 sets of 4 items resulting in a total of 192 practice items per condition. The conditions were systematically varied for phonological similarity (similar versus non-similar words), position of the minimal phonemic contrast (onset versus coda), lexicality (word versus pseudoword), and phonetic complexity (increasing versus non-systematic variation of sonority).[2] Across all six conditions, the material was designed to require specific phonological processing demands at all three levels: phonetic, sublexical and lexical. PS was trained in all conditions in order to demonstrate the specificity of the treatment effects.

It should be noted that the treatment material was different from the expressive control test material, although similar in word structure (one-syllable items) and in the distinction of words and pseudowords. Concerning syllable frequency, the control test items were less frequent than the treatment items (mean frequency based on CELEX database—control test items: words 519.83, pseudowords 0.10; treatment items: words 1087.61, pseudowords 250.53). Furthermore, the control test items were more complex in sonority than the treatment items (mean sonority quotients, Corsten et al., 2005; control test items: words .58, pseudowords .58; treatment items: words .31, pseudowords .30). All corresponding differences were significant (Mann-Whitney U-test exact, two-tailed, $p < .05$). Given these differences, improvements on control tests can be seen to indicate non-trivial transfer from practised to unpractised items.

Procedure

All exercises were computer assisted, which allowed for standardised presenta-tion. The programme contains defined mastery and break-off criteria ($P \leqslant 95$ after first trial, $P \leqslant 95$ after second trial respectively). At the beginning of each exercise, the participant was given a set of four practice items in oral as well as in written form. Each exercise consisted of three tasks concerning the four items: discrimination, identification, and reproduction. These tasks were always conducted in the same context of four multiple-choice items which were varied

---

[2] Phonetic complexity values for each item were measured in terms of sonority. According to the theory of Clements (1990), an optimal syllable of low complexity has high sonority contrast between onset and nucleus and low sonority contrast between nucleus and coda. Syllables of high phonetic complexity have the reverse sonority contrasts in onset and coda. In the condition with increasing sonority the stimuli of each set were presented from low to high complexity. Such a stepwise increase of complexity may stimulate the articulatory programming process. In all other conditions the phonetic complexity in each item set was not systematically varied.

TABLE 2
Treatment conditions: Stimulus structure, item parameters, and examples

condition (n = 48 × 4) parameters	1 Words without similarity[1]	2 Words with onset contrasts	3 Pseudowords with onset contrasts	4 Words with coda contrasts	5 Pseudowords with coda contrasts	6 Pseudowords with increasing complexity
Sonority based complexity[1]	.33 (.17)	.34 (.16)	.33 (.14)	.28 (.09)	.27 (.12)	.31 (.16)
Frequency of syllables[2]	882.28 (2346.39)	1547.63 (7787.99)	486.67 (3088.91)	832.91 (2406.62)	30.46 (144.19)	234.45 (1283.62)
Example	Punkt Brett Tanz Geld	Grad Draht Rad Krad	Plee Pree Mee Schwee	Riff Ritt Riss Rist	Futt Furf Fuls Fursch	Heet Leet Pleet Pfreet

Item parameters are given as means (SD) of each item pool.   [1]Phonetic complexity: Sonority quotients per item with 1.00 standing for most complex sonority contrast in onset and coda (cf. sonority theory of Clements, 1990).   [2]Syllable frequency: Based on 10,819 types and 9,062,607 tokens of the CELEX database (Niels Schiller, personal communication; Baayen et al., 1995). Note, that contrast of lexicality (words versus pseudowords) is confounded with differences in syllable frequency.

according to one of the six treatment conditions shown in Table 2. Thus the expected differential impact of the material was controlled by these multiple-choice sets which introduced the same phonological context for each task of one exercise.

Discrimination. The participant was asked to judge two auditorily presented items as different or the same. The interval between stimuli was fixed at 500 milliseconds (which also applied to sequential stimulation in identification and reproduction). This task was originally implemented in the treatment intended to stimulate the phonetic decoding level. Since discrimination was basically unimpaired in PS, it was used as a warm-up only; no further details will be reported on this task. Discrimination was always followed by Identification.

Identification. This task consisted of four steps (trials). During the first, the participant was asked to identify one auditorily presented item out of four written items on the screen. This was repeated five times in randomised order, i.e., one item was presented twice, in order to prevent simple exclusion strategies. In the second step the participant had to identify two auditorily presented items from the set of four items in the given order. This was repeated once with a second pair of items and the multiple-choice set presented in different order. In the third and fourth steps, the same material (each time in different order) was presented with three and four items, respectively. Across all four steps the procedure was as parallel as possible: In case of failure, the individual target was stimulated again and the whole step was repeated. Identification was followed by Reproduction.

Reproduction. This task also contained four steps. First, the multiple choice set of four items was presented both visually and acoustically and the participant had to reproduce verbally one of the four items, i.e., the participant was free to repeat and/or read aloud the stimulus (multimodal stimulation). With each new target, the order of the multiple-choice set was randomised, but the type of phonological context remained the same in order to influence the reproduction performance. On the next steps, sequences of two, three, and four items out of the multiple choice set had to be reproduced. Across all four steps, additional stimulation was provided after a failure. Failure was defined as no response, phonological and/or phonetic error, or incorrect order of sequencing.

It should be noted that the multiple-choice set of items stayed the same across tasks and trials in order to achieve material-specific practice effects. The possibility of unwanted processing by elimination was kept low by varying task demands and order of presentation.

When the participant failed a task, additional direct stimulation was given, i.e., the stimulus was immediately presented again auditorily and visually. The phonological contrast of the item set was not pointed out, nor were specific phonological cues given. In other words, the treatment tried to facilitate the correct phonological form by repeated multimodal stimulation in a constant phonological context as incorporated into the practice material. The number of necessary stimulations in each task was used as a score to document progress during treatment. The lower the score, the more additional stimulation was needed.

Experimental design

The treatment extended over nearly 6 weeks including control tests. Treatment was given twice a day, 5 days per week. The six treatment conditions (see Table 2) were provided in 16 sessions each using an alternating-treatments design (Barlow & Hayes, 1979). Two different treatment conditions were selected in each session. Every session lasted for a maximum of 60 minutes and included six exercises that corresponded to six different multiple choice sets, three for words (W) and three for pseudowords (P). Across items, the same contrast condition was practised, either onset, coda, or no similarity (W)/increasing sonority (P).[3] For motivational reasons, the order of exercises was constant, leading from easy to difficult to easy (W-P-P-W-P-W). Overall, we carried out 48 sessions on 24 days, one in the morning and one in the afternoon. In each session, two treatment conditions were covered. The total material contained 288 item sets, 48 for each condition. The same multiple-choice set of four items constituted an exercise unit with three succeeding tasks—discrimination, identification, and reproduction, as described above. Thus, intensive and material-specific practice was conducted.

Progress during treatment was monitored by the control tests (see Table 1). Baseline performance was assessed on two succeeding days immediately before treatment. During treatment, the control tests were administered four times, once after 12 sessions. A follow-up examination was conducted 3 months after treatment (maintenance test).

RESULTS

Treatment effects

We first expected a gradual increase of performance during treatment especially in those conditions that were most sensitive to the participant's general sublexical disorder, i.e., for processing pseudowords with minimal phonemic contrast in coda position. As both input and output processing were affected, the treatment effects were expected for both identification and reproduction. We applied tests for the linear trend component in a one-factorial ANOVA framework with items as observational units. This trend analysis was conducted separately for tasks, trials, and condition. We adjusted for multiple testing (Bonferroni adjustment, with a resulting p value of .008). We found significant trends that are illustrated in Figure 2.

In accordance with our expectation, PS showed significant positive linear trends in the identification tasks when processing pseudowords with contrasts in coda position. Significant trends were obtained for the identification of two-, three-, and four-item sequences ($p = .004$; $p = .006$; $p = .006$) (see upper part of Figure 2). In reproduction improvement was found for words with coda contrasts (reproduction of three-item sequences, $p = .003$) (see lower part of Figure 2) but not for pseudowords. This was not fully in line with our prediction. It should be noted that there were no other significant findings. PS did not improve in processing items with onset contrasts, nor did he improve in the condition with increasing sonority

---

[3] We introduced the no-similarity condition only for words in order to study the impact of phonological neighbourhood (Dell & Gordon, 2003; Vitevich, 2002). To study the possible impact of phonetic complexity by increasing sonority we used only pseudowords and no real words in order to minimise the influence of lexicality (cf. Maas, Barlow, Robin, & Shapiro, 2002).

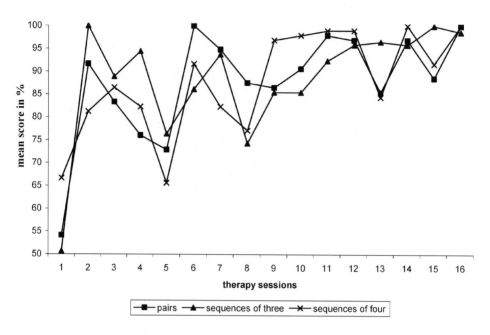

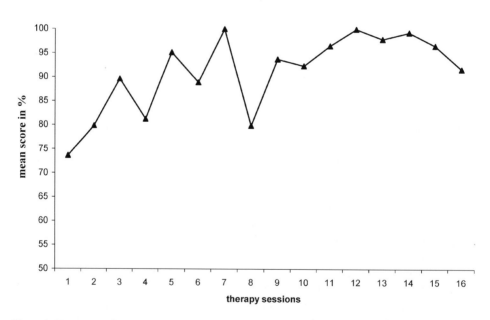

Figure 2. Treatment effects of coda contrasts in PS (all trends significant, see text) (Note that the score reflects the number of stimulations needed. The lower the score, the more additional stimulations were needed.)

and in the control condition without phonological similarity. Thus the effects must be seen as treatment specific.

Outcome and maintenance

The results of the treatment control tests (C 1–7) are shown in Table 1. During therapy we found improvement only in rhyme judgement (Page rank test, $p = .016$), which did not remain stable at 3 months post-treatment. Wilcoxon exact signed-ranks test (two-tailed) showed a significant decrease from testing immediately after treatment to the maintenance test (C6 to C7, $p = .004$). No effect was demonstrated for identification of pseudowords. This was unexpected given the improvements in the identification task during therapy.

On expressive control tests, PS demonstrated improved phonological scores on repetition of both words *and* pseudowords (Page rank test, $p < .001$; $p = .012$). As shown by the follow-up values, this improvement remained stable over the non-treatment period (see Table 1). For reading aloud, no effect was obtained, due to pre-treatment ceiling effects (P = 90).

To gain further information on output performance the oral naming test was repeated at the end of treatment. A significant increase of correct responses from 44 to 55 out of 60 was obtained (Fisher's exact test, two-tailed, $p = .05$). The remaining 5 naming errors still consisted of phonemic paraphasias (in contrast to 12 before treatment).

DISCUSSION

In accordance with the theory of different levels of phonological decoding and encoding, we found effects of therapy material in the treatment of a participant with conduction aphasia that was specified by both pre-lexical and post-lexical processing deficits. As expected, only stimuli with coda contrasts led to significant trends during training. This held true both for the input task *identification* and the output task *reproduction.* The effect was obtained in identification for pseudowords as predicted, but for words rather than pseudowords in reproduction. In addition, the improvement of reproduction was limited to sequences of three words only.

The reproduction task as implemented in our PC-assisted programme was not well suited for PS, who was able to compensate for his phonological encoding difficulties when reading aloud in contrast to pure repetition. As the reproduction training made use of spoken and written stimulation, it was not sensitive enough to the underlying phonological encoding deficit in PS. By relying on written stimuli, PS apparently was able to circumvent the phonological decoding and encoding demands of repetition. Reading aloud requires little phonological decoding and also reduces the processing demands of phonological encoding, as segmentation and sequencing are guided by graphemic information (especially with regular orthography as used in our stimuli). This graphemic compensation might have worked better when orthographic word forms were available, which would explain the unexpected significant effect for words rather than pseudowords as found for PS. In addition one has to consider the differences in short-term memory demands. They are higher for pseudowords than real words and higher for repetition than reading aloud.

The results from the control tests support the assumed dissociation between reading and repetition. When identical one-syllable words and pseudowords were presented in both tasks, reading aloud was almost unimpaired in contrast to a severely to moderate impairment of repetition. Here repetition was tested separately from reading and therefore compensation by means of graphemic information could not take place. To what extent the poor repetition performance is related to a pre- and a post-lexical deficit cannot be determined conclusively. The issue requires further examination. Possibly, the control test items were too easy for the encoding difficulties to be fully revealed. When longer and more complex post-lexical phonological processing was required, as in the oral naming task and in spontaneous language (as assessed by AAT ratings), the phonological difficulties became predominant. Thus, undoubtedly, PS was also impaired in phonological encoding. During treatment this encoding deficit was less successfully addressed than the decoding deficit either because the trained items were too easy or because compensation by means of simultaneously presented graphemic presentations took place.

The control tests demonstrated the predicted gradual improvement in repetition of both pseudowords *and* words. These gains remained stable over a 3-month period of no treatment. As it seems this involves improvement in both pre-lexical and post-lexical processing of phonological structures, an interpretation in terms of pre-lexical improvement alone is questionable given the control test results from pseudoword identification, which specifically requires pre-lexical decoding. No effect was found, although a post-hoc qualitative analysis showed a decrease of uncertainty as reflected by searching behaviour and questions for repetition. In other words, there was a slight indication of improvement of pseudoword identification outside the therapy as well. On the other hand, post-lexical improvement was clearly demonstrated by significant post-treatment improvement on the oral naming test.

In terms of model making, these data support the assumption of a functional connection between input and output phonology. A direct connection from input to output is predominantly used in repetition of pseudowords (if a lexical strategy is excluded; for discussion, see Martin & Saffran, 2002). In the case of PS, the difference in performance between repetition and reading aloud emphasises the notion that repetition performance is based on input abilities, and that errors arising from phonological decoding are fed forward to output processing. Compensation is only possible when reading and repetition co-occur. The data would appear to be incompatible with the assumption of two functionally separated phonological systems or with the idea of one single system. The lexicality effect with better repetition performance on words than on pseudowords shows that in repetition—using direct connections between input and output representations—higher-level representations are involved as well. Our results support the findings of Martin et al. (2006) who also presented evidence for at least associated processing of two separate phonological systems. Under the assumption of one single phonological system the inherent differences in short-term memory demands in repetition and reading aloud would have to be specified in addition (for a further discussion, see Martin & Saffran, 2002; R. Martin, Lesch, & Bartha, 1999).

In conclusion, our study provides further evidence for the efficacy of an impairment-specific and material-based approach to treatment of phonological processing. Furthermore, our model-based approach helps to discuss theoretical aspects of processing phonology.

REFERENCES

Abel, S., Huber, W., & Dell, G. S. (2004). Connectionist diagnosis of lexical processing in aphasia: Comparing a single- versus a dual-route model of repetition. *Brain and Language, 91*, 152–153.

Allport, D. A. (1984). Speech production and comprehension: One lexicon or two? In W. Prinz & A. F. Sanders (Eds.), *Cognitive and motor processes* (pp. 209–228). Berlin: Springer.

Baayen, R. H., Piepenbrock, R., & Gulikers, L. (1995). *The CELEX lexical database.* (Release 2) [CD ROM]. Philadelphia, PA: Linguistic Data Consortium, University of Pennsylvania.

Barlow, D. H., & Hayes, S. C. (1979). Alternating treatments design: One strategy for comparing the effects of two treatments in a single subject. *Journal of Applied Behavior Analysis, 12*(2), 199–210.

Best, W. (1996). When racquets are baskets but baskets are biscuits, where do the words come from? A single case study of formal paraphasic errors in aphasia. *Cognitive Neuropsychology, 13*, 443–480.

Blanken, G. (1990). Formal paraphasias: A single case study. *Brain and Language, 38*, 534–554.

Blanken, G., Döppler, R., & Schlenck, K. J. (1999). *Wortproduktionsprüfung.* Hofheim: NAT.

Brown, A. S. (1991). A review of the tip-of-the-tongue experience. *Psychological Bulletin, 109*, 204–223.

Caplan, D., Vanier, M., & Baker, C. (1986). A case study of reproduction conduction aphasia I: Word production. *Cognitive Neuropsychology, 3*, 99–128.

Caramazza, A., Berndt, R. S., & Basili, A. G. (1983). The selective impairment of phonological processing: A case study. *Brain and Language, 18*, 128–174.

Clements, G. N. (1990). The role of the sonority cycle in core syllabification. In J. Kingston & M. Beckman (Eds.), *Papers in laboratory phonology I. Between the grammar and physics of speech* (pp. 283–332). Cambridge, MA: MIT Press.

Connine, C. M., Titone, D., Deelman, T., & Blasko, D. (1997). Similarity mapping in spoken word recognition. *Journal of Memory and Language, 37*, 463–480.

Corsten, S., Mende, M., Cholewa, J., & Huber, W. (2004). Modellgeleitete Therapie von phonologischen Störungen bei Aphasie: Eine Einzelfallstudie zur Leitungsaphasie. *Sprachheilarbeit, 49*, 284–297.

Corsten, S., Mende, M., Cholewa, J., & Huber, W. (2005). Model-based treatment of phonetic encoding impairments: Two cases of apraxia of speech. Abstract for the Academy of Aphasia meeting, October 2005. *Brain and Language, 95*(1), 176–177.

Cutler, A., & Clifton, C. Jr. (1999). Comprehending spoken language: A blueprint for the listener. In C. Brown & P. Hagoort (Eds.), *The neurocognition of language* (pp. 123–166). Oxford, UK: Oxford University Press.

Dell, G. S. (1986). A spreading-activation theory of retrieval in sentence production. *Psychological Review, 93*, 283–321.

Dell, G. S., & Gordon, J. K. (2003). Neighbours in the lexicon: Friends or foes? In N. O. Schiller & A. S. Meyer (Eds.), *Phonetics and phonology in language comprehension and production* (pp. 9–37). Berlin: Mouton de Gruyter.

Dell, G. S., Schwartz, M. F., Martin, N., Saffran, E. M., & Gagnon, D. A. (1997). Lexical access in aphasic and non-aphasic speakers. *Psychological Review, 104*(4), 801–838.

Gow, D. W. Jr., & Caplan, D. (1996). An examination of impaired acoustic-phonetic processing in aphasia. *Brain and Language, 52*, 386–407.

Hanley, J. R., Dell, G. S., Kay, J., & Baron, R. (2004). Evidence for the involvement of a nonlexical route in the repetition of familiar words: A comparison of single and dual route models of auditory repetition. *Cognitive Neuropsychology, 21*(2/3/4), 147–158.

Härting, C., Markowitsch, H. J., Neufeld, H., Calabrese, P., Deisinger, K., & Kessler, J. (2000). *Wechsler Gedächtnis Test – Revidierte Fassung (WMS-R). Deutsche Adaptation der revidierten Fassung der Wechsler-Memory-Scale.* Bern: Huber.

Huber, W., Poeck, K., Weniger, D., & Willmes, K. (1983). *Aachener Aphasie Test (AAT).* Göttingen: Hogrefe.

Huber, W., Springer, L., & Willmes, K. (1993). Approaches to aphasia therapy in Aachen. In A. L. Holland & M. M. Forbes (Eds.), *Aphasia treatment – world publishing* (pp. 55–86). San Diego, CA: Singular Publishing Group.

Joanette, Y., Keller, E., & Lecours, A. R. (1980). Sequences of phonemic approximations in aphasia. *Brain and Language, 11*, 30–44.

Kohn, S. E. (Ed.). (1992). *Conduction aphasia.* Hillsdale, NJ: Lawrence Erlbaum Associates Inc.

Levelt, W. J. M. (2001). Spoken word production. A theory of lexical access *Proceedings of the National Academy of Sciences (PNAS), 98*, 13464–13471.

Levelt, W. J. M., Roelofs, A., & Meyer, A. S. (1999). A theory of lexical access in speech production. *Behavioral and Brain Sciences, 22*, 1–38; discussion 38–75.

Maas, E., Barlow, J., Robin, D., & Shapiro, L. (2002). Treatment of sound errors in aphasia and apraxia of speech: Effects of phonological complexity. *Aphasiology, 16*, 609–622.

Marslen-Wilson, W. D., Moss, H., & van Halen, S. (1996). Perceptual distance and competition in lexical access. *Journal of Experimental Psychology: Human Perception and Performance, 22*, 1376–1392.

Martin, N., & Saffran, E. M. (2002). The relationship of input and output phonological processing: An evaluation of models and evidence to support them. *Aphasiology, 16*, 107–150.

Martin, N., Schwartz, M. F., & Kohen, F. P. (2006). Assessment of the ability to process semantic and phonological aspects of words in aphasia: A multi-measurement approach. *Aphasiology, 20*, 154–166.

Martin, R. C., Lesch, M. F., & Bartha, M. C. (1999). Independence of input and output phonology in word processing and short-term memory. *Journal of Memory and Language, 41*, 3–29.

McClelland, J. L., & Elman, J. L. (1986). Interactive processes in speech recognition: The TRACE model. In J. L. McClelland & D. E. Rumelhart (Eds.), *Parallel distributed processing: Explorations in the microstructure of cognition* (pp. 58–121). Cambridge, MA: Bradford.

Miceli, G., Gainotti, G., Caltagirone, C., & Masullo, C. (1980). Some aspects of phonological impairment in aphasia. *Brain and Language, 11*, 159–169.

Newman, J. E., & Dell, G. S. (1978). The phonological nature of phoneme monitoring: A critique of some ambiguity studies. *Journal of Verbal Learning and Verbal Behavior, 13*, 359–374.

Nickels, L., & Howard, D. (1995). Phonological errors in naming: Comprehension monitoring and lexicality. *Cortex, 31*, 209–237.

Nickels, L., & Howard, D. (2000). When the words won't come: Relating impairments and models of spoken word production. In L. Wheeldon (Ed.), *Aspects of language production* (pp. 115–142). Hove, UK: Psychology Press.

Norris, D. (1994). Shortlist: A connectionist model of continuous speech recognition. *Cognition, 52*, 189–234.

Odell, K., McNeil, M. R., Rosenbek, J. C., & Hunter, L. (1990). Perceptual characteristics of consonant production by apraxic speakers. *Journal of Speech and Hearing Dirorders, 55*, 345–359.

Ravizza, S. M. (2001). Relating selective brain damage to impairments with voicing contrasts. *Brain and Language, 77*, 95–118.

Romani, C. (1992). Are there distinct input and output buffers? Evidence from an aphasic patient with impaired output buffer. *Language and Cognitive Processes, 7*, 131–162.

Schiller, N. O., & Meyer, A. S. (Eds.). (2003). *Phonetics and phonology in language comprehension and production*. Berlin: Mouton de Gruyter.

Shallice, T., Rumiati, R. I., & Zadini, A. (2000). The selective impairment of the phonological output buffer. *Cognitive Neuropsychology, 17*, 517–546.

Slowiaczek, L. M., McQueen, J. M., Soltana, E. G., & Lynch, M. (2000). Phonological representations in prelexical speech processing: Evidence from form-based priming. *Journal of Memory and Language, 43*, 530–560.

Vitevitch, M. (2002). The influence of phonological similarity neighbourhoods on speech production. *Journal of Experimental Psychology: Learning, Memory, and Cognition, 28*, 735–747.

Wilshire, C. E., & McCarthy, R. (1996). Experimental investigation of an impairment in phonological encoding. *Cognitive Neuropsychology, 13*, 1059–1098.

Ziegler, W. (2002). Psycholinguistic and motor theories of apraxia of speech. *Seminars in Speech and Language, 23*(4), 231–243.

APPENDIX

Response score for word and pseudoword repetition and reading aloud

Phonology score: Accuracy of phonological realisation

4	3	2	1	0
♦ correct	correct after: ♦ hesitation ♦ pause ♦ self-correction ♦ conduite d'approche with success ♦ second stimulation	♦ phonemic paraphasia (at least two third of the segments are correct) ♦ conduite d'approche with no full success	♦ phonemic neologism (less than two third of the segments are correct) ♦ conduite d'écart (phonemic drifting away from target)	♦ abstruse neologism (only one segment is correct) ♦ no responses ♦ semantic error ♦ formal paraphasia (confusions of phonological word forms) ♦ perseveration ♦ circumlotion ♦ automatism ♦ empty phrase

APHASIOLOGY, 2007, 21 (6/7/8), 604–616

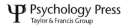

The relation between syntactic and morphological recovery in agrammatic aphasia: A case study

Michael Walsh Dickey and Cynthia K. Thompson

Northwestern University, Evanston, IL, USA

Background: Production of grammatical morphology is typically impaired in agrammatic aphasic individuals, as is their capacity to produce the syntactic structure responsible for licensing that morphology. Whether these two impairments are causally related has been an issue of long-standing debate. If morphological deficits are a side-effect of underlying syntactic ones, as has been claimed (Friedmann & Grodzinsky, 1997; Izvorski & Ullman, 1999), therapy that improves the syntactic deficit should remediate the morphological deficit as well. This paper reports a case study of one individual with such co-occurring impairments and describes their recovery in response to linguistically motivated treatment targeting his syntactic deficits.

Methods & Procedures: MD is a 56-year-old male diagnosed with non-fluent Broca's aphasia subsequent to a left-hemisphere CVA, with limited capacity to produce syntactically complex utterances and grammatical morphology. He was enrolled in therapy using Treatment of Underlying Forms (TUF; Thompson & Shapiro, 2005), targeting production of sentences involving Wh-movement (object relative clauses). MD participated in twice-weekly treatment sessions for approximately 2 months, with daily probes assessing his production of treated and untreated sentence types. In addition, probes assessing his grammatical morphology and sentence production were administered pre- and post-treatment.

Outcomes & Results: Pre-treatment scores in tests of grammatical morphology and sentence production indicated deficits in both domains. During treatment, MD successfully acquired production of a variety of sentences with Wh-movement, although this did not generalise to sentences involving a grammatically distinct movement operation (NP-movement). Post-treatment scores also indicated a lack of improvement in production of grammatical morphology.

Conclusions: The dissociation between MD's morphological and syntactic recovery indicates that the recovery of syntactic and morphological processes in aphasia may occur independently in some individuals. The result would not be predicted by approaches in which morphological and syntactic impairments are strongly and causally related in aphasia, such as the tree-pruning hypothesis (Friedmann, 2001; Friedmann & Grodzinsky, 1997). Further, these results reinforce the conclusion that aphasia treatment can lead to generalisation, but only to linguistic material that is in a subset relation to trained structures (Thompson, Shapiro, Kiran, & Sobecks, 2003).

Address correspondence to: Michael Walsh Dickey, Department of Communication Sciences and Disorders, Northwestern University, 2240 Campus Drive, Evanston, IL 60208-3540, USA.
E-mail: m-dickey@northwestern.edu

This research was supported by the NIH under grant DC-01948 to C. K. Thompson. The authors are grateful to Audrey Holland and two anonymous reviewers for their exceptionally helpful comments and suggestions. The authors are especially grateful to MD and his family for his participation in this research.

http://www.psypress.com/aphasiology   DOI: 10.1080/02687030701192059

In English and many other languages, individuals with agrammatic Broca's aphasia often have both morphological and syntactic deficits (Menn & Obler, 1990; Rochon, Saffran, Berndt, & Schwartz, 2000). They exhibit reduced syntactic complexity in their production, showing particular difficulty with production of complex sentences with syntactic movement like the ones in examples 1–3 (Ballard & Thompson, 1999; Lee & Thompson, 2004; Thompson & Shapiro, 2005).

(1) a. Who did the thief chase?   (object Wh- question)
    b. It was the artist who the thief chased.   (object cleft)
    c. I saw the artist who the thief chased.   (object relative clause)
(2) a. The artist was chased by the thief.   (passive)
    b. The thief seems to have chased the artist. (subject-raising)
(3) The man is falling.   (unaccusative)

Sentences (1a–c) all involve *Wh-movement*: the wh- element "who", the underlying object of the verb "chase", is moved to a position before the verb's grammatical subject, resulting in a non-canonical order of subject and object. Sentences (2a–b) involve *NP movement*: the surface subject has been moved from another position in the sentence. "The artist" in (2a) is moved from its underlying object position following "chased", and "the thief" in (2b) moves from the subject position of the embedded infinitival clause "to have chased the artist". Unaccusative structures like that in (3) also involve NP-movement, in which the subject of the verb is raised to its surface subject position from an underlying object position (Perlmutter, 1978, among others). Such sentences present difficulty for persons with agrammatic aphasia, even though on the surface they are simple NP-V structures (Bastiaanse & van Zonneveld, 2005; Lee & Thompson, 2004; Thompson, 2003; see also Gahl et al., 2003).

Grammatical morphology is also significantly impaired in agrammatic aphasia (Kean, 1977; Menn & Obler, 1990), especially morphemes associated with verbs and clauses. For example, inflectional suffixes such as third-person singular *-s* and *-ed* are impaired, as are free-standing auxiliaries like *was* and *is*, and clausal subordinators or complementisers such as *if*, *whether*, and *that* appear to be particularly impaired. These patterns hold for languages as diverse as English (Milman, Dickey & Thompson, 2004), Japanese, French, and Italian (Hagiwara, 1995), and Hebrew and Palestinian Arabic (Friedmann, 2001; Friedmann & Grodzinsky, 1997).

It is an issue of long-standing theoretical interest whether these two co-occurring deficits are causally related. A unified explanation of the two would be desirable for both theoretical and clinical reasons. Theoretically, such an explanation would provide a simpler and more restrictive characterisation of aphasic language disorders, and it would predict which patterns of impairment should naturally co-occur (as well as what types of impairment should be expected not to co-occur). Clinically, such a unification would open up new venues for the diagnosis and treatment of aphasic language disorders. Treatment that results in improvement in one deficit should be expected to result in improvement for the other. For example, if the morphological deficit can be reduced to a syntactic one, then treatment that remediates the syntactic deficit could be expected to remediate the morphological deficit as well.

Recently, researchers have pursued exactly this hypothesis, attempting to explain the morphological deficits in terms of underlying syntactic ones. For example, the

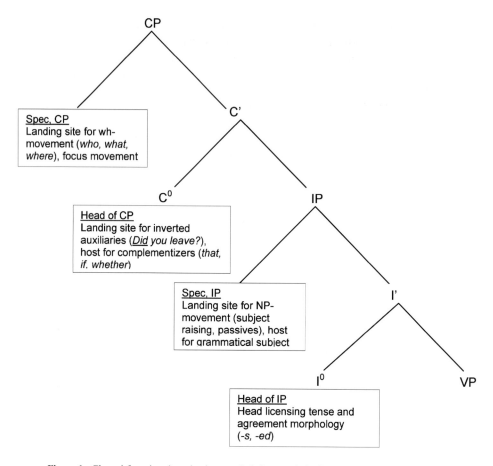

Figure 1. Clausal functional projections and their morphological and syntactic functions.

tree-pruning hypothesis (TPH; Friedmann, 2001; Friedmann & Grodzinsky, 1997) claims that individuals with agrammatic aphasia have difficulty projecting hierarchical syntactic structure. Thus, underspecified higher-level functional projections result in impairments in both morphological and syntactic deficits associated with those projections. (See Izvorski & Ullman, 1999, for a related proposal.) As illustrated by the structure in Figure 1, the different syntactic projections associated with a clause are responsible for distinct syntactic and morphological processes. The functional projection IP is responsible for tense and agreement morphology and is the position where the clause's subject appears (more generally, it serves as a landing site for NP movement, as in subject-raising, passive, and unaccusative sentences). The higher CP projection permits complementisers and fronted auxiliaries in languages like English, and it serves as a landing site for Wh-movement.

According to the TPH, "pruning" a given layer of structure disrupts both morphological and syntactic operations associated with that projection. For example, patients who are unable to generate a CP layer will be unable to license grammatical morphology associated with CP, such as complementisers, and they will also be unable to carry out syntactic operations which target CP, such as Wh-movement. Furthermore, "pruning" a given layer of structure results in impairments not only to syntactic and morphological operations associated with that layer, but all layers above it. For example, an agrammatic individual who is unable to generate an IP layer will not be able to generate a CP layer: s/he will exhibit deficits in not only IP-related morphology and syntax but CP-related morphology and syntax as well.

Under this hypothesis, syntactic and morphological deficits go hand-in-hand: a single syntactic deficit (in generating higher levels of clausal syntactic structure) explains both the syntactic and morphological impairments characteristic of agrammatic aphasia. This approach also makes a treatment-related prediction, already described above. Treatment that ameliorates the more basic deficit (in this case, the syntactic one) should result in improvement in the secondary one (in this case, the morphological one). Improving aphasic individuals' capacity to produce higher levels of syntactic structure should result in improved production of grammatical morphology associated with that syntactic structure. It is possible that the improvements in morphological production might be delayed compared to the improvements in syntactic production, an issue we will return to in the Discussion below. However, if this hypothesis is correct, improved syntactic production should in principle lead to improved morphological production, at least for some agrammatic individuals.

The TPH furthermore makes two specific predictions regarding how treatment targeting different levels of syntactic structure should generalise. First, improved production of sentences involving [Spec, CP] (such as Wh-movement sentences) should result in improved production of C, as well as the morphology licensed by C. There is some suggestion in the aphasia treatment literature in favour of this prediction: Thompson and colleagues (1997) found spontaneous production of complementisers improved following treatment of Wh-movement (targeting Spec, CP). Second, treatment that improves production of CP should result in improved production of IP as well, since IP is lower in the tree. This in turn should improve production of morphology licensed by I°, such as tense and subject-verb agreement.

This paper presents a case study testing these predictions, both the general prediction that improved syntactic production should lead to improved morphological production and the more specific predictions pertaining to the generalisation patterns noted above. MD, an individual exhibiting both morphological and syntactic impairments as a result of non-fluent Broca's-type aphasia, was trained to produce object relative clauses (a structure involving CP) using Treatment of Underlying Forms (TUF; Thompson & Shapiro, 2005). This linguistically motivated approach improves production and comprehension of Wh- and NP-movement structures, which entail access to the syntactic projections that host and license movement operations (CP and IP, respectively). MD's ability to produce a variety of CP and IP structures, both syntactic and morphological, was assessed prior to and following treatment, with the expectation that grammatical morphology associated with CP would improve. In addition, production of syntactic structures and morphological material licensed by IP was expected to improve if the TPH and its assumptions about the roots of aphasic morphological deficits are correct.

Because this is a single case report, its findings must be treated and interpreted with caution. Nevertheless, it does provide an initial look at the treatment-related predictions of the TPH, outlined above.

TABLE 1
NAVS scores (percent correct) for SPPT and SCT

	SPPT	*SCT*
Active	60%	100%
Passive	20%	60%
Yes/No Q	40%	60%
Subject Wh-Q	80%	100%
Subject Relative Clause	80%	80%
Object Wh- Q	20%	60%
Object Relative Clause	20%	100%

SPPT = Sentence Production Priming Test; SCT = Sentence Comprehension Test.

METHOD

Participant

The participant in the study, MD, was a 56-year-old, college-educated white male. He was a monolingual native English speaker who suffered a single left-hemisphere CVA. At the time of testing, MD was 48 months post-stroke and reported no previous history of speech-language or neuropsychological disorders. Results of testing using the Western Aphasia Battery (WAB; Kertesz, 1982), revealed a WAB AQ of 68.8, and a language profile consistent with non-fluent agrammatic Broca's aphasia: in spontaneous speech, he exhibited halting, effortful production with extremely reduced syntactic complexity and little or no use of grammatical morphology. In addition, testing with the Northwestern Assessment of Verbs and Sentences (NAVS; Thompson, 2005) revealed that he had difficulty comprehending and producing sentences with non-canonical Wh- and NP-movement (see Table 1).

Procedures

Measures for evaluating syntactic production. Production of semantically reversible, non-canonical Wh-movement structures (object relatives (OR), object clefts (OC), and object Wh-questions (OW), as in (1) above) and NP movement structures (subject raising (SR) and passive (PA) sentences, as in (2) above) was assessed using a 50-item probe task (10 items for each of the five sentence types). A sentence production priming paradigm was used to elicit production of target sentences, with picture pairs presented showing two versions of a single transitive action (e.g., an artist chasing a thief; a thief chasing an artist). The clinician first described one picture using one of the five sentences types and then asked MD to describe the other picture using the same type of sentence. This procedure is identical to standard probe procedures for TUF (see Thompson, 2001).

Second, MD's production of simple intransitive sentences was tested using both unaccusative verbs like *fall*, which involve NP-movement, and unergative verbs like *swim*, which do not. MD was first asked to name 25 pictures depicting intransitive events (13 unaccusatives and 12 unergatives) using a single action word, and then to describe the same pictures (presented in a different order) using a complete sentence. These pictures were adapted from picture stimuli used in a previous study of agrammatic aphasic individuals' production of unaccusative and unergative verbs (Lee & Thompson, 2004). These images elicited the anticipated verb names by control participants with 90% or higher accuracy with no differences in accuracy between unaccusative and unergative stimuli.

Measures for evaluating grammatical morpheme production. MD's production of complementisers (*n* = 20) and verb inflection (*n* = 40) was selected for testing CP and IP generated morphology, respectively. These structures were elicited in sentences using procedures developed by Thompson et al. (2006), in which pairs of cards were used for each item. One of the cards was an event card, depicting one of ten imageable transitive events (e.g., *The dog is watching the cat*). The other was a cue card, either depicting a sentential-complement verb like *ask, know, care,* or *wonder,* or the words *Nowadays* or *Yesterday.* The verb cards were intended to elicit embedded clauses introduced by complementisers, such as *if, that,* or *whether* (e.g., *They know that the dog is watching the cat*), while the *Nowadays/Yesterday* cards were intended to elicit *-s* or *-ed* marking on the transitive verb, respectively (e.g., *Nowadays the dog watches the cat, Yesterday the dog watched the cat*).

The two stimulus cards were presented to the participant. He was asked first to name the action pictured on the event card and to identify the agent and theme, and then to read the word (*Yesterday, Nowadays*) or name the action (e.g., *They wonder, They care*) pictured on the cue card. The participant was then asked to make a sentence by combining the two cards. Two practice items were presented before the test stimuli. In separate testing, these stimuli and procedures elicited *-s* and *-ed* morphemes as well as complementisers with 95% or greater accuracy in a group of eight age-matched controls.

To summarise, the study entailed a total of nine dependent variables, including both syntactic and morphological structures. Syntactic structures tested included three Wh-movement sentences (OR, OC, and OW) and three NP-movement sentences (PA, SR, and intransitive sentences with unaccusative verbs). Three morphological structures were also included: two measures of verb morphology (*-s* and *-ed*), and one measure of complementiser production.

Design

The study included pre- and post-treatment testing of all syntactic and morphological measures. In addition, five sentence types (ORs, OCs, OWs, SR, and PA forms) were tested on two separate occasions prior to treatment and administered daily throughout treatment to monitor treatment progress. This is a smaller number of baseline sessions than usual, due to time constraints for the participant, but his performance was at floor for the target Wh-movement sentence type (OR) in both sessions. Six weeks following the completion of treatment, all measures were once again administered to examine maintenance of treatment gains and generalisation patterns.

Baseline and treatment probes. Procedures identical to those used for pre-testing of OR, OC, OW, SR, and PA production were used for baseline and treatment probing. During baseline sessions, the full 50-item probe was completed. During treatment, a full probe was completed every other session (i.e., half of the probe items were presented prior to the first treatment session and the other half were presented prior to the second session, and so on until treatment was completed). Thus, data from every two sessions were combined and plotted to compare with baseline performance.

Treatment. Treatment of Underlying Forms (TUF), a linguistically motivated treatment for Wh- and NP-movement sentences, was used to train MD to produce one Wh-movement structure: object relatives (such as *The man saw the artist who the thief chased*). A total of 15 pictures of imageable transitive events were used for treatment, with each depicting two participants performing an action using a transitive verb (e.g., a thief chasing an artist), and a third participant, a man, watching. A set of corresponding sentence constituent cards were also developed for each item, with words for the agent (e.g., THE MAN), the verb (e.g., SAW), and theme (e.g., THE ARTIST) for the main clause and the agent (e.g., THE THIEF), the verb (e.g., CHASED), the theme (e.g., THE ARTIST) and a WHO card for building the embedded clause. The starting point for treatment provided an explicit model of the abstract underlying linguistic representation and derivation of object relatives, with the treatment cards arranged in two active sentences (i.e., THE MAN SAW THE ARTIST and THE THIEF CHASED THE ARTIST), with the WHO card set aside. The clinician then introduced steps required to build the target structure by thematic role identification and demonstration of the Wh-movement operation needed to arrive at the surface non-canonical word order. MD then used the cards to reassemble the sentence himself and read the sentence aloud (with assistance from the clinician when needed). Treatment was conducted twice per week for 8 weeks. Each treatment session lasted approximately 2 hours and up to fifteen treatment trials were administered per session.

RESULTS

Data derived from baseline and daily testing of Wh- and NP-movement structures are shown in Figure 2. Production of wh-movement structures—object relatives (ORs), object clefts (OCs), and object wh-questions (WHs)—is shown in the top graph and production of NP-movement structures—passives (PAs) and subject-raising sentences (SRs)—is shown in the lower graph. These data showed that MD had little or no capacity to produce any of these structures in pre-treatment or baseline (consistent with his performance in the Sentence Production Priming Test of the NAVS; see Table 1). Upon initiating treatment, he showed immediate acquisition of Wh-questions, improving from 25% in baseline to 100% by the end of treatment, as well as noticeable improvement in production of object relatives and object clefts, which rose from 0% at baseline to as high as 40% by the end of treatment. However, he showed no consistent improvement over baseline levels in production of either NP-movement structure. Follow-up probes showed retention of the gains made for all three Wh-movement sentence types at 6 weeks (from 25% in baseline to 70% for WH sentences, and from 0% and 5% to 20% for OR and OC, respectively), but no change from baseline for the two NP-movement sentences was noted.

MD's intransitve sentence production provided further data regarding the effects of treatment on syntactic structure production, for simple sentences with and without added NP-movement. Prior to treatment, MD's production of sentences with unaccusative verbs, which involve NP-movement, was impaired, and little change was noted on post testing. This result indicates that Wh-movement treatment

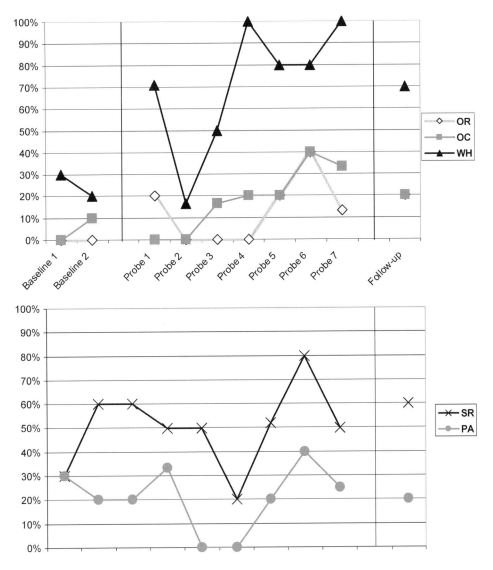

Figure 2. Baseline and daily probes from TUF treatment, with follow-up probe, Wh-movement, and NP-movement.

had no effect on simple sentences with NP-movement. However, a different pattern was noted for unergative verbs, which do not involve the same NP-movement operations. Prior to treatment, MD had little success in producing simple sentences with unergative verbs (i.e., 8% correct production). Following treatment, he showed large improvements in production of unergative sentences (i.e., 92% correct), indicating that treatment of complex sentences with movement impacted his ability to produce simple active sentences with no movement (see Table 2). Similar improvements in simple sentence production in narrative contexts following TUF treatment have been noted for other aphasic individuals, with greater numbers of verbs and greater numbers of correctly produced arguments (see Thompson & Shapiro, 2005; Thompson et al., 1997, for discussion).

TABLE 2
Accuracy

	Verb naming		Sentence production	
	Pre-treatment	Post-treatment	Pre-treatment	Post-treatment
Unaccusative (*sink*)	54%	31%	0%	15%
Unergative (*swim*)	92%	100%	8%	92%

Accuracy in verb naming and sentence production for unaccusative and unergative instransitive verbs, pre- and post-treatment.

The overall pattern of changes in MD's syntactic production is summarised in Figure 3. The Wh-movement category represents his mean performance on OR, OC, and OW sentences, the NP-movement category represents his mean performance on PA, SR, and unaccusative intransitive sentences, and the no-movement category represents his performance on unergative intransitive sentences. Wh-movement and no-movement sentences improved pre- to post-treatment, while NP-movement sentences showed no change.

With regard to grammatical morphology, MD was significantly impaired pre-treatment in production of both verbal inflection morphemes tested: -*ed* and -*s*. His errors consisted of omissions (producing a bare verb form, 8/22 errors) or inappropriate use of the -*ed* or -*s* morpheme (e.g., using -*s* with *Yesterday*, 14/22 errors). However, he produced complementisers with 100% accuracy (see Figure 4). His production of functional morphology associated with IP thus appeared to be significantly impaired pre-treatment, while his production of morphology associated with CP appeared to be intact. Post-treatment scores showed no evidence of improvement in his production of IP-related morphology: he continued to produce omission errors (8/18 errors) as well as to use -*s* and -*ed* inappropriately (10/18 errors). However, his production of CP-related morphology declined. We address this latter, unexpected finding below.

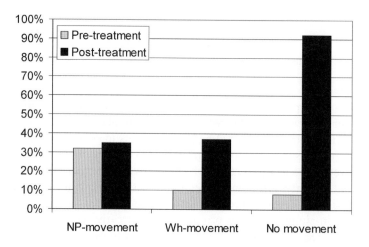

Figure 3. Mean accuracy in production of Wh-movement, NP-movement, and non-movement sentences, pre- and post-treatment.

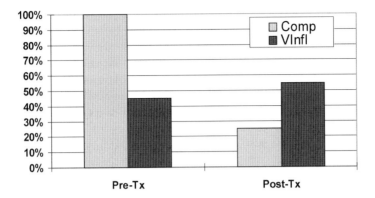

Figure 4. Mean accuracy in production of IP-related and CP-related grammatical morphemes, pre- and post-treatment.

DISCUSSION

This study examined the connection between syntactic and morphological deficits in agrammatism, looking at one agrammatic individual's patterns of recovery in response to TUF. Treatment targeting production of object relative sentences with Wh-movement improved MD's production of not only those sentences but also related sentence types, also involving Wh-movement. Further, the recovery patterns noted among Wh-movement structures showed that treatment influenced production of the least complex of the forms (i.e., wh-questions) more than production of more complex forms (object clefts). This finding is in keeping with results showing complexity effects in generalisation (Thompson et al., 2003): generalisation appears to proceed from more complex to less complex forms, provided that the forms are linguistically related to one another.

This complexity effect may underlie MD's additional improvement with simple (unergative) intransitive sentences, as well. Such sentences involve an Agent subject and a verb. OR training sentences also contained (as a subset of their more complex structure) an Agent and an eventive verb and the structure needed for producing them. Training OR sentences may thus implicitly train structures involving an Agent subject and a verb, including simple intransitives. Confirmation of this explanation would come from generalisation from OR training to other simple sentences that are a subset of OR structures, such as canonical SVO active sentences. Improvement in the production of canonical active sentences has been noted in narrative production following TUF (Thompson et al., 1997), and generalisation from object-relative training to simple active production has been found for second-language learners (Eckman, Bell, & Nelson, 1988). However, further work explicitly testing this possibility is needed to support this explanation of MD's improvement with simple intransitives.

It is unclear why greater improvement was not noted for the directly trained OR structure. Based on Thompson et al.'s (2003) complexity account of treatment and generalisation, improvement in all wh-movement structures would have been expected: training on the most complex structures (object relatives) should have resulted in acquisition of the trained structure as well as generalisation to less complex structures (object clefts and object Wh-questions). Why MD did not exhibit this recovery pattern remains unresolved. One possibility is that MD has additional, independent impairments, which interfered with his acquisition of the more complex sentences. Such additional/independent impairments may also be the explanation for the small number of individuals who have not shown the expected TUF generalisation patterns (see Thompson et al., 2003, for discussion). Nevertheless, MD's striking improvement in his production of Wh-questions shows that treatment generalised to sentences with different words but similar abstract structure. These data thus indicate that MD's ability to generate CP-level syntactic structure was improved with treatment.

However, MD's results also showed that Wh-treatment did not generalise to sentences involving NP-movement: subject raising or passive sentences, as well as simple, active intransitive sentences with unaccusative verbs. That is, the treatment and generalisation effects were linguistically specific, with acquisition of Wh-movement structures having no effect on constructions with NP-movement. These results also replicate previous TUF findings (Ballard & Thompson, 1999; Thompson & Shapiro, 1995, 2005; Thompson et al., 2003). Further, they show that while CP-level syntax is higher in the syntactic tree than IP-level syntax, position in the tree alone does not predict a structure's improvement following treatment, as would be expected based on strongly tree-based accounts of agrammatism like the TPH.

MD's production of grammatical morphology also did not improve with treatment: complementisers and verbal inflection were produced at only 24% and 46% accuracy, respectively, on post-treatment testing. Compared to baseline performance, these data show that his production of verb inflections was unchanged. However, his production of complementisers actually declined. These patterns are inconsistent with both the general and the specific predictions of the TPH outlined above: improving production of the CP-level material did not improve production of morphology associated with C^0 immediately below it, nor did it result in improved production of verbal morphology associated with the more deeply embedded IP layer. Treatment that demonstrably improved production of even the highest level of clausal syntactic structure thus did not appear to help with production of grammatical morphology, at any level of hierarchical syntactic structure. This seems inconsistent with attempts to reduce morphological deficits in agrammatism to syntactic ones (Friedmann, 2001; Friedmann & Grodzinsky, 1997; Izvorski & Ullman, 1999). More generally, these results indicate that syntactic and morphological recovery may proceed independently in aphasia.

There is at least one aspect of the current results that merits further attention: MD's unexpected decline in complementiser production following treatment. This result is not consistent with previous TUF results (e.g., Thompson et al., 1997). One possible explanation is that MD's pre-treatment performance with complementisers did not reflect his capacity to produce morphemes located in C^0. Consistent with this is his relatively poor performance in production of yes–no questions on the NAVS (Table 1: 40% correct), which involve the sentence-initial auxiliary "did" (also located in C^0). Another possibility is that the decline in complementiser production is an example of antagonistic recovery of CP. Focusing on Wh-movement (which targets Spec, CP) inhibited his performance with complementisers (which reside in C^0). Further testing with other agrammatic individuals is needed to decide between these possibilities.

As noted above, these results must be treated with caution. They are from one agrammatic individual, whose behaviour may not be typical. Potentially consistent with this is MD's good performance on some subtests of the NAVS (such as object-relative comprehension) and on the initial complementiser production probes (although these results are at odds with his NAVS performance, as discussed above). However, MD's recovery patterns do provide an initial test of the relationship between recovery in the syntactic and morphological domains in response to treatment, as well as the treatment-related predictions of the TPH. As such, they provide a starting point for further research. Additional testing is needed to determine whether MD's pattern holds for a larger sample of agrammatic individuals.

Further data are also needed to test another possibility described above: that morphological recovery may be delayed compared to syntactic recovery. Perhaps syntactic recovery proceeds as suggested by the TPH, with recovery of higher-level syntactic projections (like CP) entailing recovery of lower-level ones (like IP), and with morphological recovery following sometime later. It is possible that MD's morphological production may have recovered further following his syntactic recovery, given sufficient time. It is worth noting that MD's morphological production had not improved by the time of his post-testing 6 weeks following treatment. However, additional and more extended testing is needed to determine whether such delayed morphological improvement would occur for other individuals trained to produce Wh-movement sentences (and with them, CP-level structure).

CONCLUSION

In conclusion, the current results provide evidence that the syntactic and morphological impairments characteristic of agrammatism cannot be reduced to a single underlying deficit. In particular, they cast doubt on attempts to reduce the morphological deficit to a syntactic one. As indicated above, this conclusion must be treated with caution, as these data are from a single agrammatic individual. However, these results do suggest that the relation between syntactic and morphological processes in aphasia and aphasia recovery isn't a simple one. Training one will not automatically improve the other. The ability to generate complex syntactic structure is likely a necessary condition for producing related grammatical morphology, but it does not appear to be a sufficient one. Rather, the operations required to produce functional morphology must be trained separately (cf. Thompson et al., 2006).

REFERENCES

Ballard, K., & Thompson, C. K. (1999). Treatment and generalisation of complex sentence production in agrammatism. *Journal of Speech, Language, and Hearing Research, 42*, 690–707.

Bastiaanse, R., & van Zonneveld, R. (2005). Sentence production with verbs of alternating transitivity in agrammatic Broca's aphasia. *Journal of Neurolinguistics, 18*, 57–66.

Eckman, R., Bell, L., & Nelson, D. (1988). On the generalisation of relative clause instruction in The acquisition of English as a second language. *Applied Linguistics, 9*, 1–20.

Friedmann, N. (2001). Agrammatism and the psychological reality of the syntactic tree. *Journal of Psycholinguistic Research, 30*, 71–88.

Friedmann, N., & Grodzinsky, Y. (1997). Tense and agreement in agrammatic production: Pruning the syntactic tree. *Brain and Language, 56*, 397–425.

Gahl, S., Menn, L., Ramsberger, G., Jurafsky, D., Elder, E., & Rewega, M. et al. (2003). Syntactic frame and verb bias in aphasia: Plausibility judgments of undergoer-subject sentences. *Brain and Cognition, 53*, 223–228.

Hagiwara, H. (1995). The breakdown of functional categories and the economy of derivation. *Brain and Language, 50*, 92–116.

Izvorski, R., & Ullman, M. (1999). Verb inflection and the hierarchy of functional categories in agrammatic anterior aphasia. *Brain and Language, 69*, 288–291.

Kean, M-L. (1977). The linguistic interpretation of aphasic syndromes. *Cognition, 5*, 9–46.

Kertesz, A. (1982). *Western Aphasia Battery.* New York: Grune & Stratton.

Lee, M., & Thompson, C. K. (2004). Agrammatic aphasic production and comprehension of unaccusative verbs in sentence contexts. *Journal of Neurolinguistics, 17*, 315–330.

Menn, L., & Obler, L. K. (1990). *Agrammatic aphasia.* Amsterdam: John Benjamins.

Milman, L. H., Dickey, M. W., & Thompson, C. K. (2004). Production of functional categories in agrammatic narratives: An IRT analysis. *Brain and Language, 91*, 126–127.

Perlmutter, D. M. (1978). Impersonal passives and the unaccusative hypothesis. *Berkeley Linguistics Society, 4*, 157–189.

Rochon, E., Saffran, E. M., Berndt, R. S., & Schwartz, M. F. (2000). Quantitative analysis of aphasic sentence production: Further development and new data. *Brain and Language, 72*, 193–218.

Thompson, C. K. (2001). Treatment of underlying forms: A linguistic specific approach for sentence production deficits in agrammatic aphasia. In R. Chapey (Ed.), *Language intervention strategies in adult aphasia* (4th ed., pp. 605–628). Baltimore: Williams & Wilkins.

Thompson, C. K. (2003). Unaccusative verb production in agrammatic aphasia: The argument structure complexity hypothesis. *Journal of Neurolinguistics, 16*, 151–167.

Thompson, C. K. (2005). *The Northwestern Assessment of Verbs and Sentences.* Unpublished manuscript, Northwestern University, Evanston, IL, USA.

Thompson, C. K., Milman, L. H., Dickey, M. W., O'Connor, J. E., Arcuri, D. A., & Choy, J. J. (2006). Treatment and generalisation of functional category production in agrammatic aphasia. *Brain and Language, 99*, 69–71.

Thompson, C. K., & Shapiro, L. P. (1995). Training sentence production in agrammatism: Implications for normal and disordered language. *Brain and Language, 50*, 201–224.

Thompson, C. K., & Shapiro, L. P. (2005). Treating agrammatic aphasia within a linguistic framework: Treatment of Underlying Forms. *Aphasiology, 19*, 1021–1036.

Thompson, C. K., Shapiro, L. P., Ballard, K. J., Jacobs, B. J., Schneider, S. L., Tait, M., et al. (1997). Training and generalised production of wh- and NP-Movement structures in agrammatic aphasia. *Journal of Speech, Language, and Hearing Research, 40*, 228–244.

Thompson, C. K., Shapiro, L. P., Kiran, S., & Sobecks, J. (2003). The role of syntactic complexity in treatment of sentence deficits in agrammatic aphasia: The complexity account of treatment efficacy (CATE). *Journal of Speech, Language, and Hearing Research, 46*, 591–607.

APHASIOLOGY, 2007, 21 (6/7/8), 617–631

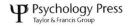

Lexical influences on single word repetition in acquired spoken output impairment: A cross language comparison

Nicole Lallini, Nick Miller and David Howard

University of Newcastle upon Tyne, UK

Background: Among the many factors that may affect speech production, phonological neighbourhood density (ND) and phonotactic probability (PROB) have displayed effects on speech and language performance in healthy speakers. What is not clear is if they show an effect in impaired speech output after stroke and if they do, whether this effect is facilitatory or inhibitory.
Aims: To determine whether ND and/or PROB play a role in speech production accuracy in acquired output impairment after stroke. To compare the performance of English vs German speakers on a matched set of words in order to tease out language-specific and language-independent factors affecting impaired speech output.
Methods & Procedures: Seven English and seven German native speakers with acquired output impairment after stroke repeated in their respective languages 509 real words that are (near) homophones across German and English (e.g., leader–Lieder; vine–Wein). Responses were transcribed phonetically and scored as correct or incorrect.
Results & Outcomes: There was a small correlation between accuracy on near-homophones between English and German speakers ($r = .201$; $p < .001$). Correlating accuracy for speakers combined across both languages with language-independent factors (i.e., number of phonemes, syllables, clusters) showed significant independent effects of number of phonemes and clusters in the target, but multiple regressions did not show an effect of number of syllables. Within-language correspondence was greater than between-language correspondence (9.4% vs 4%; $p < .00001$). Correlating differences in accuracy in English/German with differences in language-specific factors (i.e., word and syllable frequency, PROB, ND) multiple regression displayed a significant independent effect of the target's word frequency but not of the target's ND, PROB, or syllable frequency.
Conclusions: The small but significant correlation between accuracy on (near) homophones for English and German speakers suggests there are language-independent determinants of production accuracy, whereas greater within-language correspondence indicates language-specific determinants of performance. Only word frequency appears to have a significant (facilitatory) effect on response accuracy. Neither ND nor PROB had a significant effect on response accuracy in this study. The results are discussed in light of theoretical and methodological issues within the study.

After stroke or other neurological illness people may experience difficulties in speaking which range from a slight unnaturalness about speech, through mild intelligibility problems, to muteness. Such difficulties are generally subsumed under

Address correspondence to: Nicole Lallini, Speech and Language Sciences, King George VI Building, University of Newcastle upon Tyne, Newcastle upon Tyne NE1 7RU, UK.
E-mail: Nicole.Lallini@ncl.ac.uk

© 2007 Psychology Press, an imprint of the Taylor & Francis Group, an informa business
http://www.psypress.com/aphasiology   DOI: 10.1080/02687030701192067

the diagnostic labels dysarthria, apraxia of speech (AoS), and phonemic paraphasia (PhPa). Dysarthria arises from changes to muscle tone, power, and coordination, whereas AoS and PhPa represent problems of speech programming and/or phonologic encoding. AoS is taken to be a "phonetic-motoric disorder of speech production caused by inefficiencies in the translation of a well-formed and filled phonologic frame to previously learned kinematic parameters assembled for carrying out the intended movement ..." (McNeil, Robin, & Schmidt, 1997, p. 329). By contrast PhPa is understood as a disruption to the retrieval of elements of and assembly of this phonological frame. Of course all this begs many questions, concerning what precisely the frames are frames of; what is retrieved and assembled, and how; what processes are involved in affecting the translation of frame specifications into motoric control; and what is the nature of the interface between these apparent subsystems. Debates directed at these issues have spawned much controversy (Ballard, Granier, & Robin, 2000; McNeil, 2001; Miller, 2002; Ziegler, 2002). It is not the aim to address or settle any of these issues here.

A means of contributing to this debate has been to determine which variables influence performance in people with acquired output impairment after stroke. Many variables influence speech output, such as word phoneme length and frequency (Nickels & Howard, 1995). Two additional factors that deserve consideration based on the literature on typical spoken language production are phonological neighbourhood density and phonotactic probability. Phonological neighbourhood density is a measure of the number of neighbours of a target. A neighbour, based on the single-phoneme edit distance (Luce, 1986), differs from its target by exactly one phoneme through substitution, deletion, or addition (e.g., cat → catch, at, hat, mat, kit ...). Words may come from dense phonological neighbourhoods where the target has many neighbours (e.g., cat) or from sparse neighbourhoods with very few or no neighbours at all (e.g., elf). Phonotactic probability refers to the (positional) frequency of phonemes/sequences of phonemes in a particular language. Sequences can have high phonotactic probability (e.g., st- in stuck) or low probability (e.g., sv- in svelte).

This study seeks to establish whether these variables play a role in determining accuracy in speakers with output problems following stroke. Phonological neighbourhood density and phonotactic probability have been shown to predict performance in spoken language comprehension and production tasks among typical speakers. Significant effects of both variables have been found on response accuracy in speech perception (e.g., wordlikeness judgements: Bailey & Hahn, 2001; Frisch, Large, & Pisoni, 2000; lexical decision: Luce & Pisoni, 1998; Vitevitch & Luce, 1999; speeded same–different judgements: Luce & Large, 2001; Vitevitch & Luce, 1999). On the output side evidence is not so abundant, but preliminary indications are that phonotactic probability and phonological neighbourhood density also play a significant role (e.g., vowel production: Munson & Solomon, 2004; repetition: Vitevitch & Luce, 1998; primed production: Stemberger, 2004). As it stands, both variables tend to have a facilitatory effect in speech production but an inhibitory effect in speech perception (comprehension and recognition). Consequently, healthy speakers repeat targets with high phonotactic probability/ phonological neighbourhood density more quickly than those with low probability/ density. In contrast, healthy speakers tend to require longer response times for high probability/density items in a lexical decision task. Studies done with impaired speakers have shown the same pattern of effect compared to healthy speakers in regard to phonological neighbourhood density in that a competition effect is noted for speech perception tasks but a facilitatory one for spoken production (e.g., Boyczuk & Baum, 1999; Gordon, 2002).

A major hurdle in examining speech output variables is their strongly interconnected nature, with measures being highly confounded with one another. For instance, words with more phonemes tend to have lower frequency, fewer neighbours, and lower phonemic probability (see Table 4 below). We present a novel way of addressing these issues though a cross-language study of speech output in aphasia.

English and German share many phonetically identical or similar words— homophones and near-homophones (e.g., leader–Lieder; vine–Wein). These words have the same number of phonemes and syllables and are equal in the complexity of their articulatory gestures (language-independent properties); yet they differ in word frequency, the number of neighbours, and phonological predictability, because these are language-specific. Thus, when we investigate the effects of differences in these factors on the differences in the accuracy of their production by English- and German-speaking participants, we can explore the effects of their language-specific properties independent from their language-independent properties. Thus, by examining the differences in the accuracy of German and English speakers with disorders of speech output planning, it should be possible to determine whether language-specific factors (e.g., word frequency, neighbourhood density, phonotactic predictability) or language-independent factors (e.g., number of phonemes, phoneme sequence) play a greater role in influencing speech output. If language-specific variables play a dominant role, then there should be little correlation between German and English speakers in the susceptibility of (near) homophones to error; if there are strong correlations, then it would suggest a greater role of language-independent factors in determining accuracy. As a consequence, the study specifically examined the effects of the target's number of syllables, phonemes, and clusters (language-independent factors), and the target's phonotactic probability, phonological neighbourhood density, and word and syllable frequency (language-specific variables) on accuracy rate..

Specifically we asked the following questions:

- Is there a significant association between response accuracy and language independent factors (i.e., target's number of syllables, clusters, and phonemes) across languages?
- Is there a significant association between response accuracy and language-specific measures (i.e., target's word frequency, syllable frequency, phonotactic probability, and phonological neighbourhood density) across languages?

METHOD

Participants

Seven native English and seven native German speakers were matched for their achieved scores in their performance on the Token and Naming subtests of the Aachener Aphasia Test (AAT; Huber, Poeck, Weniger, & Willmes, 1983) and the English version of this (Miller, Willmes , & De Bleser, 2000). Both English and German participants met the following inclusion criteria: (1) viable attention, memory, visual, and auditory-perceptive skills enabling the participants to correctly follow simple auditory commands necessary to complete the repetition task, understand the purpose of the study, and sign a consent form; (2) monolingual native speakers of either English or German; (3) at least 4 months post onset of their stroke; (4) speech output impairment evidenced by perceived production errors including perceived omission, substitution, addition, transposition, and distortion errors during spontaneous speech production and/or reading aloud. Participant details are given in Table 1. Table 2 displays the matched pairs of English and German speakers and their performance in the Naming and Token Test of the AAT, and Table 3 shows the characteristics of the participants' spoken output.

Presence of a speech output impairment was determined perceptually. Dysarthria was excluded on the basis of standard clinical speech motor examination. There was no loss of range, strength, or speed of articulatory movement in nonverbal, speechlike (diadochokinetic), or speech tasks, and where mild facial or lingual hemiparesis existed it was insufficient to explain either the degree or pattern of articulatory breakdown. Speakers showed no fatigue effects on maximum performance tasks and no dysarthrophonia.

The following characteristics were taken to provide evidence that the individual had AoS: perceived errors of articulation included substitutions, omissions, additions, distortions, and, crucially, distorted substitutions and additions; perceived blurring of voiced–voiceless distinctions in stop production (in spontaneous speech and in contrasting diadochokinetic tasks, e.g., pea–bee); inconsistencies of error (a target sound was not always wrongly produced; on different occasions it may be misarticulated in a variety of ways); altered rhythm and prosody; presence of syllabification; preparatory and intra- and inter-word struggle to achieve target sounds and transitions. Speakers are usually labelled as having PhPa if diadochokinetic rates and rate of intact stretches in spontaneous speech are of normal rate; there are no alterations to prosody and rhythm in intact speech

TABLE 1
Participant information

Participant	Gender	Age	Language	Months post onset	Location of CVA
CM	M	37	German	30	Left middle cerebral artery
CJ	F	51	German	105	Left middle cerebral artery
MSch	F	42	German	167	Left internal carotid artery
ES	M	58	German	5	Left middle cerebral artery
CK	M	61	German	4	Left middle cerebral artery
LW	F	76	German	132	Left middle cerebral artery
JL	F	67	German	6	Left middle cerebral artery
CT	M	69	English	21	Diffuse mild cortical atrophy; aneurysm left internal carotid
JOV	M	75	English	8	Left middle cerebral artery
PS	M	48	English	8	Left middle cerebral artery
AY	F	55	English	31	Left anterior cerebral territory & possible left parietal region
PJ	F	56	English	77	Left frontal parietal
YB	F	45	English	36	Left hemisphere
JS	F	63	English	17	CVA following retromastoid craniotomy

TABLE 2
Participants' test scores

English participant	German participant	EAAT Token Test % rank	AAT Token Test % rank	EAAT Naming Test % rank	AAT Naming Test % rank
CT	CM	86	81	73	89
JOV	CJ	55	53	55	75
PS	MSch	19	28	15	15
AY	ES	89	81	65	79
PJ	CK	49	33	35	35
YB	LW	70	79	60	63
JS	JL	89	81	61	81

stretches; substitutions, transpositions, perseverations, anticipations, and additions are undistorted.

Given the shades of opinion that exist concerning the differential diagnosis of AoS and PhPa, and in order not to preclude the possibility that speakers with these different output disorders may respond differently to the variables under study, we included in the first instance speakers who might traditionally be labelled as having either AoS or PhPa. However, a later stage of this study (not reported in detail here) asks whether there are differences according to the variables studied in relation to diagnostic group or impairment profile.

Stimuli

A list of 509 real words was compiled, to all intents homophones or near-homophones in English and German (e.g., house–Haus, leader–Lieder). Words containing sounds or sequences of sounds not found in the other language were excluded: thus, German words containing initial/medial /r/, medial/final /x/, final /ç/ and/or word initial /ʃp/ and /ʃt/ were excluded, as were English items with word-initial and post-consonantal /r/ and /w/. The real-word stimuli included nouns, adjectives, prepositions, adverbs, articles (e.g., an), and numbers, and consisted of one ($N = 259$, e.g., eye/Ei), two ($N = 226$, e.g., abbey/Abi), three ($N = 21$, e.g., commissar/Kommissar), or four syllables ($N = 2$). Syllable frames covered V, CV/VC, to CCVC/VCCV syllable structure. Words were matched for form, not meaning, although 171 items (33%) had the same meaning in both languages.

Measures for the number of phonemes, syllables, clusters, phonological neighbours, word frequency, syllable frequency, and phonotactic probability for each of the stimulus items were derived from the CELEX database of British English and German (Baayen, Piepenbrock, & Gulikers, 1995). Probability was defined as the sum of the log-transformed conditional probabilities of the next phoneme given the previous phoneme; phoneme position within the onset, nucleus, and coda of a syllable was taken into account on this calculation. Neighbourhood density was computed based on the single-edit distance definition. A neighbour was obtained by substituting, deleting, or adding exactly one phoneme of the target.

To record the English stimuli one male and one female healthy adult native British English speaker were recruited from the speech accent area in which the

TABLE 3
Participants' speech characteristics

	Substitutions; omissions; additions; distortions	Distorted substitutions/additions	Inconsistency of error	Altered rhythm/prosody	Syllabification	Struggle	Transpositions; perseverations; anticipations
CM	✓						✓
CJ	✓	✓✓	✓	✓✓		✓✓	
MSch	✓	✓✓✓✓	✓				
ES	✓		✓				
CK	✓	✓✓✓✓	✓	✓✓✓		✓	✓
LW	✓	✓	✓	✓		✓	✓
JL	✓		✓				
CT	✓	✓	✓		✓		
JOV	✓		✓				
PS	✓	✓✓✓✓	✓		✓✓✓	✓✓	✓✓✓
AY	✓		✓			✓✓	
PJ	✓	✓	✓		✓	✓✓	✓
YB	✓		✓		✓	✓	
JS	✓	✓	✓	✓			

TABLE 4

Correlations between properties of the words, and with repetition accuracy by German and English participants with output impairment

	Number of syllables	Number of phonemes	Number of clusters	English log word frequency	English phonological neighbours	English log phonological predictability	German log word frequency	German phonological neighbours	German log phonological predictability	English proportion correct	German proportion correct
Number of phonemes	0.730*										
Number of clusters	−0.246*	0.288*									
English log word frequency	−0.274*	−0.294*	−0.102*								
English phonological neighbours	−0.671*	−0.777*	−0.222*	0.323*							
English log phonological predictability	−0.697*	−0.840*	−0.172*	0.298*	0.771*						
German log word frequency	−0.180*	−0.235*	−0.103*	0.125*	0.187*	0.230*					
German phonological neighbours	−0.360*	−0.499*	−0.168*	0.064	0.539*	0.559*	0.258*				
German log phonological predictability	−0.598*	−0.750*	−0.162*	0.209*	0.620*	0.776*	0.324*	0.625*			
English proportion correct	−0.066	−0.321*	−0.335*	0.245*	0.266*	0.327*	0.059	0.194*	0.254*		
German proportion correct	−0.244*	−0.363*	−0.165*	0.121*	0.305*	0.331*	0.339*	0.261*	0.327*	0.202*	
Combined proportion correct	−0.190*	−0.438*	−0.330*	0.242*	0.365*	0.424*	0.241*	0.289*	0.370*	0.815*	.732*

* $p < .01$.

participants lived. In order to delete excessive noise (e.g., coughing), minimise hiss, and increase the volume to a comfortable listening level the recording was edited using the SoundWave97 computer program. The recording used with the German-speaking participants was produced in the same manner as the English recording and was completed using male and female adult healthy native German speakers with a standard high German accent.

A pilot investigation with healthy native British English speakers was conducted to determine whether the recorded stimuli could be clearly understood and words correctly recognised. The speakers' productions were analysed according to whether the speakers correctly perceived the intended target stimuli. A total of 25 stimuli were not correctly perceived and thus re-recorded. The 25 re-recorded stimuli were then presented to the healthy speakers who participated in the pilot study. All speakers correctly perceived the 25 stimuli. The stimuli recorded for the German-speaking participants underwent an identical pilot study. During this pilot study 26 items were re-recorded, which were then correctly perceived by the healthy German speakers taking part in the pilot study.

Task

The speakers with speech output problems repeated each word in the same order. Repetition was chosen in favour of other elicitation methods due to the difficulty in obtaining representable pictures, drawings, or objects for sufficient stimuli. Secondly, it was chosen to minimise confounding effects of reading problems on output. Repetition was also chosen to minimise the effects of possible semantic impairment on output.

Participants were assessed individually. Each participant was asked to repeat each stimulus, which was presented via headphones. After the verbal explanation of the task, headphones were placed on the participant and on the investigator. A Stereo Mini T adaptor was used to enable the investigator to hear the stimuli simultaneously with the participants. After each stimulus the minidisk player was paused in order not to place any time constraints on the participants' production of the stimuli. The participants could make as many attempts as they wanted to produce each stimulus, but they heard the stimulus only once. The participants' responses were recorded. No form of direct feedback was given to the participants on the productions of the stimuli, only general encouragement to maintain motivation.

Scoring

Each response was scored as either correct or incorrect. A response was scored as incorrect if it contained any substituted, deleted, added, or distorted phoneme(s) compared to the target stimulus. Suprasegmental aberrations, hesitations, and intra-word and intra-syllable pauses did not constitute an error if they occurred without a phonemic error. The investigator listened to the same responses on a different day to establish intra-rater reliability, which was 93.1%. Of the recorded responses, 20% were independently transcribed by a second transcriber who was an experienced speech and language therapist. Inter-rater agreement was 88.3%. The first attempt to produce the entire target (where that attempt was a possible phonological word in English or German) was scored as a response.

Data analysis

Chance-corrected correspondence between participants within one language and across German and English was obtained by computing the kappa statistic. To investigate the effects of variables common to both English and German on production accuracy we took, as a first step, the mean accuracy rate combined across both languages. As a second step we completed multiple regression analyses in which the dependent variable was the mean response accuracy (proportion correct) combined across both languages, and the predictor variables were language-independent factors—number of syllables, phonemes, and clusters in the target. In order to answer the question whether language-specific variables affect production accuracy, we ran another set of multiple regressions. The dependent variable in the second set was the difference in response accuracy in English/German with the predictor language-specific variables—phonological neighbourhood density, phonotactic probability, word frequency, and syllable frequency.

RESULTS

Chance-corrected correspondence was calculated between all pairs of speakers. Of the 42 within-language comparisons 30 were individually significant, compared to 11 of the 49 between-language comparisons. Reflecting this, the overall within-language chance-corrected correspondence was on average greater than between-language correspondence (9.7% vs 4.0%; $p < .00001$). This correspondence, while significant, is low. This may reflect day-to-day variability of participants' performance, or that different participants in the groups are having difficulties for different reasons, resulting in different kinds of items attracting errors.

Table 4 shows the correlations between word properties and their relationship to repetition accuracy in German and English. Reflecting the low item-level consistency between participants, the correlation between English and German participants' accuracy is small but significant ($r = .202$, $p < .001$). The combined proportion correct was significantly related to all of the independent variables with the best predictor being the number of phonemes in the target. However, there are substantial correlations between many of the independent variables, as discussed in the introduction. For example, the number of phonemes in the target has a significant correlation with all the other independent variables, with particularly high correlations with phonological predictability and neighbourhood density in both languages. There is a substantial correlation ($r = .776$) between phonological predictability in the two languages, reflecting their shared phonotactic properties that in turn relate to their common origin. Neighbourhood density is also quite strongly correlated across languages, but the relationship for word frequency is weaker because two thirds of the stimuli are not translation equivalents.

It is noteworthy that, considering the language-specific factors (neighbourhood density, phonological predictability, and word frequency), the correlation between participants' performance accuracy and these properties is always higher for the speaker's language than for the same property in the other language. So, for example, English participants' repetition accuracy is more strongly related to English word frequency than German word frequency ($r = .245$ vs $r = .059$). This gives us some confidence that language-specific factors are important in determining participants' repetition accuracy. However, proper analysis (given below) will need to account for the effects of confounding variables.

Effects of language-independent variables on response accuracy combined across English and German

The first question of this study concerned factors that are common to both English and German—the target's number of syllables, phonemes, and clusters. The aim was to establish whether these language-independent variables significantly affect production accuracy in speakers with output impairment. At a second step we sought to establish whether language-specific variables accounted for any additional variance in repetition accuracy after language-specific variables have been accounted for.

Simultaneous multiple regression, with combined accuracy as the dependent variable, using number of syllables, phonemes, and clusters as the independent variables showed that there were statistically significant independent effects for the number of phonemes in the target ($\beta = -.474$, $p < .001$) and the number of clusters ($\beta = -.165$, $p = .004$) in a target. There was no significant effect of number of syllables in a word ($\beta = -.115$, $p = .15$). Between them, these three variables accounted for 24.0% of the variance in the participants' repetition accuracy combined over languages.

A second stage in the regression considered the effects of word frequency, by entering both English and German log-transformed frequency as a block. These variables accounted for a further 3.3% of the variance, with both English and German frequency ($\beta = -.124$, $p = .002$, and $\beta = -.136$, $p = .001$, respectively) having significant independent effects.

As a third stage, we explored the effects of including either the number of neighbours or the phonological predictability of the target in the regression, including both English and German measures at each stage. The number of neighbours accounted for a further 0.6% of the variance, and this was not significant ($p = .14$). In contrast, phonological predictability, when added after both frequency and the phonological properties had been entered, accounted for a further 1.7% of the variance ($p = .003$). When added after the number of phonological neighbours, the effect was also significant, accounting for 1.2% of the variance ($p = .015$). This shows that there is a very small effect of phonological predictability that is statistically independent of the effects of the number of phonemes, syllables, and clusters, word frequency, and the number of neighbours.

Effects of language-specific variables on difference in response accuracy in English and German

A second main question of the study was whether factors specific to English and German (i.e., language-specific factors like frequency of "Wiese" vs "visa") determine the response accuracy in speakers with acquired output impairment. To investigate this, we explored the relationship between the difference of production accuracy (proportion correct) between the English and German participants, and the difference of the target's phonotactic probability, phonological neighbourhood density, and word and syllable frequency in English and German using multiple regression analysis. As the previous analyses showed, there are language-specific factors that determine the accuracy of people with output impairments.

Because the effects of syllable frequency can only be compared with items with the same number of syllables, we conducted three analyses. All of these analyses take advantage of the near-homophone stimuli across the two languages. As a result there is no confounding with word syllable or phoneme length, number of clusters, or complexity of the articulatory gestures. The first analysis took the difference in accuracy for German and English participants as the independent variable and related it to differences between German and English in the number of neighbours, phonological predictability, and word frequency using simultaneous multiple regression. The second analysis used only one-syllable targets, but added differences between English and German in syllable frequency to the predictors. The third analysis was confined to two-syllable words and considered differences in number of phonological neighbours, phonological predictability, word frequency, and first and second syllable frequency between German and English in determining the differences in accuracy of repetition in participants using the two languages, using multiple regression.

Table 5 shows the relationships between differences between the German and English stimuli and their language-specific properties. In contrast to the picture in Table 4, the independent variables show relatively low correlations with each other, reducing the problems associated with intercorrelated predictors in multiple regression. Only differences in word frequency show a significant relationship with differences in accuracy. That is, a (near) homophone with higher frequency in German than in English is more likely to be repeated correctly by a German speaker than an English speaker with an acquired output impairment.

The first simultaneous regression considered differences in frequency, phonological predictability, and number of phonological neighbours as predictors of differences in accuracy between the speakers of English and German. There was a significant effect of the difference in log frequency ($\beta = .24$, $p < .001$, accounting uniquely for 5.3% of the variance). There were no effects of differences in the number of phonological neighbours ($\beta = -.04$, $p = .39$, accounting uniquely for 0.1% of the variance) or differences in phonological predictability ($\beta = .04$, $p = .39$, accounting uniquely for 0.1% of the variance).

The second analysis considered only the one-syllable targets, but included in addition log syllable frequency. Again, in simultaneous multiple regression there was a significant effect of difference in log word frequency ($\beta = .18$, $p = .033$), but not of differences in number of phonological neighbours ($\beta = .03$, $p = .63$), log phonological predictability ($\beta = .08$, $p = .27$), or log syllable frequency ($\beta = .01$, $p = .88$).

TABLE 5
Correlations among differences between English and German

	Difference in log word frequency	Difference in number of phonological neighbours	Difference in log phonological probability
Difference in number of phonological neighbours	0.237*		
Difference in log phonological probability	0.201*	0.201*	
Difference in proportion correct	0.239*	0.025	0.080

* $p < .01$.

The third analysis including only two-syllable targets produced a similar pattern of results: in simultaneous multiple regression there was a significant effect of difference in log word frequency ($\beta = .30$, $p < .001$), but not of differences in number of phonological neighbours ($\beta = .10$, $p = .17$), log phonological predictability ($\beta = .01$, $p = .93$), or log syllable frequency for the first syllable ($\beta = -.05$, $p = .50$) or the second syllable ($\beta = -.07$, $p = .41$).

In summary, the results of these analyses are clear and consistent. When considering differences in accuracy between English and German speakers using a set of homophonic stimuli, only differences in word frequency are a reliable predictor. There is no evidence for any effect of phonological predictability, number of phonological neighbours, or syllable frequency.

DISCUSSION

The reason for conducting this investigation was to address the question of the linguistic variables that influence the accuracy of output in individuals with acquired output impairment after stroke. Previous investigations into these issues have been hampered by the notorious confoundedness of the predictor variables. However, this unique cross-language study enabled us to investigate both the effects of language-independent variables and those that are more closely tied to the properties of a specific language.

The results in regard to the language-independent variables (i.e., number of syllables, clusters, phonemes) suggest that they can account for about 24% of the output variability of our participants, which leaves a great amount of variance still unexplained. The source of this variability is unclear; it may reflect differences between patients—there was not substantial consistency between participants in the items that they found difficult—or it may reflect day-to-day item variability for individual participants. Our current data do not differentiate these possibilities. Word frequency accounted for a further 3.3% of the variance, and there was a significant—although arguably minimal—effect of phonological predictability (accounting uniquely for just 1.2% of the variance). Utilising the cross-language design we were able to determine which of the language-specific variables could predict differences across languages in response accuracy in a repetition task: word frequency differences had a consistent though small effect, but there was no evidence of any significant effect of differences in phonological predictability, number of phonological neighbours, or syllable frequency. Others have found effects of such variables (e.g., Laganaro, 2005, for syllable frequency; or Gordon, 2002, for neighbourhood density) for people with aphasia. However, unlike this study, these findings did not take into account the effects of the full range of possible confounding variables. For instance, Gordon (2002), in investigating the effects of the number of phonological neighbours, controlled for the number of syllables but not for the effects of the number of phonemes or phonological predictability. Within a syllable length, words with more phonemes have fewer neighbours ("it" has more neighbours than "splint", for example). The effects of number of neighbours that she claims, are more likely—in the light of our results—to be due to the number of phonemes in the target.

The finding that language-independent factors (numbers of phonemes, syllables, and clusters) do influence accuracy patterns, at least on a repetition task such as employed here, is in keeping with Nickels and Howard (2004), who also noted an effect of number of phonemes. Based on this, Nickels and Howard argued that any model of speech production should include a level of phonemes. With regard to the potency of the number of phonemes, the speech production model proposed by Levelt, Roelofs, and Meyer (1999) offers an account for some of our findings. In this model phonemes are selected and placed into metrical frames according to whether they represent an onset, nucleus, or coda within a syllable. In addition, the selected phonemes do not receive feedback from the lexical level. As a consequence, the more phonemes to be placed into the appropriate slots in a frame, the higher the chance of an error.

Given the substantial between-participant variability, the language-independent variables account for a rather high proportion of the variance. That there was, in addition, an effect of language-specific variables affecting response accuracy in our participants was shown by the greater within- than between-language consistency in our participants. However, only one of the language-specific variables, word frequency, was a significant predictor of differences in response accuracy across languages. The significant independent effect was in the expected direction, with more accuracy on higher- than lower-frequency words. This facilitatory effect, which is seen in healthy speakers, can be taken as evidence to support the notion that our participants have an intact or at least partial access to the word form—an intact morphophonological encoding and syllabification process referring to Levelt et al.'s (1999) model.

There were no substantial independent effects of probability, neighbourhood density, or syllable frequency observed. However, this does not fully exclude that they have a role, since word frequency, density, and probabilistic phonotactics are highly correlated with each other. However, our data make it unlikely that the effect of these variables is substantial for many participants. It *may* be the case that there are *some* individual people with acquired output impairments for whom these variables are important independent predictors of accuracy. Previous research (e.g., Aichert & Ziegler, 2004; Gordon, 2002; Levelt & Wheeldon, 1994) has suggested such effects might be found, although in none of these cases has the full range of possible confounds been taken into account. The absence of an effect of the target's phonological neighbourhood density suggests that interaction between lexical phonological representations and output phonological processes, if it occurs, is not a major determinant of response accuracy in our subjects (see Dell & Gordon, 2002). The absence of a significant effect of syllable frequency is in agreement with the results of Nickels and Howard (2004), who did not detect such an effect in their study with individuals with aphasia in a repetition task. This result is in contrast to Levelt et al.'s (1999) model, which predicts a syllable frequency effect on response production based on the inclusion of the so-called syllabary.

The effects of phonological neighbourhood density and phonotactic probability were not significant in this investigation despite a large number of items (509) and a large number of participants (14). Our results suggest that the effects of these variables for people with output impairment are generally small, accounting for a very small proportion of the variance. This does not, of course, preclude the possibility that there are speakers with impaired output for whom these factors are major determinants of accuracy in repetition. Our participants did not constitute a homogeneous group, as evidenced by their low inter-participant consistency in response accuracy—this could have had an impact on observing a significant effect of either phonotactic probability or phonological neighbourhood density on response accuracy. In addition, the severity of the participants' acquired output impairment varied. These factors might offer explanations for the absence of a significant effect of probability and/or neighbourhood density on repetition accuracy.

In conclusion, this study shows that the major determinants of the repetition accuracy of people with output impairment are the number of phonemes and the number of clusters in the target. The effect of other variables is small, although there is strong evidence for an effect of word frequency. There is no evidence for any substantial effect of phonological predictability, neighbourhood density, or syllable frequency when the effects of confounding variables are taken into account.

REFERENCES

Aichert, I., & Ziegler, W. (2004). Syllable frequency and syllable structure in apraxia of speech. *Brain and Language, 88,* 148–159.

Baayen, R. H., Piepenbrock, R., & Gulikers, L. (1995). *The CELEX lexical database (Release 2) [CD-ROM].* Philadelphia, PA: Linguistic Data Consortium, University of Pennsylvania.

Bailey, T. M., & Hahn, U. (2001). Determinants of wordlikeness: Phonotactic or lexical neighbourhoods? *Journal of Memory and Language, 44,* 568–591.

Ballard, K. J., Granier, J. P., & Robin, D. A. (2000). Understanding the nature of apraxia of speech: Theory, analysis, and treatment. *Aphasiology, 14,* 969–995.

Boyczuk, J. P., & Baum, S. R. (1999). The influence of neighborhood density on phonetic categorization in aphasia. *Brain and Language, 67,* 46–70.

Dell, G. S., & Gordon, J. K. (2002). Neighbors in the lexicon: Friends or foes? In N. O. Schiller & A. S. Meyer (Eds.), *Phonetics and phonology in language comprehension and production: Differences and similarities.* New York: Mouton de Gruyter.

Frisch, S. A., Large, N. R., & Pisoni, D. B. (2000). Perception of wordlikeness: Effects of segment probability and length on the processing of nonwords. *Journal of Memory and Language, 42,* 481–496.

Gordon, J. K. (2002). Phonological neighborhood effects in aphasic speech errors: spontaneous and structured contexts. *Brain and Language, 82,* 113–145.

Huber, W., Poeck, K., Weniger, D., & Willmes, K. (1983). *Aachener Aphasie Test (AAT).* Göttingen: Hogrefe.

Laganaro, M. (2005). Syllable frequency effect in speech production: Evidence from aphasia. *Journal of Neurolinguistics, 18,* 221–235.

Levelt, W. J. M., Roelofs, A., & Meyer, A. S. (1999). A theory of lexical access in speech production. *Behavioral and Brain Sciences, 22,* 1–38.

Levelt, W. J. M., & Wheeldon, L. (1994). Do speakers have access to a mental syllabary? *Cognition, 50,* 239–269.

Luce, P. A. (1986). *Neighborhoods of words in the mental lexicon. Research on Speech Perception Progress Report, No. 6.* Speech Research Lab., Psychology Department, Indiana University.

Luce, P. A., & Large, N. R. (2001). Phonotactics, density, and entropy in spoken word recognition. *Language and Cognitive Processes, 16,* 565–581.

Luce, P. A., & Pisoni, D. B. (1998). Recognizing spoken words: The neighbourhood activation model. *Ear and Hearing, 19,* 1–36.

McNeil, M. R. (2001). The assiduous challenge of defining and explaining apraxia of speech. *Proceedings of the 4th International Speech Motor Conference* (pp. 337–342). Nijmegen, The Netherlands: Uitgeverij Vantilt.

McNeil, M. R., Robin, D. A., & Schmidt, R. A. (1997). Apraxia of speech: Definition, differentiation, and treatment. In M. R. McNeil (Ed.), *Clinical management of sensorimotor speech disorders* (pp. 311–344). New York: Thieme.

Miller, N. (2002). The neurological bases of apraxia of speech. *Seminars in Speech and Language, 23,* 223–230.

Miller, N., Willmes, K., & De Bleser, R. (2000). Psychometric properties of the English Aachen Aphasia Test. *Aphasiology, 14,* 683–722.

Munson, B., & Solomon, N. P. (2004). The effect of phonological neighborhood density on vowel articulation. *Journal of Speech, Language, and Hearing Research, 47,* 1048–1058.

Nickels, L. A., & Howard, D. (1995). Aphasic naming: What matters? *Neuropsychologia, 33,* 1281–1303.

Nickels, L. A., & Howard, D. (2004). Dissociating effects of number of phonemes, number of syllables and syllable complexity on word production in aphasia: It's the number of phonemes that counts. *Cognitive Neuropsychology, 21,* 57–78.

Stemberger, J. P. (2004). Apparent anti-frequency effects in language production: The addition bias and phonological underspecification. *Journal of Memory and Language, 30,* 161–185.

Vitevitch, M. S., & Luce, P. A. (1998). When words compete: Levels of processing in spoken word perception. *Psychological Science, 9,* 325–329.

Vitevitch, M. S., & Luce, P. A. (1999). Probabilistic phonotactics and spoken word recognition. *Journal of Memory and Language, 40,* 374–408.

Ziegler, W. (2002). Psycholinguistic and motor theories of apraxia of speech. *Seminars in Speech and Language, 23,* 231–244.

APHASIOLOGY, 2007, 21 (6/7/8), 632–642

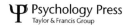

Improved effects of word-retrieval treatments subsequent to addition of the orthographic form

Julie L. Wambaugh

VA Salt Lake City Healthcare System and
University of Utah, Salt Lake City, UT, USA

Sandra Wright

VA Salt Lake City Healthcare System, Salt Lake City, UT, USA

Background: The participant, an individual with moderate–severe Wernicke's aphasia, had not benefited from two word-retrieval cueing treatments in a previous investigation. The participant insisted that her performance would have been improved if the written word had been provided as part of the cueing process.

Aims: The purpose of this investigation was to examine the effects of adding the orthographic form of targeted action names to a semantic cueing treatment (SCT) and a phonologic cueing treatment (PCT).

Methods & Procedures: The participant received SCT and PCT applied to the retrieval of action names. The treatments both provided the written word form paired with the pictured action in conjunction with cueing hierarchies. Two, sequential multiple baseline designs across behaviours were employed to examine the acquisition and response generalisation effects of treatment.

Outcomes & Results: Improved accuracy of action naming was found for both treatments. Gains were limited to trained items; no changes were observed in naming of untrained actions.

Conclusions: It appeared that the participant utilised the orthographic word form to develop associations between the visual object recognition system and the orthographic input lexicon, thus facilitating access to the phonological output lexicon.

This investigation was designed to examine the effects of two word-retrieval cueing treatments that were modified to include provision of the orthographic form of the target action. The modification was made at the suggestion of the participant, who had shown negligible improvements in naming in response to both treatments in a previous investigation (Wambaugh, Nessler, Cameron, & Wright, 2007).

During the course of testing the relative effects of a semantic cueing treatment (SCT) and a phonologic cueing treatment (PCT) (Wambaugh et al., 2007), a participant, MA, insisted that her response to the treatments would be much better if she were provided with the written form of the word. The treatment protocol could

---

Address correspondence to: Julie L. Wambaugh PhD, 151 A Foothill Blvd., Salt Lake City, UT 84148, USA. E-mail: julie.wambaugh@health.utah.edu

This research was supported by Department of Veterans Affairs, Rehabilitation Research and Development.

---

http://www.psypress.com/aphasiology   DOI: 10.1080/02687030701192133

not be adjusted during the course of that investigation to accommodate her request. Following completion of that investigation a decision was made to conduct an indirect replication of the initial investigation, with the interest of potentially improving the effects of treatment by capitalising on MA's insights. Extensive pre-treatment testing prior to this second investigation revealed little evidence to suggest that the addition of the orthographic form would improve performance (see below).

The development and testing of word-retrieval treatments for aphasia has generally focused on approaches that have targeted either the semantic or phonologic levels of processing (Nickels, 2002a). There have been relatively few studies in which orthographic approaches have been studied and positive effects on naming have been reported. Most often, letter to sound correspondences have been trained to facilitate self-cueing (see Nickels, 2002a, for a review), but letter cues alone have also been used (Herbert, Best, Hickin, Howard, & Osborne, 2001). An underlying assumption of such strategies is that knowledge of the written form is relatively intact, which, as noted by Nickels (2002a), may rarely occur. This may account for the limited study of the impact of orthographic stimuli in the treatment of word retrieval.

The present investigation was designed to examine the potential benefits of adding the orthographic form to the treatments that had produced insignificant effects for MA. A series of two experimental designs were implemented to examine the effects of the modified treatments on MA's verbal naming of actions.

METHOD

Participant

The participant, MA, was a 62-year-old female who was 9 years post evacuation of a left temporal haematoma secondary to head injury. She evidenced moderate–severe Wernicke's aphasia, with significant word-retrieval difficulties (Table 1). MA had served as a participant in a prior investigation examining the effects of two treatments for verb retrieval. In that investigation, semantic cueing treatment (SCT) and phonologic cueing treatment (PCT) were each applied to two lists of verbs in the context of a multiple-baseline, crossover design. Table 2 displays a summary of MA's probe performance in response to those treatments. Both treatments resulted in negligible improvement in oral naming of actions. As seen in Table 2, immediately following treatment, MA's naming of trained actions improved by 18–44% across the four lists. These gains were not maintained in follow-up probes.

Pre-treatment assessment results suggested that MA's word-retrieval difficulties stemmed from disruptions in both semantic and phonological levels of processing (Table 1). Although MA insisted that she would benefit from provision of the orthographic form of the target word, there was little evidence to suggest that this would be the case. Specifically, her written word to picture matching performance was poorer than her spoken word to picture matching, her oral reading was severely impaired, and her letter naming and matching skills were significantly disrupted. However, MA performed remarkably well on visual, lexical decision tasks (i.e., deciding if printed letter strings represented words), indicating that her "orthographic input lexicon" (Kay, Lesser, & Coltheart, 1992) was relatively intact.

Table 1
Pre-treatment assessment results

Measure	Score
Test of Adolescent/Adult Word Finding (German, 1990)	
Total Raw Score	0/107
Comprehension	74%
Coloured Progressive Matrices (Raven, Raven & Court, 1998)	
Total Score	33/36
Pyramids & Palm Trees (Howard & Patterson, 1992)	
Total Raw Score	47/52
An Object and Action Naming Battery (Druks & Masterson, 2000)	
Total objects	1/81
Total actions	7/100
Western Aphasia Battery (Kertesz, 1982)	
Aphasia Quotient	32.2
Classification	Wernicke's
Porch Index of Communicative Abilities, 4th Ed. (Porch, 2001)	
Overall Percentile	35th
Psycholinguistic Assessment of Language Processes in Aphasia (Kay et al., 1992)	
Auditory Rep. Gramm. Class	
Nouns	0/15
Verbs	0/15
Adjectives	0/15
Functors	0/15
Lexical Morphology & Rep.	
Regularly inflected	0/15
Derived	0/15
Irregularly inflected	0/15
Regular infl. Control	0/15
Derivational control	1/15
Irregular infl. Control	1/15
Grammatical Class Reading	
Nouns	0/20
Adjectives	0/20
Verbs	0/20
Functors	0/20
Spoken Word–Pic. Matching	27/40
Auditory Synonym Judgements	
Hi Image	20/30
Lo Image	15/30
Word Semantic Association	
Hi Image	4/15
Lo Image	3/15
Aud. Comp. of Verbs & Adj.	
Form 1	26/41
Form 2	22/41
Letter Naming & Sounding	
Lower case letter naming	11/26
Upper case letter naming	12/26

(Continued)

Table 1
(Continued)

Measure	Score
Spoken Letter-Written Letter Matching	12/26
Visual Lexical Decision with "Illegal" Nonwords	
Exception words	12/15
Regular words	14/15
Nonwords	30/30
Imageability & Frequency Visual Lexical Decision	
High imageability/high frequency	12/15
High imageability/low frequency	11/15
Low imageability/high frequency	13/15
Low imageability/low frequency	6/15
Nonwords	46/60
Letter Length Reading	0/24
Syllable Length Reading	
One-syllable	1/8
Two-syllable	0/8
Three-syllable	0/8
Spoken Word–Picture Matching	28/40
Errors ($n = 12$): Close semantic:	10/40
Distant semantic:	0/40
Visual:	0/40
Unrelated:	2/40
Written Word–Picture Matching	18/40
Errors ($n = 22$): Close semantic:	9/40
Distant semantic:	3/40
Visual:	6/40
Unrelated:	4/40
Picture Naming	
Spoken Naming	1/40
Written Naming	0/40
Oral Reading	7/40
Repetition	8/40
Written Spelling	0/40

Experimental design

Two sequential multiple-baseline designs (MBDs) across behaviours were employed
to examine the effects of treatment. In each design, naming of two sets of verbs was
repeatedly measured in a baseline phase. Then one treatment was applied
sequentially to the verb sets. In the first design, a semantic cueing treatment (with
orthographic cues) was applied. In the second design, a phonologic cueing treatment
(with orthographic cues) was applied. Follow-up probes were conducted at 2 and 6
weeks post-treatment.

Table 2
Performance in previous study: Percent correct naming of actions

	Baseline average	End tx.	3 week follow-up	6 week follow-up
List 1 (Semantic Tx.)	13%	47%	30%	20%
List 2 (Phonologic Tx.)	22%	40%	30%	20%
List 3 (Semantic Tx.)	20%	47%	40%	30%
List 4 (Phonologic Tx.)	26%	70%	50%	40%

This investigation was initially designed to explore the effects of adding the orthographic word form to one treatment only (i.e., SCT). When it became apparent that treatment effects were positive, the decision was made to conduct an indirect replication using PCT. Consequently, two sequential MBDs, each with two baselines, were utilised. Although one MBD with four baselines may have offered advantages such as counterbalancing of the treatments, other benefits were gained by conducting the experiments sequentially. For example, the numbers of true baseline sessions were identical across treatments and the numbers of extended baseline sessions were similar (i.e., 23 and 21 for SCT and PCT, respectively; two additional probes were conducted for SCT to ensure behavioural stability). Controlling the number of baseline exposures may be important in word-retrieval investigations for two reasons: (1) repeated exposure may lead to improved naming independent of treatment (Nickels, 2002b), and (2) repeated incorrect, unconsequented naming attempts may cause stimulus items to become resistant to treatment (Wambaugh, Cameron, Kalinyak-Fliszar, Nessler, & Wright, 2004).

Experimental stimuli

Two sets of actions were selected for each design on the basis of performance on *An Object and Action Naming Battery* (OANB; Druks & Masterson, 2000). Specifically, for each list, eight items were named incorrectly and two items were named correctly on the *OANB*. A total of 40 items were selected, with 10 items designated per set (Appendix A). Items had not received treatment in the preceding study. Furthermore, items were selected to allow for balancing for familiarity, number of arguments, homophonous noun roots, and image agreement across the sets of experimental items (Appendix B). For familiarity and image agreement, the normative data from the *OANB* were utilised. For the determination of number of arguments, the verb classifications provided by the *OANB* were used, with adjustments made when classifications appeared to be inaccurate or inappropriate for the picture stimuli—e.g., "sewing" was listed as intransitive (one argument) by the *OANB*, but was classified as a transitive verb (two arguments) for this investigation. The ad hoc addition of the second experimental design to this investigation resulted in an inability to balance argument structure across PCT and SCT sets. That is, argument structure was balanced as closely as possible across lists *within* design, but there were a limited number of *OANB* verbs remaining for selection for the PCT treatment (recall that verbs had been trained in the previous investigation). Consequently, more one-place verbs were employed in the second MBD (PCT treatment).

The stimuli for the previous investigation were selected in a similar manner. In conducting an indirect replication of that study, it was considered important to attempt to equate the stimuli across investigations. The four action lists in that investigation were comparable to the stimuli in the present investigation in terms of familiarity, image agreement, and noun roots. Importantly, argument structure was also similar in that two of the four lists comprised two 1-place verbs and eight 2-place verbs, and the remaining two lists were composed of three 1-place verbs and seven 2-place verbs. All of the selected actions were depicted in black and white line drawings.

Dependent variable

Correct naming of the target actions within 15 seconds of presentation of the line drawing in probes constituted the behaviour of interest. Probes were conducted in which the 20 pictures depicting the actions were presented one at a time, in random order. No written stimuli were provided with the pictures. MA was instructed to "tell me an action word, a verb that tells what's happening". No feedback concerning accuracy of naming was given during probes. All probes were audio recorded.

Probes were scored online by the investigator who administered treatment (SW). Audio recordings were used to verify scoring. A multidimensional scoring system was utilised (Appendix C), with scores following at "7" or higher considered correct. As seen in Appendix C, self-corrections and errors in inflection were not penalised.

Baseline probes were conducted two to three times per week (five in total for each design). Probes conducted during the treatment phase were completed prior to each day's treatment session.

Treatment

The same treatments that were utilised in the previous investigation, SCT and PCT, were studied, with one modification: the written form of the word was printed below the drawings used in treatment. The present progressive form of the verb ("-ing inflected verb, *without* am/is/are) served as the written stimuli (e.g., climbing, flying). MA was *not* asked to read the word aloud, and no attention was drawn to the printed word. Please note that the orthographic form was *not* included on the probe stimuli used to measure treatment effects.

Both treatments included a pre-stimulation phase, wherein MA was asked to choose the target item from a field of four pictures. For SCT, the foils included two semantically related items and one unrelated item (e.g., target = "peeling"; foils = "grating", "squeezing", "diving"). For PCT, the foils included two items beginning with the same sound and one unrelated item (e.g., target = "sitting"; foils = "sailing", "sawing", "marching"). Upon presentation of the four picture choices, the experimenter provided a phrase and asked MA to choose the picture corresponding to the phrase. For SCT, the phrase was a description of the action (e.g., target = "peeling"; description = "to strip off an outer layer"). For PCT, the phrase was a presentation of a nonword rhyme (e.g., target = "sitting"; rhyme = "it rhymes with ditting"). Upon a correct pointing response, the target was then submitted to the corresponding cueing hierarchy. Contingencies were available for provision of an incorrect response in the form of repetition of the phrase followed by a pointing model.

Following pre-stimulation, the cueing hierarchy was applied to the target picture. The target picture was presented with the orthographic word form printed below the picture. As noted above, no attention was drawn to the printed word, and MA was never asked to read the word aloud. The picture and printed word remained in front of MA for all steps of the cueing hierarchies.

Each cueing hierarchy had five levels of cueing, with levels providing progressively "stronger" cues. The application of the levels of the hierarchy was response contingent. That is, the steps were applied sequentially until a correct naming response was provided. Then, the order of the steps was *reversed*, to elicit correct responses at each of the preceding steps. Upon an incorrect response during the hierarchy reversal, the order of hierarchy steps was again reversed until a correct response was produced. Verbal feedback was provided following each naming attempt.

The cueing hierarchy in SCT comprised the following steps: (1) request for verbal naming response upon presentation of the picture and printed word form; (2) provision of a verbal description of the target with a request for naming [target = flying – "to move through the air using wings"]; (3) provision of a semantically non-specific sentence completion phrase with a request for naming [target = flying – "the birds are …"]; (4) provision of a semantically loaded sentence completion phrase with a request for naming [target = flying – " to go south in the winter, the flock of birds is …"]; and (5) verbal model of the target word with a request for repetition.

The cueing hierarchy for PCT consisted of the following steps: (1) request for verbal naming response upon presentation of the picture and printed word forms; (2) provision of a nonword rhyme with a request for naming [target = riding – "it rhymes with piding"]; (3) provision of first sound cue with request for naming [target = riding – "it starts with r …"]; (4) provision of a sentence completion phrase that included the rhyme and the sound cue with a naming response requested [target = riding – "what he's doing rhymes with piding; he is r …"]; (5) verbal model of the target word with a request for repetition.

Each of the 10 pictures was presented individually in random order (one trial), with the pre-stimulation and cueing hierarchy applied to that picture prior to the presentation of the next picture.

A treatment session consisted of four applications of treatment to each picture (four trials). Sessions were conducted three times per week by an ASHA-certified SLP. The criteria for termination of treatment were (1) 90% accuracy of naming on three consecutive probes, or (2) a maximum of 15 treatment sessions.

MA did not participate in any other speech/language treatment during the course of this investigation. The therapist who provided therapy also provided treatment in the previous study.

Reliability

Dependent variable. A total of 25% of all probes sessions were re-scored from audiotapes by an individual who had not conducted the original scoring. Probes for re-scoring were selected randomly from all phases of the study (baseline, treatment, withdrawal). Point-to-point agreement for scoring of correct/incorrect ranged from 95% to 100% for each probe session, with an average of 99% agreement across the 19 re-scored sessions.

Independent variable. Accuracy of application of the steps of treatment was evaluated for eight treatment sessions (14% of treatment sessions; two sessions per treatment application) by an individual who had not administered treatment. The following represents the percentage of trials for which treatment was applied as per the protocol for each of the treatment steps: (1) presentation of pre-stimulation with appropriated feedback = 99.6%; (2) sequential presentation of hierarchy until correct response was obtained = 100%; (3) provision of appropriated feedback after each response = 99%; (4) reversal of hierarchy upon correct response = 100%; (5) reversal of hierarchy upon incorrect response = 100%.

RESULTS

Figures 1 and 2 depict MA's accuracy of naming in probes in response to *SCT + orthographic* and *PCT + orthographic*, respectively. MA demonstrated stable

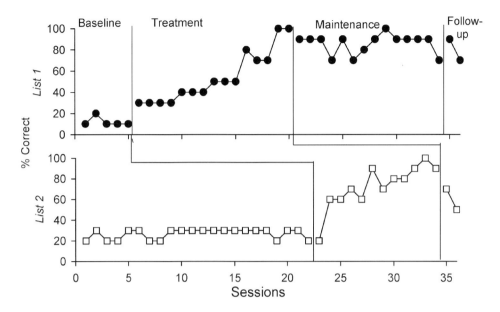

Figure 1. Probe performance is response to SCT+ orthographic

responding prior to the application of treatment for all lists, with correct responding ranging from 10% to 30% accuracy. Obvious improvements in naming were observed following application of treatment to each list of items.

MA's response to both treatments was similar (i.e., there was no apparent treatment preference). She met the performance criterion within 15 sessions for all except the first SCT treatment set (and she reached 100% accuracy over two sessions for that set).

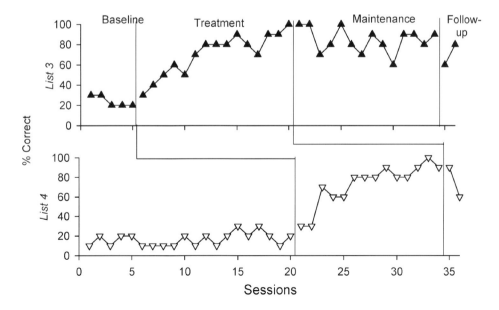

Figure 2. Probe performance is response to PCT+ orthographic

Positive treatment effects were limited to trained items; no generalisation to untrained items was noted for either treatment. Treatment gains were maintained through the withdrawal period, with some decreases observed at 2 and 6 weeks post treatment probes.

DISCUSSION

MA's response to the modified treatments was clearly superior to her response to the original treatments. Unfortunately, it is impossible to determine if order effects might have played a role in the obtained results. That is, the positive effects obtained in these investigations may have been due to the prior application of treatment. However, the previous investigation involved two applications of each treatment, and prior experience with the treatment did not improve results in that investigation.

MA's response to inclusion of the written form was enthusiastic, which is not surprising considering that this treatment modification was her idea. As reported previously, MA was not asked to read the written words aloud, and no attention was drawn to the written words. Consequently, MA's utilisation of the printed form could not be verified. However, it was noted that MA frequently attempted to read aloud letters of the printed words in treatment, although she was often incorrect in those self-initiated attempts. Interestingly, MA is currently participating in another investigation and repeatedly requests provision of the written word form.

If the provision of the orthographic form was responsible for the improved naming performance, it is likely that the improvements were mediated by associations formed between the visual object recognition system and the orthographic input lexicon, with the phonological output lexicon being accessed through the orthographic input lexicon. During probes, the orthographic form was not available, suggesting that MA was able to recall the orthographic form upon picture presentation (allowing access to the phonological output lexicon).

Although the preceding explanation would appear to be the most parsimonious with observed results, it is possible that treatment served to indirectly strengthen connections in the direct naming route. Conceivably, direct route processing was attempted simultaneously with orthographic processing, and the success achieved provided an error-reduced environment conducive to facilitation of direct route processing.

It could also be argued that correct activation of the phonological form via the orthographic output lexicon may have strengthened weak direct route connections through bidirectional processing mechanisms (Dell, Schwartz, Martin, Saffran, & Gagnon, 1997). However, provision of the phonological form occurred with both treatments in the previous investigation with little impact.

Regardless of which route was potentially strengthened, the impact was obviously item specific. That is, there was no general improvement in word retrieval as evidenced by the lack of generalisation to untrained items. This was consistent with the observation that MA's only strength with respect to orthographic stimuli was her ability to recognise real from non-real words. That is, utilisation of this treatment approach as a strategy for generalised naming of untrained items would necessitate *recall* of the orthographic form of those untrained items, and MA's abilities were limited to *recognition.* As hypothesised above, treatment had likely promoted recall for the trained items.

Two additional explanations may account for MA's improved naming performance in this study. It may simply be the case that more is better—additional stimulation in any form may have resulted in gains in naming. Alternatively, the addition of the orthographic word form at MA's suggestion may have had a placebo effect—MA was so insistent that she would benefit from the written word that gains were likely.

Regardless of the mechanism(s) for change, this investigation highlights the benefit of being responsive to the insights of individuals receiving treatment for aphasia. Additionally, the findings suggest that even limited residual orthographic processing skills may be capitalised upon to facilitate improved word-retrieval.

REFERENCES

Dell, G. S., Schwartz, M. F., Martin, N., Saffran, E. M., & Gagnon, D. A. (1997). Lexical access in aphasic and non aphasic speakers. *Psychological Review, 104*, 801–838.

Druks, J., & Masterson, J. (2000). *An object & action naming battery*. Philadelphia: Taylor & Francis.

German, D. (1990). *Test of adolescent/adult word finding*. Allen, TX: DLM.

Herbert, R., Best, W., Hickin, J., Howard, D., & Osborne, F. (2001). Phonological and orthographic approaches to the treatment of word retrieval in aphasia. *International Journal of Language and Communication Disorders, 36*, 7–12.

Howard, D., & Patterson, K. (1992). *The Pyramids and Palm Trees Test*. Bury St Edmunds, UK: Thames Valley Test Company.

Kay, J., Lesser, R., & Coltheart, M. (1992). *Psycholinguistic assessment of language processes in aphasia (PALPA)*. Hove, UK: Lawrence Erlbaum Associates Ltd.

Kertesz, A. (1982). *The Western aphasia battery*. New York: Grune & Stratton.

Nickels, L. (2002a). Therapy for naming disorders: Revisiting, revising, and reviewing. *Aphasiology, 16*(10/11), 935–979.

Nickels, L. (2002b). Improving word finding: Practice makes (closer to) perfect? *Aphasiology, 16*(10/11), 1047–1060.

Porch, B. (2001). *Porch index of communicative ability [Vol. 2]. Administration, scoring, and interpretation*. (4th ed.). Albuquerque, NM: PICA Programs.

Raven, J., Raven, J. C., & Court, J. H. (1998). *Coloured progressive matrices*. Oxford, UK: Oxford Psychologists Press, Ltd.

Wambaugh, J. L., Cameron, R., Kalinyak-Fliszar, M., Nessler, C., & Wright, S. (2004). Retrieval of action names in aphasia: Effects of two cueing treatments. *Aphasiology, 18*(11), 979–1004.

Wambaugh, J. L., Nessler, C., Cameron, R., & Wright, S. (2007). *Effects of cueing treatments on action naming in fluent and non fluent aphasia*. Manuscript in preparation.

APPENDIX A

Experimental stimuli: Verb lists

Semantic treatment		Phonologic treatment	
List 1	*List 2*	*List 1*	*List 2*
climbing	catching	bleeding	blowing
flying	dancing	dripping	diving
folding	drawing	pointing	licking
lighting	jumping	raining	pouring
peeling	melting	running	praying
shaving	playing	sewing	pulling
tying	pushing	tickling	snowing
waving	typing	yawning	watching
driving	reading	riding	ironing
eating	walking	sitting	sleeping

APPENDIX B

Balancing of verb lists

List	Number of verbs by argument structure	Familiarity (average)	Homophonous noun root	Image agreement (average)
Semantic treatment				
List 1	1 place – 1	4.55	10/10	4.36
	2 place – 9			
	3 place – 0			
List 2	1 place – 2	4.53	9/10	4.38
	2 place – 8			
	3 place – 0			
Phonologic treatment				
List 1	1 place – 5	4.31	8/10	4.43
	2 place – 5			
	3 place – 0			
List 2	1 place – 4	4.29	8/10	4.24
	2 place – 5			
	3 place – 1			

APPENDIX C

Multidimensional scoring system: Verbs

Score	Description
9	Accurate, immediate ($<$ 5 seconds)
8	Accurate, delayed ($>$ 5 and $<$ 15 seconds)
7.5	Correct verb root, uninflected or incorrectly inflected
7	Self-corrected
6A	Phonemic paraphasia (single phoneme substitution)
6B	Phonemic paraphasia (recognisable word with more than one sound substitution; at least 50% of phonemes correct, excluding inflection)
5.5	Partial retrieval (word embedded in more complex form)
5	Noun for verb semantic paraphasia
4.5	Semantic paraphasia containing phonemic paraphasia
4	Appropriate gestural or written response
3	Circumlocution
2.5	Tangential speech
2	Neologism or unintelligible word
1	Perseveration
0	No response or "I don't know"

APHASIOLOGY, 2007, 21 (6/7/8), 643–657

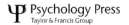

A contextual approach to facilitating word retrieval in agrammatic aphasia

Jean K. Gordon

University of Iowa, Iowa City, IA, USA

Background: Although virtually all individuals with aphasia demonstrate problems with word retrieval, this symptom might arise for different reasons in individuals with different types of aphasia. A trade-off of dependence on semantic and syntactic information is hypothesised to underlie dissociations in word retrieval shown by fluent anomic and non-fluent agrammatic speakers. This division of labour predicts that strengthening semantic input will improve word retrieval for those with anomic aphasia, whereas strengthening syntactic input through contextual cues will improve word retrieval for those with agrammatic aphasia.
Aims: To explore the outcome of a new treatment approach that proposes to improve word retrieval in individuals with agrammatic aphasia by implicitly strengthening the links between target words and associated words which co-occur in a connected speech context.
Methods & Procedures: The outcomes of two therapy approaches were examined in two participants with agrammatic aphasia. One therapy approach focused on explicitly training semantic features of target words; the other, more novel, approach focused on implicitly strengthening contextual associations through story telling and retelling. It was predicted that the latter approach would result in greater benefits for the two agrammatic participants.
Outcomes & Results: Although both therapy approaches appeared to be effective, the predicted advantage of the contextually based approach was not found. The evolution of the error patterns throughout the treatment was examined to help understand the mechanisms underlying the improvements shown for each participant.
Conclusions: A novel treatment involving training words in a story context was shown to result in improved word retrieval for two participants with agrammatic aphasia. The merits of the approach are discussed, relative to more traditional explicit word retrieval therapy approaches.

Although all individuals with aphasia have difficulty retrieving words, patterns of lexical access impairment vary in different types of aphasia. The ease with which words are retrieved depends on many factors, including characteristics of the words themselves and the eliciting stimuli, and characteristics of the speaker's aphasia

Address correspondence to: Jean K. Gordon, 125 B, WJSHC, 250 Hawkins Drive, University of Iowa, Iowa City, IA 52242, USA. E-mail: jean-k-gordon@uiowa.edu

I would like to thank the two participants in this study for their patience and perseverance. Several students helped with the collection and analysis of data, particularly (in chronological order) Rebekah Abel, Michelle Bullock, Ellen Marschner, Becky Bartlett, and Anna Happ. Finally, I would like to express my gratitude to ASHA's special interest Division 2 for the financial and moral support provided to carry out this study.

DOI: 10.1080/02687030701192141

profile. One factor that is receiving an increasing amount of attention is the context in which words are retrieved. It has been noted that people with non-fluent aphasia have more difficulty retrieving the same words in connected speech than in naming tasks, whereas those with fluent aphasia often show the opposite pattern (e.g., Pashek & Tompkins, 2002; Schwartz & Hodgson, 2002; Williams & Canter, 1982). This dissociation can be explained by a difference in the underlying impairment that gives rise to word retrieval difficulties in non-fluent and fluent aphasia. One explanation is that word retrieval in naming relies primarily on input from the semantic features of the target word, and that this semantic input is disrupted in fluent (particularly anomic) aphasia; by contrast, word retrieval in connected speech relies more heavily on input from syntactic-sequential cues—that is, the syntactic requirements of the sentence frame, and word association cues from the context— and this input is hypothesised to be disrupted in non-fluent (particularly agrammatic) aphasia.

The theory that types of aphasia dissociate along semantic–syntactic dimensions dates back at least as far as Jakobson's (1971) dichotomy between "similarity" and "contiguity" disorders. A similarity disorder affects the ability of the speaker to select an appropriate word in isolation, while cues from the context of connected speech facilitate production: "The more his utterances are dependent on the context, the better he copes with his verbal task" (Jakobson, 1971, p. 78). With a contiguity disorder, the ability to conjoin words in a syntactic context is impaired, such that "the less a word depends grammatically on the context, the stronger its tenacity" (Jakobson, 1971, p. 86). This trade-off in the importance of context can account for a number of observed dissociations between fluent and non-fluent aphasias. In contrast to people with anomic aphasia (a similarity disorder), speakers with agrammatism (a contiguity disorder) tend to produce more content words than function words, since function words play a primarily syntactic role (Goodglass, Kaplan, & Barresi, 2001a). Others (e.g., Bird, Franklin, & Howard, 2002) have noted that this grammatical class dissociation is not absolute, and attribute the paucity of function words to their lack of semantic richness.

Dissociations within the class of content words have also been hypothesised to arise from differences in semantic or syntactic complexity. Much research has shown that verbs are more difficult to produce than nouns for many with aphasia, but particularly those with agrammatism (e.g., Bastiaanse & Jonkers, 1998; Miceli, Silveri, Villa, & Caramazza, 1984; Zingeser & Berndt, 1990; see Druks, 2002, for a review). Kim and colleagues found that syntactic complexity impairs verb retrieval in non-fluent aphasia (Kim & Thompson, 2004). Breedin, Saffran, and Schwartz (1998), on the other hand, found that verbs that were more semantically rich were easier to produce for three of their four participants with agrammatism, while semantically simple verbs were easier to produce for both of their participants with anomia. This semantic dimension, sometimes called semantic complexity or "heaviness", is generally defined by the number of semantic features that specify the word. For example, the verb *go*, a so-called "light" verb, may be specified by the feature of motion, whereas the heavy verbs *run* and *fly* specify motion as well as the manner of motion and the agents that can carry out that particular manner of motion. The heavy verb advantage in agrammatism found by Breedin and colleagues was recently replicated in a larger study comparing 12 participants with agrammatic aphasia to 11 with non-agrammatic aphasia (Barde, Schwartz, & Boronat, 2006).

To help explain these contrasts, it has been hypothesised that there is a continuum of dependence of lexical production on syntax and semantics, with words like determiners at one end (almost purely syntactic), concrete nouns and heavy verbs at the other (almost purely semantic), and light verbs at an intermediate point. Gordon and Dell (2003) constructed a connectionist model to simulate this trade-off, or division of labour, between syntactic and semantic information. Using as its input a set of semantic and syntactic features corresponding to sentence-level messages, the model learned to produce sentences containing either heavy verbs or light verbs. In the course of training, the model learned to rely primarily on semantic features to predict the heavy verbs and nouns in the sentence, but on syntactic input to predict light verbs and function words. Thus, when either semantic or syntactic input was eliminated, simulating anomia and agrammatism respectively, the model's sentence production was remarkably similar to the behaviour of speakers with the corresponding aphasia syndrome, showing a heavy-verb advantage with syntactic lesions, and a light-verb advantage with semantic lesions. A naming task was then simulated by providing the trained model only with input relevant to a single word. When lesioned, the naming model again showed a double dissociation between heavy and light verbs. A task dissociation was also observed, whereby the syntactically lesioned model retrieved words significantly more accurately in naming than in sentence production, a finding that also replicates behavioural results, as described above.

In addition to clarifying the nature of the impairments underlying aphasic deficits, the concept that a given task is accomplished by dividing the labour between alternate sources of information also provides some direction for therapy. The hypothesis that anomic aphasia arises from reduced input from a word's semantic features supports therapeutic efforts that focus on the strengthening of semantic interconnections (e.g., Boyle & Coelho, 1995). By analogy, a therapy designed to strengthen a word's syntactic-sequential cues should improve the ability of agrammatic speakers to retrieve words. These syntactic-sequential cues come from the syntactic context in which the word is presented; henceforth they will be referred to as "contextual".

To test these hypotheses, the current study compares the outcomes of two therapy approaches on lexical access deficits in agrammatic aphasia. It is proposed that a treatment approach that strengthens the relationships among words in context should improve lexical access in agrammatic speakers more than a treatment approach designed to strengthen only the semantic relationships of a target word. (Similarly, the word retrieval impairment in anomic aphasia should be ameliorated more by focusing on the weakened semantic input than on syntactic-sequential cues, although this hypothesis remains to be addressed in a future study.) Whereas strengthening semantic input is expected to generalise to untreated items in the same semantic categories, strengthening contextual input is expected to generalise to improved retrieval of treated items in connected speech tasks.

THERAPY PROTOCOL

Participants

In this Phase I therapy study, response to the two therapy approaches was tested consecutively in two participants with agrammatic Broca's aphasia, diagnosed using the Boston Diagnostic Aphasia Exam (BDAE, Goodglass, Kaplan, & Barresi, 2001b). Agrammatism was identified according to characteristics described by Goodglass and colleagues: a paucity of inflectional markers and function words relative to content words, simplified syntactic structures, and the "loss of indicators or relations between words" (Goodglass et al., 2001a, p. 9). Demographic information about the two participants is provided in Table 1.

The first participant (Ag1) is a young woman who was 18 years old at the time of the study. She had suffered a left hemisphere CVA a little over a year prior to the onset of the study, resulting in moderately severe Broca's aphasia. Her output consisted primarily of single words and short automatic phrases. Following is a sample of her connected speech, a description of the Cookie Theft picture:

> Drink. All o– [gestures]. Uh-oh. Stair, uh-oh. Down. Cookie. Yeah, this, yes. Um, yes. This, ok. Whoa! [gestures falling] Mom. Cookie. "Oh well". All done. Well, no, but here. Slippin', slippin', water slippin'. Oh-oh. Cookie both. Cookie there. Mom. Cootie, budder and sisser.

Features of agrammatism are evident in elliptical utterances such as "Cookie both", in the lack of inflectional morphemes and function words, and in the relative preponderance of nouns compared to verbs. Symptoms of word retrieval problems include semantic and phonological paraphasias ("stair" for "stool", "slipping" for

TABLE 1
Participant information

Demographics	Participant 1 (Ag1)		Participant 2 (Ag2)	
Gender	Female		Male	
Age	18 years		44.5 years	
Education	10 years		13 years	
Aetiology	large left MCA stroke		left fronto-temporo-parietal head injury	
TPO	14 months		9 years, 2 months	
Diagnosis	Broca's aphasia		Broca's aphasia with apraxia of speech	
BDAE severity	1–2 (moderate-to-severe)		3 (moderate)	
BDAE Subtest	Pre-Test	Post-Test	Pre-Test	Post-Test
AC-Word Discrimination	28/37 76 %	35/37 95 %	32/37 86 %	33/37 89 %
AC-Complex Ideational Material	7/12 58 %	8/12 67 %	11/12 92 %	12/12 100 %
AC-Syntactic Processing	16/32 50 %	15/32 47 %	14/32 44 %	19/32 59 %
Verbal Agility	5/14 36 %	9/14 64 %	2/14 14 %	3/14 21 %
Word Repetition	5/10 50 %	6/10 60 %	3/10 30 %	3/10 30 %
Sentence Repetition	0/10 0 %	0/10 0 %	0/10 0 %	0/10 0 %
Responsive Naming	9/20 45 %	11/20 55 %	11/20 55 %	11/20 55 %
Written Word-Picture Matching	10/10 100 %	8/10 80 %	9/10 90 %	8/10 80 %
RC-Sentences & Paragraphs	5/10 50 %	4/10 40 %	7/10 70 %	8/10 80 %
Mechanics of Writing-	18/27 67 %	22/27 81 %	19/27 70 %	22/27 81 %
Letter Choice	NA NA	NA NA	3/12 25 %	2/12 17 %
Written Naming of Pictures				

"overflowing", "cootie" for "cookie"), and in the substitution of sound effects and gestures for words.

Participant 2 (Ag2) sustained a left fronto-temporo-parietal brain injury 9 years prior to the onset of the study. At the time of the study, he displayed moderate Broca's aphasia characterised by agrammatic expression and apraxia of speech. The following Cookie Theft picture description illustrates his tendency to circumlocute in the face of word retrieval difficulties, as well as his frequent omission of grammatical morphemes.

> Well looks like mom and sisters and brothers and all ... Like, you cook there um ... It like you go there and cook there. ... People, though, there um, look like mom, she too much, eat too much pill; she high! No, sorry ... And, like, water all there. Her, um, daughter or son, all worry, but she don't care. She don't, so so she um ... Mom, she um [gestures] try ... Oh, water here, but water fall. It full, too much full, okay and um ... Her sisters, too much sweet stuff, mom. Brother's okay. She wants there, but he he not think. He's um, he fall too. He fall.

Although verbs are relatively more frequent in Ag2's than in Ag1's speech, some verb omission is noted (e.g., "water all there", "It full"), while pronouns and empty words (e.g., "stuff") frequently substitute for nouns. Gestures are also common in Ag2's expression.

Pre- and post-testing

The Boston Diagnostic Aphasia Examination (Goodglass et al., 2001b) and a story-retelling task were conducted before and after the treatment phase, in order to obtain a descriptive profile of language skills for each participant, and an index of general improvement over the therapy treatment period. Performance on representative BDAE subtests is illustrated in Table 1 for both participants. Ag1 obtained lower auditory and reading comprehension scores for sentences and paragraphs than Ag2, although both were significantly impaired in processing syntactically complex sentences. On the other hand, Ag1 showed better performance than Ag2 on tests highlighting articulatory skill (verbal agility and word repetition). Despite these differences, the two participants were remarkably similar on tests of single-word processing, both receptively (word discrimination) and expressively (responsive naming).

Following an established protocol used by several authors (e.g., Saffran, Berndt, & Schwartz, 1989), the story-retelling task involved the participants being told the Cinderella story using a picture book with no words, then retelling the story with the aid of the picture book but no other cueing. This task was used to supplement the sample of spontaneous speech elicited with the Cookie Theft picture, because it has been suggested that story retelling may elicit more natural and coherent samples of discourse than do descriptions of single pictures (e.g., Olness, 2006; Saffran et al., 1989). The proportion of content words (nouns, verbs, and adjectives) relative to total words was measured on this task as an index of word retrieval ability.

Baseline naming

Before beginning treatment, a baseline phase was conducted in order to establish the stability of word retrieval ability in the two participants. Each session began with a

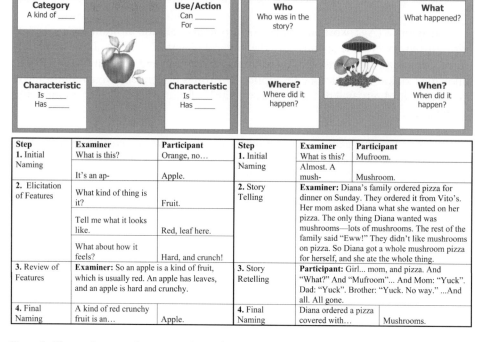

Figure 1. Therapy layout and sequence of steps for sample items in Semantic (left) and Contextual (right) treatment approaches.

naming test that included black and white line drawings from three sources: the Object and Action Naming Test (O&A, Druks & Masterson, 2000), the Philadelphia Naming Test (PNT, Roach, Schwartz, Martin, Grewal, & Brecher, 1996), and the Snodgrass and Vanderwart-like (S&V) picture set (Rossion & Pourtois, 2004). In total, there were 124 nouns and 20 verbs, which were divided evenly among the baseline testing sessions. Although baseline measures of naming are typically gathered from the experimental set of items, the decision was made here to use a separate set of items, to avoid the likelihood that repeated exposure to and attempts to name the items during the baseline phase would influence performance during the treatment phase.

Therapy conditions

The Semantic Treatment condition, similar to Semantic Feature Analysis (e.g., Boyle & Coelho, 1995), explicitly focused on strengthening the associations between a target word and its prototypical semantic characteristics. Participants first named a colour drawing of the target word, then described some of its characteristics, prompted by written cues (see sample in Figure 1) or cues from the clinician. Once elicited, these features were reviewed aloud by the clinician, and the participant was asked to name the picture again, using the elicited features as a sentence completion cue. Figure 1 is an example of the progression through these steps for the illustrated item. In the Contextual Treatment condition, a similar protocol was followed but, instead of describing the item's semantic features, participants listened to a story about the target word, then attempted to retell the story, with cueing as required from the clinician. Listening to the story, then retelling the story, which involves generating the target words in a realistic syntactic context, were hypothesised to implicitly strengthen the target word's syntactic and semantic associations with other words in the story. (Note that targets may also be produced in context in the Semantic Treatment, e.g., "An apple is a kind of fruit". However, the production of targets is not *encouraged* as it is by the Contextual Treatment, and the context itself is hypothesised to be less representative of everyday language use.) An example of the stimuli and the sequence of steps for one item are shown in Figure 1.

Aside from the critical difference of focusing on explicit semantic features in one and implicit contextual associations in the other, the two treatments were designed to be as similar as possible. Both began with a confrontation-naming trial and ended with a sentence completion cued response. During the intermediate steps, every attempt was made to equate the number of times the target was presented across the two conditions. In the Contextual stories, each target appeared four times, and the clinician aimed to produce the Semantic targets four times each during the review of features. Treatment occurred twice weekly, and both treatments were administered in each session, their order counterbalanced.

Stimulus characteristics

A complete list of the stimuli is provided in the Appendix. Each therapy condition included 50 words, divided into five semantic categories with 10 exemplars in each category. The categories in the Semantic Treatment were different from the categories in the Contextual Treatment, to minimise the potential for generalisation across treatment conditions, but were balanced by semantic characteristics across the two conditions (e.g., one treatment condition contained a set of fruit, the other a set of vegetables). In addition, the stimuli in the two conditions were matched on frequency of occurrence and length. In each condition, a subset of the items were treated and the rest were untreated, to provide a test of within-category generalisation. Each treated item appeared six times throughout the therapy phase.

Treatment probes

All 100 items were probed in a confrontation-naming format at the beginning, halfway point, and end of the treatment period. During the probes, each item was presented in isolation; no cues or feedback were provided by the examiner. Maintenance of treatment effects was assessed by administering another probe at least 6 weeks after the end of the therapy phase. Performance on these probes, which were videotaped, provided the primary data assessing the hypotheses. Following the protocol of the PNT (Roach et al., 1996), the accuracy of the first complete response (not counting word fragments) and the final response (from repeated attempts or self-corrections) were recorded. Outcome measures were based on the accuracy of either the initial or final response; that is, whether the participant produced a correct response at any point during a given trial. First complete responses were also coded as either correct (including synonymous variations of the target and phonetic distortions); semantic paraphasias; phonological paraphasias (defined as sharing at least two phonemes with the target, or one phoneme in the same position); mixed errors (semantically and phonologically related); unrelated errors; and other responses (circumlocutions, visual errors, and no responses).

Accuracy in the probe sessions was scored by the clinician on-line and double-checked later against the videotape. The reliability of scoring was determined by having a second rater transcribe all responses from the video recordings, identify the first complete response, and score its accuracy. The inter-rater reliability of these two scores was 97% for Ag1 and 98% for Ag2. The second rater also coded the error types of the first responses. Reliability of the error coding, determined by a third rater scoring a randomly chosen 20% of the responses from each probe session, was 82% for Ag1 and 89% for Ag2.

It was hypothesised that both of the participants might benefit from the Semantic Treatment, since Coelho and colleagues have shown beneficial effects of SFA for non-fluent aphasic subjects (Boyle & Coelho, 1995; Conley & Coelho, 2003). The Contextual Treatment, however, was predicted to facilitate *greater* gains in the retrieval of treated items than the Semantic Treatment, to the extent that it directly addresses the root of the word retrieval impairment in agrammatic aphasia; that is, by strengthening the associations between target words and the other words with which they co-occur. Participants were also expected to show generalisation of these benefits to untreated items in the same semantic categories (see Conley & Coelho, 2003), through their shared semantic features. However, improvement—if achieved—was not expected to generalise to connected speech tasks. For contextually treated items, generalisation was not expected to untreated items within the same semantic categories, since semantic features were not explicitly trained, but this treatment was expected to facilitate the retrieval of content words in connected speech. This was assessed by analysing the retrieval of content words in picture description and story-retelling tasks.

AG1: PROCEDURE AND RESULTS

Ag1 was treated on 8 items in each semantic category, for a total of 40 treated items in each of the Semantic and Contextual conditions, leaving 10 untreated in each condition (2 in each semantic category). *T*-tests demonstrated that items in the two conditions did not differ significantly in lemma frequency (Francis & Kučera, 1982) ($p = .80$), or in number of syllables ($p = .66$). Within each condition, treated items were not significantly different from untreated items, either in frequency ($p = .97$ for semantic items; $p = .58$ for contextual items) or in length ($p = .24$ for semantic items; $p = .31$ for contextual items).

Baseline naming ability, assessed in three sessions over 3 weeks, showed accuracy scores of 23%, 32%, and 22%, respectively. Although this demonstrates some fluctuation over the three sessions, no systematic improvement was shown. The therapy phase involved a total of 17 sessions including probes, and lasted 12½ weeks.

Accuracy of naming from each probe session is presented in Figure 2 (top graph). During the initial probe, Ag1 was able to name 45% of Semantic items and 38% of Contextual items. By the end of treatment, her naming had improved to 68% for the Semantically Treated items and 55% for the Contextually Treated items. These gains dropped slightly, to 65% and 53% respectively, by the maintenance probe 2 months later. Untreated items in the Semantic condition also improved from baseline (20% to 50%), but untreated items in the Contextual condition did not (50% initial, 40% final), as predicted. Clearly, however, the reliability of the generalisation effects is

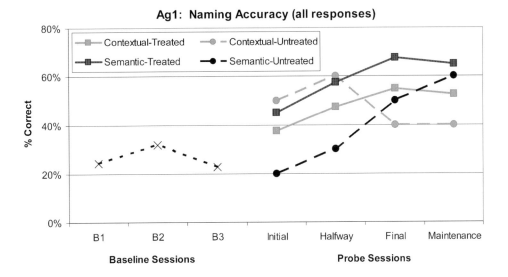

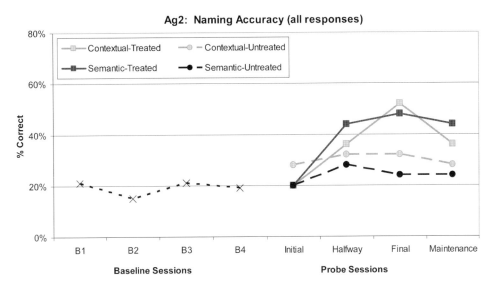

Figure 2. Naming performance of Ag1 and Ag 2 across stimulus sets.

limited by the fact that there were only 10 items in each set. In connected speech tasks (Cookie Theft picture description, Cinderella story retelling), Ag1 did not show the expected improvement in production of content words: the proportions of content words produced were 61% in pre-testing and 56% in post-testing for picture description, and 37% and 40%, respectively, for story telling. This may be due to the fact that the content words required for these tasks were not the same ones trained. Improvements in post-testing were noted in spoken word recognition (20th to 60th percentile); verbal agility (20th to 50th percentile); and a slight improvement in responsive naming (30th to 35th percentile), changes that might be expected to have generalised from either treatment.

By visual inspection of the data, both treatment approaches appeared to be effective for Ag1, as predicted. However, contrary to expectations, the Semantic Treatment resulted in an outcome as beneficial as the Contextual Treatment. It was encouraging to find that word retrieval was facilitated by the previously untested Contextual Treatment. However, confidence in these results is limited by having so few items in the untreated conditions, and by the lack of a connected speech task containing treated words.

AG2: PROCEDURE AND RESULTS

With Ag2, shortcomings in the original protocol were addressed to increase the reliability of the generalisation effects. The main protocol change was to increase the number of untreated items, allowing a more reliable assessment of generalisation. The same 100 items were used for Ag2, but only 5 items in each semantic category were treated, leaving 5 untreated. In total, then, there were 25 treated items and 25 untreated items in each condition. As with Ag1, these sets were balanced for frequency and length: items in the Semantic condition were not significantly different from those in the Contextual condition on either lemma frequency ($p = .50$) or length ($p = .49$); within each set, treated items were not significantly different from untreated items in terms of their frequency (Semantic: $p = .56$; Contextual: $p = .80$) or length (Semantic: $p = .89$; Contextual: $p = .63$).

In addition, a new task was added to the pre- and post-testing battery to enable direct testing of the hypothesis that improved naming of words treated in the Contextual condition would generalise to improved retrieval of those words in a spontaneous speech task. A set of five composite pictures was developed, each of which showed a scene with four naming targets embedded. Of the 20 items included, 10 were from the semantically treated set, and 10 from the contextually treated set (identified in the Appendix). The items selected from each set were not significantly different in frequency ($p = .31$) or length ($p = .41$). Ag2 was simply asked to describe these pictures at pre- and post-test; his attention was not drawn to the targeted items (although they were no doubt more salient following the treatment phase).

The baseline schedule was also altered slightly for Ag2. Tasks were conducted in four sessions spread over 2 weeks. Accuracy of naming across the four baseline sessions was 21%, 15%, 21%, and 19% respectively, demonstrating stability of word retrieval ability. For Ag2, the treatment took 15 sessions (counting probe sessions), and lasted for 8 weeks.

Naming accuracy of items in each treatment condition across the probe sessions are presented in the bottom graph in Figure 2. In the initial probe, Ag2's performance was fairly consistent across the sets of items, providing a more controlled comparison of change. Both the Semantic and Contextual Treatment items were named at 20% accuracy initially. In the final probe session, naming of Semantic Treatment items had improved to 52%, and Contextual Treatment items to 48%. By the maintenance probe 6 weeks later, these gains had dropped considerably for the Contextually treated items (36%), although improvement on the Semantically treated items was fairly well maintained (44%). Untreated sets, on the other hand, improved minimally—from 20% initially to 24% on the final probe for the Semantic control items, and from 28% to 32% for the Contextual control items. Although expected for the Contextual condition, the lack of significant generalisation from treated to untreated items was contrary to predictions for the Semantic condition.

In the Contextual condition, improvement was expected to generalise to the retrieval of treated items in spontaneous speech, as assessed in the composite picture descriptions. An improvement was noted in the number of Contextually treated targets attempted in this task, from 40% in pre-testing to 90% in post-testing, but the accuracy of the target attempts improved only marginally, from 20% to 30% (i.e., one more target was produced correctly). Semantically treated targets also showed minimal improvement in the composite picture description task: target attempts improved from 70% to 90%; target accuracy improved from 20% to 40%. Thus, the expected advantage for Contextually treated items in this task was not shown, except perhaps in increasing their salience, resulting in a greater increase in Contextual targets attempted. Again, the reliability of these results is limited by the small number of items in the generalisation set.

DISCUSSION

For both participants, improvement in word retrieval ability was shown across the therapy phase for both sets of treated items. In the Semantic Treatment condition, the expected generalisation to untreated items in the same semantic categories was shown for only one of the two participants (Ag1). In the Contextual Treatment condition, generalisation to semantically related items was not shown for either participant, as hypothesised. Generalisation of treated items across contexts was only assessed for one of the participants (Ag2) through the composite picture description task. Retrieval of the target words in this context showed minimal improvement in both therapy conditions, contrary to predictions. However, Ag2's pattern of performance in the composite picture description task did show some similarity to the naming task: more target-related attempts were noted in both tasks following therapy, which might represent sub-clinical improvements, i.e., improvements not yet consolidated enough to show up in the accuracy measures. These conclusions remain speculative, however, given the small number of items in the generalisation conditions.

Although the improved retrieval of contextually treated items was predicted, results did not show the predicted advantage for these items over the semantically treated items. There are several possible reasons for such an outcome. One is that the words treated in the current study did not vary sufficiently in their relative reliance on semantic and syntactic input, with the result that significant differential effects of the two therapy approaches could not be obtained. In this study, only nouns were treated, on the assumption that their retrieval relies on a variable combination of semantic and syntactic input. However, this assumption was based on previous research showing a division of labour between semantic and syntactic cues for verbs (Barde et al., 2006; Breedin et al., 1998; Gordon & Dell, 2003). Showing differences between the two treatments might require the use of other types of words, such as verbs, which vary more on the extent to which they rely on semantic and syntactic input. Another possibility, suggested by a reviewer, is that administering both treatments in the same session might have caused some cross-contamination, and administering them consecutively might have helped to separate their effects.

The lack of differences between the two therapy approaches might also call into question either the hypothesised deficit underlying word retrieval impairments in agrammatic aphasia, or the hypothesised mechanisms of the two therapy approaches. It may be, for example, that the outcomes of both treatments rely on the same mechanism, such as the repetition of the target word during treatment, or the strengthening of semantic-associational cues provided by both treatments. One way to explore the hypothesised mechanism of the therapy is to examine the evolution of the participants' error patterns throughout the course of the treatment. If improved retrieval of treated items is related to their repeated production in response to the pictures, it can be supposed that this effect occurs through strengthening the connections between an item's semantic representation and its phonological label. If this were the case, one might expect an increase in phonologically related errors, relative to unrelated errors, as the links are being strengthened. On the other hand, if the semantic-associational cues among related words retrieved explicitly during the Semantic Treatment and implicitly during story telling in the Contextual Treatment are being strengthened, one might expect an increase in the proportions of semantically related errors or circumlocutions (categorised in the "other" category).

Figure 3 shows the evolution of error patterns for Ag1 (top graph) and Ag2 (bottom graph) throughout the probe sessions. For Ag1, the proportion of semantic errors initially increased, perhaps due to interference from semantically related items elicited during the Semantic Treatment, then fell back to the initial level. Increases in correct responses ultimately appear to have resulted from declines in phonological, mixed, and unrelated errors. For Ag1, then, the treatment appears to have improved the phonological proximity of the errors to their targets—from unrelated to related, or from related to correct. Ag2 showed an increase in the proportion of phonological errors throughout treatment, even as accuracy increased. Semantic errors decreased modestly, but the largest reduction was in "other" responses. These consisted primarily of circumlocutions and non-responses, both of which declined considerably. For Ag2, then, the treatment facilitated the production of target-related attempts. A more fine-grained error analysis might illustrate differential mechanisms of the two treatments, although there weren't enough instances of each error type to permit a reliable analysis of this question in the current study.

Given the similar improvements stimulated by the two treatments, what considerations might influence the choice between them? As speech-language pathologists, our goal is not simply to improve the accuracy of word retrieval, but also to facilitate the ways in which people with aphasia can compensate for their word-finding difficulties. This might be done by achieving a closer proximity between errors and targets, or by explicitly training compensatory strategies such as circumlocution or gesture. Both of these efforts have the aim of making the unsuccessful word retrieval attempt more transparent to the listener, so that the message is at least partially conveyed. Therapy approaches based on Semantic Feature Analysis (Boyle & Coelho, 1995) have the advantage of training the purposeful production of words semantically related to the target. In the absence of accurate word retrieval, these can help cue the listener about the intended word (e.g., "I can't remember what you call it, but you eat it, and it's red."), or even provide a self-cue for the aphasic speaker. A potential disadvantage of this approach, though, is that learning such a strategy requires considerable metalinguistic skill.

The Contextual approach, by contrast, is proposed to rely on implicit learning, as in most natural language learning contexts, to facilitate language production. (Although the target words were explicit in this treatment, the contextual associations hypothetically being strengthened were not.) Recent evidence has shown that ageing involves a decrement in tasks that require explicit learning, while

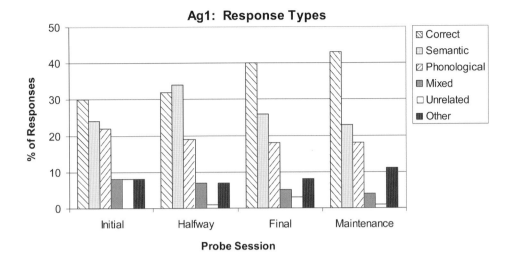

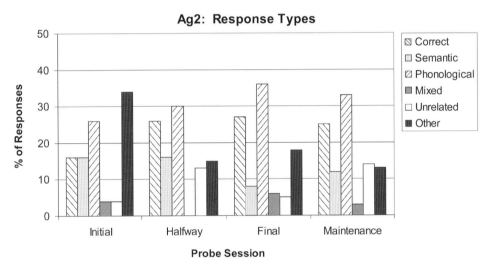

Figure 3. First complete responses categorised by error type for Ag1 and Ag2.

implicit learning is generally maintained (e.g., Howard & Howard, 1997; Midford & Kirsner, 2005). That the two participants in the current study were both under 50 years of age might help to explain why they performed equally well with the more explicit Semantic Treatment and the more implicit Contextual Treatment. For more typical (i.e., older) individuals with aphasia, the explicitness of a treatment might be an important influence on its potential effectiveness. Further study can address this question in older participants with aphasia.

In conclusion, the current study provides preliminary evidence in support of a novel treatment—a contextually based approach—for word-retrieval deficits in agrammatic aphasia. Although no evidence was found for the superiority of this approach over semantically based approaches, the contextual approach is arguably more representative of actual language use. Further study is required, with careful specification of generalisation conditions, and qualitative analyses of performance, to help understand the mechanism by which the approach exerts its effect. In addition, the approach should be attempted with participants with other types of aphasia. In particular, the outcome of the Contextual approach relative to semantic-feature-based therapies needs to be examined in participants with anomic aphasia, whose word retrieval impairments are hypothesised to arise from decreased semantic input.

REFERENCES

Barde, L. H. F., Schwartz, M. F., & Boronat, C. B. (2006). Semantic weight and verb retrieval in aphasia. *Brain and Language, 97*(3), 266–278.

Bastiaanse, R., & Jonkers, R. (1998). Verb retrieval in action naming and spontaneous speech in agrammatic and anomic aphasia. *Aphasiology, 12*(11), 951–969.

Bird, H., Franklin, S., & Howard, D. (2002). "Little words" – not really: function and content words in normal and aphasic speech. *Journal of Neurolinguistics, 15*(3–5), 209–237.

Boyle, M., & Coelho, C. A. (1995). Application of semantic feature analysis as a treatment for aphasic dysnomia. *American Journal of Speech-Language Pathology, 4*, 94–98.

Breedin, S. D., Saffran, E. M., & Schwartz, M. F. (1998). Semantic factors in verb retrieval: An effect of complexity. *Brain and Language, 63*, 1–31.

Conley, A., & Coelho, C. A. (2003). Treatment of word retrieval impairment in chronic Broca's aphasia. *Aphasiology, 17*(3), 203–211.

Druks, J. (2002). Verbs and nouns: A review of the literature. *Journal of Neurolinguistics, 15*(3–5), 289–315.

Druks, J., & Masterson, J. (2000). *An object and action naming battery.* Philadelphia, PA: Taylor & Francis.

Francis, W. N., & Kučera, H. (1982). *Frequency analysis of English usage.* Boston, MA: Houghton Mifflin Company.

Goodglass, H., Kaplan, E., & Barresi, B. (2001a). *The Assessment of Aphasia and Related Disorders* (3rd ed.). Philadelphia, PA: Lippincott, Williams & Wilkins.

Goodglass, H., Kaplan, E., & Barresi, B. (2001b). *Boston Diagnostic Aphasia Examination* (3rd ed.). Philadelphia, PA: Lippincott, Williams & Wilkins.

Gordon, J. K., & Dell, G. S. (2003). Learning to divide the labor: An account of deficits in light and heavy verb production. *Cognitive Science, 27*, 1–40.

Howard, J. H. Jr., & Howard, D. V. (1997). Age differences in implicit learning of higher order dependencies in serial patterns. *Psychology and Aging, 12*(4), 634–656.

Jakobson, R. (1971). Two aspects of language and two types of aphasic disturbances. In R. Jakobson & M. Halle (Eds.), *Fundamentals of language* [previous edition 1956]. The Hague: Mouton.

Kim, M., & Thompson, C. K. (2004). Verb deficits in Alzheimer's disease and agrammatism: Implications for lexical organisation. *Brain and Language, 88*(1), 1–20.

Miceli, G., Silveri, M. C., Villa, G., & Caramazza, A. (1984). On the basis for the agrammatic's difficulty in producing main verbs. *Cortex, 20*, 207–220.

Midford, R., & Kirsner, K. (2005). Implicit and explicit learning in aged and young adults. *Aging, Neuropsychology, and Cognition, 12*, 359–387.

Olness, G. S. (2006). Genre, verb, and coherence in picture-elicited discourse of adults with aphasia. *Aphasiology, 20*(2/3/4), 175–187.

Pashek, G. V., & Tompkins, C. A. (2002). Context and word class influences on lexical retrieval in aphasia. *Aphasiology, 16*(3), 261–286.

Roach, A., Schwartz, M. F., Martin, N., Grewal, R. S., & Brecher, A. (1996). The Philadelphia Naming Test: Scoring and rationale. *Clinical Aphasiology, 24*, 121–133.

Rossion, B., & Pourtois, G. (2004). Revisiting Snodgrass and Vanderwart's object set: The role of surface detail in basic-level object recognition. *Perception, 33*, 217–236.

Saffran, E. M., Berndt, R. S., & Schwartz, M. F. (1989). The quantitative analysis of agrammatic production: Procedure and data. *Brain and Language, 37*, 440–479.

Schwartz, M. F., & Hodgson, C. (2002). A new multiword naming deficit: Evidence and interpretation. *Cognitive Neuropsychology*, *19*(3), 263–288.

Williams, S. E., & Canter, G. J. (1982). The influence of situational context on naming performance in aphasic syndromes. *Brain and Language*, *17*, 92–106.

Zingeser, L. B., & Berndt, R. S. (1990). Retrieval of nouns and verbs in agrammatism and anomia. *Brain and Language*, *39*(1), 14–32.

APPENDIX

Stimulus items

Semantic treatment		Contextual treatment	
Treated items	*Untreated items*	*Treated items*	*Untreated items*
Land animals		*Water animals*	
tiger [2]	zebra	dolphin	seal
elephant	monkey	penguin [2]	(alli)gator
giraffe [2]	rhinoceros	whale	duck
cat [2]	lion [1]	turtle [2]	lobster [1]
bear	dog [1]	fish [2]	frog [1]
Fruits		*Vegetables*	
banana [2]	apple	celery	peas
cherry [2]	orange	carrot [2]	pepper
pear	peach	potato	broccoli
grape(s) [1]	strawberry	mushroom	corn [1]
pineapple [1]	lemon	onion [2]	lettuce [1]
Clothing		*Body parts*	
belt	coat	lips	tongue
hat [2]	dress	leg	toe
shoe(s)	shirt	hair [2]	finger
suit [2]	sweater	moustache [2]	nose [1]
skirt [1]	shorts [1]	thumb	ear [1]
Appliances		*Transportation*	
(re)frig(erator)	(tele)phone	(air)plane [2]	(heli)copter
TV [2]	hair dryer	blimp	car
vacuum (cleaner)	washer	motorcycle/bike	truck
clock	stove [1]	(sail)boat [2]	bus [1]
iron [2]	computer [1]	train	wagon [1]
Occupations		*Sports*	
chef/cook [2]	photographer	soccer	football
fireman	butcher	basketball	baseball
teacher	waitress	tennis	(ice) skating
astronaut/spaceman	doctor	skiing	volleyball [1]
dentist [1]	nurse [1]	golf [2]	bowling [1]

[1] untreated items for Ag1.　　[2] generalisation item for Ag2.

APHASIOLOGY, 2007, 21 (6/7/8), 658–669

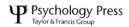

Self-correction in apraxia of speech: The effect of treatment

Anita van der Merwe

University of Pretoria, South Africa

Background: Overt attempts at self-correction of speech errors reflect conscious monitoring of speech output. The ability to monitor speech reveals something about the dynamics of motor control. Speakers with apraxia of speech (AOS) attempt to self-correct speech, but systematic analyses of self-correction in AOS have rarely been done.
Aims: The aims of the study were to determine the effect of treatment on the number of overt attempted self-corrections during the course of treatment, on the number of overt attempted self-corrections as a percentage of the total number of incorrect productions, and on successful self-corrections as a percentage of the total number of self-corrections.
Methods & Procedures: One speaker with AOS was treated for a period of 18 months. Self-corrections were noted during three repetitions of 110 words and 110 nonwords. Three pre-treatment baseline probes and four subsequent probes, spanning the treatment period, were performed.
Outcomes & Results: The number of attempted self-corrections decreased and the percentage of successful self-corrections increased during treatment. However, attempted self-corrections as a percentage of the total number of incorrect productions remained fairly stable during treatment.
Conclusions: The results indicate that success of overt self-corrections improved during treatment. However, the almost unchanged number of self-corrections as a percentage of the total number of incorrect productions suggests that the process of internal predictive control remained dysfunctional. The inadvertent occurrence of speech errors points towards a loss or dysfunction of volitional control of speech production. Mental practice as a complementary treatment technique may need to be considered. A continuum of volitional control of speech is presented to explain AOS.

Speakers can monitor almost any aspect of their own communication (Levelt, 1995), and speech monitoring can reveal something about the dynamics of speech motor control. Overt attempts at self-correction of incorrect speech production reflect conscious monitoring of speech output and an awareness of overt speech errors. Speakers with apraxia of speech (AOS) attempt to self-correct speech errors (Duffy, 2005; McNeil, Robin, & Schmidt, 1997; Wertz, LaPointe, & Rosenbek, 1984), but very little is known about the nature of these self-corrections and which variables may influence the ability to monitor speech output. An analysis of changes in the pattern of self-correction during a period of treatment may elucidate speech monitoring processes in speakers with AOS.

Systematic analyses of the prediction and attempts at self-correction of apraxic speech errors have rarely been done. Deal and Darley (1972) examined the ability to

Address correspondence to: Anita van der Merwe PhD, Department of Communication Pathology, University of Pretoria, Pretoria 0002, South Africa. E-mail: anita.vandermerwe@up.ac.za

DOI: 10.1080/02687030701192174

predict speech errors in AOS and found that these speakers were able to predict upcoming errors, but that more errors occurred than were predicted. The speakers who participated in their study were able to point out the errors they had made, and thus displayed an awareness of speech errors after output. Duffy (2005) also reports that patients can predict errors, that some speak slowly to prevent errors, that some recognise errors that were made, and that some are surprised by unpredicted errors that occurred in otherwise fluent speech.

Van der Merwe, Uys, Loots, and Grimbeek (1988) studied successful and unsuccessful self-correction of speech errors in five speakers with speech apraxia. Four speakers met the diagnostic criteria for AOS as suggested by McNeil et al (1997), and the fifth was a child with childhood apraxia of speech. The participants had all received treatment with the Speech Motor Learning Program (Van der Merwe, 1985) (which will be described under Method), but for different lengths of time and from different clinicians. The data were based on a nonword repetition task in which the speakers with speech apraxia had to repeat 40 nonwords, six times consecutively. The nonwords varied in consonant (C) and vowel (V) structure (CVCV, CVC, CVCVC, and CVCVCVC) but conformed to the phonotactic rules of the first language of the speakers (English or Afrikaans). The type of errors that the speakers attempted to self-correct was also noted. A total of 19 successful self-corrections and 13 unsuccessful self-corrections occurred. Of the total of 32 attempted self-corrections, 9 were on CVCV nonwords, 1 on a CVC nonword, and 22 on CVCVC and CVCVCVC nonwords. The majority of self-corrections therefore occurred on the longer utterances, which by nature provide a greater opportunity for more errors. Self-correction of phoneme substitutions and distorted substitutions were observed, but not distortions, slow rate, syllable segregation, or segmental lengthening, even though these errors were in the majority (214 substitutions and distorted substitutions versus 2021 motor-level errors). The lack of motor-level attempted self-corrections (all errors other than phoneme substitutions and distorted substitutions) by the participants in that study may indicate a lack of awareness of these errors or the perception that motor-level errors are not amenable to self-correction.

Self-correction of linguistic errors has been analysed by several researchers, and theoretical models for linguistic monitoring have been proposed (Levelt, 1995; Oomen & Postma, 2001). Natural and experimentally induced "slips" are analysed to explore the nature of linguistic monitoring (Baars, 1992; Oomen & Postma, 2001). The perceptual loop theory proposed by Levelt (1995) is widely accepted as an explanatory model (Oomen & Postma, 2001) that accounts for linguistic, including phonological, self-monitoring of speech output. According to this theory the phonetic plan (internal speech according to Levelt) and overt speech are relayed to a speech *comprehension* system via an internal and external loop. Levelt (1995) uses the words "speech" comprehension system and "language" comprehension system alternatively, but indicates the intended meaning by stating that this comprehension system can "detect deviations from linguistic standards" (Levelt, 1995, p.470). It seems logical to assume that a language comprehension system can detect linguistic (e.g., phonological, syntactic, morphological) errors, but not errors in articulatory precision, rate, fluency, and voicing characteristics. Clarification of the monitoring of motor speech output could more logically be found in speech production models.

The Four Level Framework of speech sensorimotor control (Van der Merwe, 1997) offers some clarification of the nature of speech monitoring. According to this framework the outcome of production can be monitored by means of response-produced feedback of tactile-kinaesthetic and auditory stimuli. This type of feedback may result in overt self-correction of speech errors. However, self-correction may also occur before speech is executed. During speech motor planning the speaker can centrally monitor the efference (reference) copy of the planned utterance through internal feedback. For accurate production of the speech sound, a comparison with an internal model of the motor plan in the sensorimotor memory may take place (Van der Merwe, 1997). Internal feedback and internal predictive control may perform an error-correction function before speech is produced (Kawato & Gomi, 1992; Keele, 1982; Kelso, 1982; Van der Merwe, 1997).

The questions addressed in the current study relate to changes in self-monitoring during a period of treatment that resulted in improved speech production ability in a speaker with AOS (Van der Merwe, 1998; Van der Merwe, Tesner, Groenewald & Moore, 1998). The specific aims of the current study were to determine the effect of treatment on the *number* of overt attempted self-corrections during the course of treatment, on the number of overt attempted self-corrections as a *percentage* of the total number of incorrect productions, and on *successful* self-corrections as a percentage of the total number of self-corrections. It was predicted that the number of attempted self-corrections would decrease and the percentage of successful self-corrections would increase as speech improved (total number of incorrect productions decline) during treatment. It was also predicted that the number of overt attempted self-corrections as a percentage of the total number of errors would decrease during treatment. A decrease in the percentage of overt attempted self-corrections may indicate a shift from externally manifested (overt) self-corrections based on response-produced feedback to error correction of upcoming speech errors based on internal feedback. If internal predictive control (Kawato & Gomi, 1992; Keele, 1982; Kelso, 1982; Van der Merwe, 1997) improves, the percentage of overt attempted self-corrections may decline. Answers to these questions may contribute to a better understanding of speech monitoring and speech motor control in AOS.

METHOD

The current study was part of a larger study on the outcomes of the Speech Motor Learning (SML) Program (Van der Merwe, 1985). The SML Program targets speech sound treatment in nonwords and words and incorporates motor learning principles such as variability in practice, augmented feedback on some productions, and blocked and random practice. Production drill of series of nonwords is continued until utterances become 80% correct, speech rate approaches normal, and no start–restart and groping behaviours occur. Data from the larger study showed that the number of incorrect productions and the number of perceptual errors decreased during treatment of the same speaker with AOS who participated in this study. The number of incorrect productions was determined by two independent raters. A total of 5940 productions of words and nonwords were analysed and a point-to-point agreement score of 89% was reached (Van der Merwe, 1998; Van der Merwe et al., 1998). In the current study the data were further analysed with regard to self-corrections.

Participant

The participant was a university trained, bilingual, right-handed male who suffered an embolic stroke at the age of 52 years. The study started 30 months post-onset.

The Boston Diagnostic Aphasia Examination (an informally translated Afrikaans version) showed no problems other than in fluency. The participant had normal hearing, normal voice quality and resonance, and no facial or tongue weakness. He was not hemiplegic, but did show tactile agnosia of the right hand. Radiological reports (MRI and CT) revealed small lesions near Broca's area and the left parietal-occipital and right occipital areas of the brain. He displayed slow speech rate, lengthened segmental duration, lengthened intersegment durations, sound distortions, substitutions, distorted substitutions, articulatory groping, awareness of errors, and increasing errors with increasing word length. The diagnosis was consistent with AOS without aphasia. At the start of treatment his speech was very slow, struggling, and highly unintelligible. At the time Probe 4 was administered his speech had become much more fluent and not as slow as previously. He used words that he knew he could produce well for communication, and therefore he was much more intelligible. He had once again become independent in all aspects of his life.

The participant had signed informed consent to take part in the study, and for the data collected during the three baseline and four following probes to be used at scientific meetings and in scientific publications. He was free to withdraw from the study at any stage. He continued treatment for 18 months and then withdrew from the study.

Procedures

The SML Program (Van der Merwe, 1985) was applied for 18 months. The treatment was provided twice a week for an hour by the author. Three baseline probes (B1 to B3) were completed before treatment commenced. Throughout the course of treatment, multiple probes were administered. The data for four of these probes, spanning the treatment period, were analysed in the present study. Each word or nonword was printed on a separate card and presented to the participant one at a time. All responses were read. The clinician did not pace the three responses, and no time restriction was imposed. The instruction was to repeat each word and nonword three times consecutively. This procedure differed from that followed during scoring of the total number of incorrect productions (Van der Merwe, 1998; Van der Merwe et al., 1998) where only a single utterance of the target was allowed. The three repetitions were requested to foster attempted self-correction. The environment and procedures followed were similar for all baseline and subsequent probes.

Materials

The probe stimuli consisted of 110 Afrikaans words and 110 nonwords that complied with the phonological rules of Afrikaans. Afrikaaans was the native language of the participant. Three repetitions of each of the 220 target utterances were scored for each baseline and each subsequent probe. Probe stimuli were not part of the treatment stimuli but were representative of the type of material used during treatment. The probe stimuli were identical for all probes. The probe stimuli contained 15 different consonants (C), 10 vowels (V), and eight consonant clusters in CVCV, CVC, CVCVC, and CVCVCVC (or initial CC) syllable structures. The speech sounds represented easy and difficult sounds as perceived by the participant. All sounds except the consonant clusters had been treated.

Attempted self-corrections were judged perceptually by the author. These data were scored from tape recordings. The production of words and nonwords was regarded as incorrect when distortion, substitution, or distorted substitution of any speech sound occurred. The three repetitions of a target word or nonword were scored as a *single opportunity* to self-correct production. To differentiate between audible trial-and-error groping (Duffy, 2005) and attempted self-correction, attempted self-correction was identified as such only if the client had produced the entire word or nonword (incorrectly) and then displayed a pause or start–restart behaviour and attempted to change the utterance. The total number of times a word or nonword was said also guided the decision that attempted self-correction had been displayed.

Production of a target utterance was scored as *one* of the following: (1) Three correct repetitions of the target utterance. (2) Incorrect with no attempt to self-correct when *one or more* of the three repetitions were produced incorrectly with no pauses or start–restart behaviour and no attempt to change production. (3) Successful self-correction when the *incorrect production of the target word or nonword was followed* by a successful attempt to correct a sound substitution, a sound distortion, or a distorted substitution; if a successful self-correction was followed by an error on the same target utterance during a next repetition, it was still accepted as an instance of successful self-correction. (4) Unsuccessful self-correction under same circumstances as successful.

Reliability

The rating system developed by the author was verified by a second rater. Data from the first baseline (B1) were analysed by consensus to refine the formulation of the different ratings. The judgements made by consensus were then compared point-to-point to the ratings of the first rater. An agreement score of 85% was reached. The data of B1 were re-analysed by the first rater and an intra-rater point-to-point agreement score of 87% was achieved.

RESULTS

The total number of incorrect productions of words and nonwords as determined in the larger study (Van der Merwe, 1998; Van der Merwe et al., 1998) is displayed in Figure 1 to provide an indication of the nature of speech changes during the period that was analysed with regard to self-corrections. The data show that the total number of incorrect productions declined across the 18-month treatment period. The number of incorrect productions demonstrated some improvement during the baseline probes, and improvement continued during treatment but subsequently seemed to reach a plateau.

The number of attempted self-corrections showed no improvement during the baseline probes but then decreased during treatment and then also reached a plateau (see Figure 2). Self-corrections as a percentage of the total number of incorrect productions remained fairly stable during treatment (see Figure 3). There is some improvement displayed during Probe 2 for words and Probe 3 for nonwords, but thereafter the percentage appears to remain relatively stable. The percentage of successful self-corrections for both words and nonwords (see Figure 4) increased across time. A plateau was not reached in this regard. Nonwords followed the same

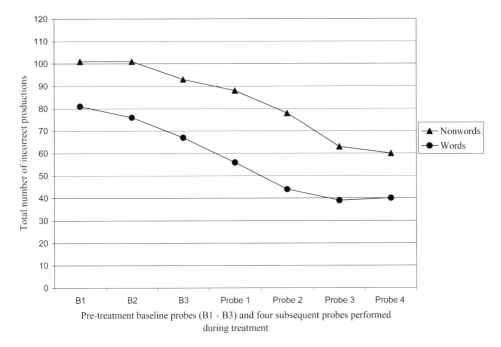

Figure 1. Total number of incorrect productions of nonwords and words.

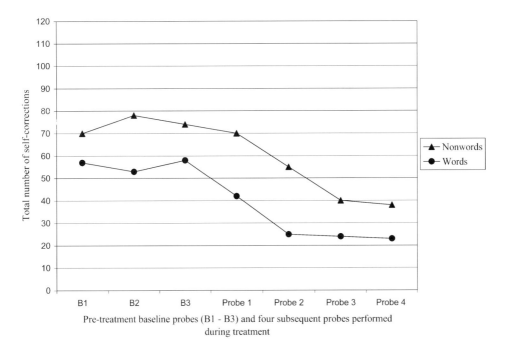

Figure 2. Total number of attempted self-corrections of nonwords and words.

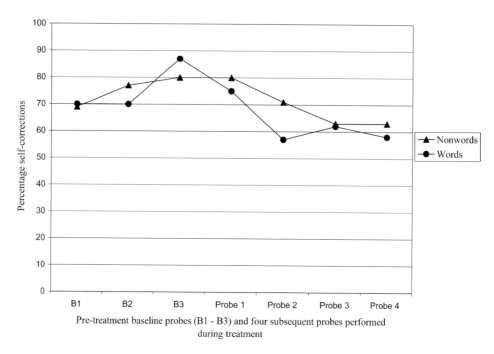

Figure 3. Attempted self-corrections as a percentage of the total number of incorrect productions.

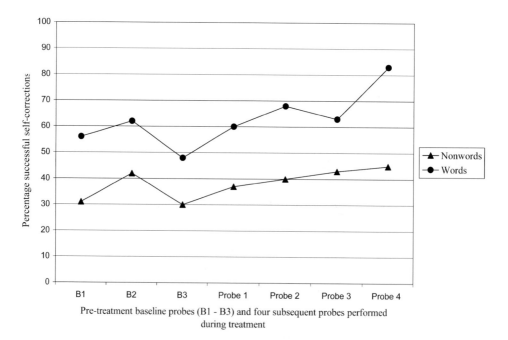

Figure 4. Successful self-corrections of nonwords and words as a percentage of the total number of self-corrections.

trend as words, but not as pronounced. A greater number of successful self-corrections occurred on words than on nonwords.

DISCUSSION

The decrease in number of incorrect productions and number of overt attempted self-corrections together with the increase in the percentage of successful self-corrections seem to suggest that this client's speech production ability and his ability to monitor speech through overt self-corrections improved during treatment. As the participant's speech improved, the need for self-correction declined, and therefore the percentage of self-corrections declined. However, the almost unchanged number of attempted self-corrections as a percentage of total number of incorrect productions suggests that prediction of upcoming errors and the ability to prevent these errors did not improve. Speech errors continued to occur inadvertently, and the mode of speech motor monitoring seems unchanged. This result suggests that the process of internal predictive control remained dysfunctional in this speaker with AOS. These findings are supported by Van der Merwe and Grimbeek (2006), who noted inadvertent errors in a study of five speakers with speech apraxia. In that study the variability of voice onset time of the speakers with speech apraxia was found to be less variable than that of the control speakers. Despite the smaller range of variability and mostly correct voice onset times, occasional voice onset time errors occurred during six consecutive repetitions of nonwords. These results concur with the observation of unpredicted speech errors by patients with AOS as cited by Duffy (2005).

The inadvertent occurrence of speech errors that are not amenable to internal predictive control reveals something about the underlying nature of speech motor control in AOS. Inadvertent speech errors may be comparable to linguistic (e.g., morphological and phonological) "slips" that occur in normal communication. "Slips" reflect a momentary loss of volitional control and are "in essence a mismatch between intention and performance" (Baars, 1992, p. 4). The loss of volitional control of speech production has traditionally been integral to early definitions of AOS (Wertz et al., 1984). Later conceptualisations of AOS place greater emphasis on the nature of the breakdown in speech motor planning and/or programming (McNeil et al., 1997; Van der Merwe, 1997). The integration of a theory of volitional control of speech production with a comprehensive conceptualisation of the nature of breakdown in speech motor planning (or programming) (Van der Merwe, 1997) may contribute to a more comprehensive definition of this intriguing and not well understood disorder.

In Table 1 a continuum of volitional control of speech motor output is presented. This continuum may elucidate the underlying nature of some speech errors in AOS, including unpredicted errors that are not prevented by internal predictive control. The continuum portrays speech motor control as being mediated along a continuum ranging from highly controlled processing to a mode of automatic processing. The hypothesised continuum is in accord with current theories of motor control of movement and of speech output (Duffy, 2005; Schmidt & Lee, 1999). During highly controlled processing, speech monitoring occurs via response feedback. As processing becomes more automatic, internal predictive control becomes operational. Fully automatised utterances are probably produced without reliance on internal feedback cues. Automatic processing is "faster and many processes can be

TABLE 1
Continuum of volitional control of speech motor planning and programming: A guide to understanding apraxia of speech

	Highly controlled processing →	Controlled processing →	Automatic processing
Continuum of volitional motor control	Speech is produced with attention and volitional monitoring. May occur during motor learning of novel utterances and during production of long and/or phonetically complex utterances. Monitoring may occur via response feedback and closed loop control is operational. Utilisation of internal feedback cues and predictive control is not yet effective. The mode of coalition of neural structures that control speech output is adapted to accommodate highly controlled processing (Van der Merwe, 1997).	Speech motor planning and programming is more automatic and the speaker becomes more skilled at utilisation of internal feedback cues and therefore more capable of predictive motor control. Open loop control becomes operational. Utilisation of internal feedback cues and predictive control becomes more effective. The mode of coalition of neural structures that control speech output is adapted to accommodate controlled processing (Van der Merwe, 1997).	Speech motor planning and programming is mediated via automatic processing where open loop control is operational and there is little reliance on internal feedback and predictive control. Such processing is "faster and many processes can be done in parallel" (Schmidt & Lee, 1999, p. 69) and control may be mediated by progressively "lower" levels (p. 374) in the central nervous system. This mode of control is operational during production of frequently used words, phrases, syllables, and automatised utterances such as counting.
Disorder in volitional motor control	A disorder in volitional motor control may result in a loss of, or dysfunction in, volitional speech motor planning and programming, or in ineffective volitional access to motor plans in the sensorimotor memory. A disorder may affect all speech utterances and cause severe apraxia of speech or it may affect certain speech sounds, syllable structures, words, a second/third language or long utterances that the apraxic speaker finds motorically complex. Predicted and unpredicted errors may occur and articulation is slow and groping. Groping may reflect the underlying disorder and/or attempts to monitor speech.	A disorder in volitional motor control may result in a dysfunction in volitional speech motor planning and programming, or in ineffective volitional access to motor plans in the sensorimotor memory. A disorder may cause moderate apraxia of speech of most utterances or may affect certain speech sounds, syllable structures, words, a second/third language or long utterances that the apraxic speaker finds motorically complex to produce. Predicted and unpredicted errors may occur and articulation is slow and groping. Normal speakers who produce novel or difficult utterances may show slow careful articulation.	A loss of automatised control of speech motor planning and programming may be momentary and inadvertent. Unpredicted spatial, temporal and inter-articulatory synchronisation errors may occur resulting in speech sound distortion and disrupted fluency. In the apraxic speaker a loss of automatised control and/or reliance on automatised control that is no longer operational, may lead to unpredicted errors. Even in the normal speaker a momentary loss of automatised motor control may occur.

done in parallel" (Schmidt & Lee, 1999, p. 69), and control may be mediated by progressively "lower" levels (Schmidt & Lee, 1999, p. 374) in the central nervous system. Motor planning and programming of speech movements (Van der Merwe, 1997) is probably imbedded within a volitional control system with different levels of conscious processing—highly controlled to automatic. Execution and even phonological planning are probably also under volitional control, but the current focus is on planning and programming, as these are probably the stages in speech motor control which are dysfunctional in AOS.

Different speech utterances might be controlled at different levels of controlled processing in the adult speaker. The contextual factors as portrayed in the Four Level Framework (Van der Merwe, 1997) may clarify the nature of speech utterances that are controlled consciously or automatically. The contextual factors are hypothesised to be the level of automaticity of the utterance (volitional versus automatised), motor complexity of the utterance, syllable structure of the utterance, length of the utterance, familiarity with the utterance (novel versus well known), and the required rate of production. It is hypothesised in the framework that contextual factors influence the mode of coalition of neural structures and the skill required from the planning, programming, and execution mechanisms. Motorically complex, long, novel utterances and an increase in speech rate may require more attention and controlled processing during production.

Signs of disorders along the continuum of volitional control will probably differ (see Table 1). A loss of volitional control and/or lost volitional access to the sensorimotor memory and/or a loss of previously automatic processing, may cause a speaker to divert to *highly conscious processing* and reliance on response-produced feedback for speech monitoring. Such a disorder may result in severe apraxia of speech of all utterances, or it may affect certain speech sounds, syllable structures, words, longer utterances, or speech in second/third languages. Groping and trial-and-error articulation may be evident. Groping may reflect the underlying disorder and/or attempts to monitor speech. Predicted and unpredicted errors may occur. A less severe disorder in volitional control may lead to *controlled processing*. Some measure of automatic processing and internal predictive control is possible. A disorder at this point in the continuum may result in moderate AOS or may affect certain speech sounds, syllable structures, words, a second/third language, or long utterances that the speaker finds motorically complex. Predicted and unpredicted errors may occur. A loss of *automatic processing* of speech motor planning and programming may be momentary and inadvertent. Unpredicted spatial, temporal, and inter-articulatory synchronisation errors may occur and result in speech sound distortion and disrupted fluency. In the speaker with AOS a loss of automatic processing and/or (momentary) reliance on automatic processing that is no longer operational may lead to inadvertent speech errors. Even in normal speakers such momentary loss of automatised motor control may occur. Motor-based "slips" are traditionally not the focus of study. However, analyses of such phenomena may contribute to a better understanding of speech motor control.

The automatised processing of speech utterances and the prevention of unpredicted speech errors in speakers with speech apraxia should be addressed in clinical practice. Overlearning of movement sequences enhances automaticity (Schmidt & Lee, 1999), while mental practice or mental imagery (i.e., imagining the movements without any overt actions) turn the attention of the learner to the predicted outcomes and the possible avoidance of errors (Schmidt & Lee, 1999). In the SML Program overlearning and delayed responses with mental preparation of production during the delay period are two of the techniques that are applied. However, it may be necessary to place more emphasis on mental imagery during treatment and to direct the attention of the learner to the prevention of errors. The point in time during which this motor learning principle is applied will have to be considered carefully. It is also important to bear in mind that mental imagery can in no instance replace the value of rehearsal of overt speech production.

In conclusion the present study suggests that internal predictive control of speech and the ability to prevent speech errors did not improve in this particular speaker with AOS even though his success in repairing these errors did improve over the course of treatment. The inadvertent occurrence of speech errors points towards a loss or dysfunction of volitional control of speech production. A comprehensive definition of the nature of AOS may need to incorporate the loss or dysfunction in volitional control of speech.

REFERENCES

Baars, B. J. (1992). The many uses of error: Twelve steps to a unified framework. In B. J. Baars (Ed.), *Experimental slips and human error: Exploring the architecture of volition* (pp. 3–34). New York: Plenum Press.

Deal, J. L., & Darley, F. L. (1972). The influence of linguistic and situational variables on phonemic accuracy in apraxia of speech. *Journal of Speech and Hearing Research, 15,* 639–653.

Duffy, J. R. (2005). *Motor speech disorders: Substrates, differential diagnosis, and management.* Missouri: Elsevier Mosby.

Kawato, M., & Gomi, H. (1992). The cerebellum and VOR/OKR learning models. *Trends in Neurosciences, 15,* 445–453.

Keele, S. W. (1982). Learning and control of coordinated motor patterns: The programming perspective. In J. A. S. Kelso (Ed.), *Human motor behavior: An introduction* (pp. 161–188). Hillside, NJ: Lawrence Erlbaum Associates, Inc.

Kelso, J. A. S. (1982). Concepts and issues in human motor behavior: Coming to grips with the jargon. In J. A. S. Kelso (Ed.), *Human motor behavior: An introduction* (pp. 21–62). Hillside, NJ: Lawrence Erlbaum Associates, Inc.

Levelt, W. J. M. (1995). *Speaking: From intention to articulation.* Cambridge, MA: The MIT Press.

McNeil, M. R., Robin, D. A., & Schmidt, R. A. (1997). Apraxia of speech: Definition, differentiation, and treatment. In M. R. McNeil (Ed.), *Clinical management of sensorimotor speech disorders.* New York: Thieme Medical Publishers.

Oomen, C. C. E., & Postma, A. (2001). Effects of time pressure on mechanisms of speech production and self-monitoring. *Journal of Psycholinguistic Research, 30,* 163–184.

Schmidt, R. A., & Lee, T. D. (1999). *Motor control and learning: A behavioral emphasis.* Champaign, IL: Human Kinetics.

Van der Merwe, A. (1985). *Treatment program for developmental apraxia of speech and other speech disorders* [title translated]. Publication of the University of Pretoria, South Africa.

Van der Merwe, A. (1997). A theoretical framework for the characterization of pathological speech sensorimotor control. In M. R. McNeil (Ed.), *Clinical management of sensorimotor speech disorders.* New York: Thieme Medical Publishers.

Van der Merwe, A. (1998). *Speech motor learning in apraxia of speech: Report on a single subject experimental study.* Paper presented at the 8th International Aphasia Rehabilitation Conference. Kwa Maritane, Pilanesberg National Park, S.A.

Van der Merwe, A., & Grimbeek, R. J. (2006). Variability of voice onset time, vowel duration and utterance duration in apraxia of speech. *Stem-, Spraak- en Taalpathologie: 5th International Conference on Speech Motor Control Nijmegen: Abstracts, 14,* Supplement June, 72.

Van der Merwe, A., Tesner, H., Groenewald, E., & Moore, C. A. (1998). *Successive level intervention in apraxia of speech: Status report on a single subject experimental study*. Paper presented at the Ninth Biennial Conference on Motor Speech: Motor Speech Disorders and Speech Motor Control, Tucson, Arizona, USA.

Van der Merwe, A., Uys, I. C., Loots, J. M., & Grimbeek, R. J. (1988). Perceptual errors in apraxia of speech: Indications of the nature of the disorder. *South African Journal of Communication Disorders, 35*, 45–54.

Wertz, R. T., LaPointe, L. L., & Rosenbek, J. C. (1984). *Apraxia of speech in adults: The disorder and its management*. New York: Grune & Stratton.

APHASIOLOGY, 2007, 21 (6/7/8), 670–686

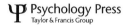

Orthographic cueing in anomic aphasia: How does it work?

Antje Lorenz and Lyndsey Nickels

Potsdam University, Germany, and Macquarie University, Sydney, Australia

Background: Both orthographic and phonological information from the target word can be appropriate cues in anomia treatment. Furthermore, both types of cues are used very frequently in clinical practice, although their underlying mechanisms of effectiveness and stability are still a matter of debate (e.g., Basso, Marangolo, Piras, & Galluzzi, 2001; Best, Herbert, Hickin, Osborne, & Howard, 2002; Howard & Harding, 1998).

Aims: The aim of the study was to examine the mechanisms by which orthographic cues are effective in detail. The study addresses two questions. First, what is the relationship between sublexical transcoding ability and the effectiveness of orthographic cues? And second, what is the relationship between effectiveness of orthographic cues and effectiveness of phonological cues?

Methods & Procedures: Three people with chronic aphasia and moderate to severe anomia participated in facilitation of spoken naming, using either the initial phoneme or initial letter of the target word. Both immediate and delayed effects were assessed over six facilitation sessions. Orthographic and phonological cue effects were investigated with regard to regularity of orthographic-phonological conversion (OPC) of the target's initial letter, and with regard to sub-lexical and lexical reading and repetition in the participants using a multiple single-case design (cf. Howard, 2003).

Outcomes & Results: In one participant both phonological and orthographic cues produced similar effects. In the other two participants, orthographic cueing effects were present in the absence of phonological cueing effects. With regard to regularity of the initial letter-phoneme conversion in the orthographic condition, a similar pattern overall was present for regular, ambiguous, and irregular target words, e.g., initial letter cues seemed to be similarly effective in words such as KNIFE (irregular OPC of initial *letter*) as in words such as KING or DOLL.

Conclusions: Initial letter cues are appropriate cues for the effective treatment of anomia as they may produce strong and long-lasting effects. In contrast to earlier predictions (e.g., Bruce & Howard, 1988), initial letter cues may be effective even in participants where the initial phoneme cue remains totally ineffective. There are likely to be various mechanisms of effectiveness underpinning orthographic cue effects: a sub-lexical mechanism and a lexical mechanism of effectiveness.

Address correspondence to: Antje Lorenz, Potsdam University, Department of Linguistics, Karl-Liebknecht-Str. 24–25, 14476 Golm, Germany. E-mail: lorenz@ling.uni-potsdam.de

We would like to thank JUE, KCC, and MCB for their participation in this study. Furthermore, many thanks are due to Belinda McDonald, Kate Makin, and Melanie Moses for their support in recruitment of participants.

This research was supported by an NHMRC Senior Research Fellowship to Lyndsey Nickels and an Endeavour Australia Postdoctoral Research Fellowship and a MACCS visiting scholar grant to Antje Lorenz.

http://www.psypress.com/aphasiology   DOI: 10.1080/02687030701192182

Difficulty in recalling the words needed to communicate is a common symptom of aphasia. This word retrieval impairment can be severe and cause frustration and social isolation. While it is amenable to treatment, there is controversy regarding the most appropriate treatment task (Nickels, 2002).

Both phonological and orthographic information from the target word (e.g., initial phoneme or letter of the target word) can be appropriate and effective cues in the treatment of anomia. Furthermore, both types of cues are used very frequently in clinical practice, although neither phonological nor orthographic cues have been found to be universally effective for all individuals with impaired word retrieval (e.g., Best et al., 2002; Bruce & Howard, 1988; Howard, Patterson, Franklin, Orchard-Lisle, & Morton, 1985). Furthermore, with regard to stability of effects, different outcomes have been found. Originally, word-form-specific cues, such as the initial sound or rhyme, were found to produce only very short-lasting effects on spoken naming. Even a few minutes after application of the cue, effects were no longer observable (e.g., Howard et al., 1985; Patterson, Purell, & Morton, 1983). In contrast, some more recent studies have shown that both phonological and orthographic cues may produce effects that last for at least 10 minutes (Best et al., 2002). Furthermore, it is well known today that those cues—if applied repeatedly over several sessions within one set of items in therapy—can produce stable improvement that lasts for up to several weeks post treatment. (e.g., Hickin, Herbert, Best, & Howard, 2002; Wambaugh et al., 2001). The effectiveness of these different types of cue may depend on the underlying functional deficit of the person with anomia.

There have been a number of different accounts of how phonological cues may be effective (e.g., Monsell, 1987), some suggesting a lexical and others a sublexical mechanism. Best et al. (2002) found no correspondence between the ability of their aphasic participants to convert input to output phonology (e.g., in nonword repetition) and the effectiveness of phonological cues. They therefore argued that phonological cues are effective using a lexical mechanism: the auditory cue activates all stimuli in the phonological input lexicon corresponding to the cue, which in turn activate their corresponding representations in the phonological output lexicon. Retrieval of the target is facilitated by the additional activation from the cue combining with the partial activation from semantic processing.

For orthographic cues, different assumptions have been made regarding the relationship between sublexical processing abilities for written materials (the ability to read aloud nonwords and/or to sound out individual letters) and the effectiveness of the orthographic cues (e.g., Best et al., 2002; Howard & Harding, 1998). Several authors have pointed out a direct relationship between preserved nonword reading and effectiveness of orthographic cues (e.g., Best et al., 2002; Nickels, 1992). This relationship suggests that orthographic cues are effective through the written cue activating the corresponding phonological segment(s) (via a sublexical reading route), which in turn feeds back to the phonological representation. This facilitates retrieval by further activating the already partially activated target. However, other authors have found significant benefit from orthographic cues in patients without sublexical transcoding abilities for written materials (e.g., Howard & Harding, 1998; Lorenz, 2004), suggesting that there are additional mechanisms by which these cues may be effective. There has also been debate regarding the relationship between the effectiveness of orthographic and phonological cues. For example, Bruce and Howard (1988) argue that, in order for letter cues to be effective, phonological cues must also be effective for the person with aphasia. This prediction has received remarkably little attention.

The goal of this study is to examine the factors affecting the efficacy of orthographic and phonological cues in anomia treatment. We focus on two main points of debate:

1. The relationship between sublexical transcoding ability and the effectiveness of orthographic cues.
2. The relationship between effectiveness of orthographic cues and effectiveness of phonological cues.

CASE HISTORIES

We present data from two women and one man with chronic anomic aphasia. All three participants were monolingual speakers of English and had suffered a left hemisphere cerebro-vascular accident between 3 and 6 years prior to the start of the study. Word-finding difficulties formed a major aspect of the aphasia for all three individuals: when naming a set of 224 pictures of objects the participants produced between 31% and 65% correct responses. All participants had normal or corrected-to-normal vision, and none had major hearing loss, severe apraxia of speech, or dysarthria. A summary of background information for the participants is given in Table 1.

Prior to the start of the treatment study, the language-processing abilities of each participant were assessed in detail (cf. Best et al., 2002) (see Tables 2, 3, and 4).

PROCESSING OF SINGLE PHONEMES AND LETTERS

Auditory processing of single phonemes was assessed in an auditory discrimination task using the same phonemes that were later used as cues in the facilitation phases. A total of 25 phonemes were spoken, recorded, and the corresponding wav-files were implemented into the Universal Data Acquisition Program (UDAP; Zierdt, 1998–2005). A total of 50 pairs of phonemes were presented. Half of the pairs consisted of the same and half of different phonemes. The phonemes in the different pairs differed by one phonetic feature only (voicing, or place of articulation; manner was held constant).

All participants were able to identify all same pairs as *same*. Between two and four errors were made with different pairs. The pair /m/ – /n/, which was presented twice in different sequences, was classified as *same* by every participant. Unfortunately no

TABLE 1
Background information

Initials	Gender	Age (years)	Time post onset (years; months)	Aetiology	Speech output
MCB	F	63	3;2	left CVA	fluent
KCC	M	66	6	left CVA	non-fluent
JUE	F	33	4;9	left CVA	non-fluent

The table shows gender, years of age, and time post onset at start of a person's involvement in the study, their aetiology, type of speech output as assessed by clinical judgement.

TABLE 2
Background assessments: Processing of single letters and phonemes

PALPA test no.	Task	n-items	MCB	KCC	JUE
	Auditory discrimination, single phonemes (Lorenz, unpublished)	50	48 (96)	46 (92)	48 (96)
	same pairs	25	25	25	25
	different pairs	25	23	22	23
	repetition, single phonemes (Lorenz, unpublished)	25	21* (84)	13* (52)	22* (88)
22	naming, single graphemes	26	11* (42.3)	16* (61.5)	12* (46.1)
22	sounding out, single graphemes	26	3 * (11.5)	1* (3.8)	11* (42.3)

The table shows absolute number correct and percent correct in parentheses.
*Impaired performance.

control data are available from language-unimpaired participants. However, it seems quite likely that it is very hard to discriminate between /n/ and /m/ when no mouth-shape information is given. Both JUE and MCB were correct for all other stimulus pairs. Similarly, KCC produced only one further error with the pair /d/ – /t/. Therefore, it seems very unlikely that they have major auditory discrimination deficits for single phonemes.

In repetition of single phonemes KCC was moderately, and MCB and JUE were mildly, impaired (see Table 2). No mouth-shape information was given in this task. Providing letter names for single graphemes was moderately to severely impaired in all participants. Sounding out single graphemes was significantly worse than finding letter names for KCC and MCB—sounding vs naming letters: Fisher exact (two-tailed): KCC: $p < .0001$, MCB: $p < .05$—whereas JUE achieved similar scores in both tasks (see Table 2).

AUDITORY WORD PROCESSING

Auditory lexical decision was mildly impaired in all participants, which points to a mild functional deficit of the auditory input lexicon. Both JUE and MCB classified a significant number of nonwords as words, while fewer errors were made for words. Neither frequency nor imageability influenced their responses. In contrast, KCC's responses were significantly influenced by imageability, Fisher-exact (one-tailed): $p < .05$. In contrast, frequency was not a significant predictor of accuracy for KCC.

Repetition of words was mildly to moderately impaired for these participants. JUE performed significantly better with high-imageability than with low-imageability words, and KCC and MCB showed a trend towards an effect, Fisher exact (one-tailed): JUE: $p < .01$, KCC $p = .05$, MCB: $p = .08$. Word frequency was not a significant predictor of repetition accuracy for any of the participants.

Repetition of nonwords was significantly worse than repetition of words in all participants, which points to a functional deficit of auditory-phonological conversion for all participants—Fisher exact (two-tailed): MCB: $z = 3.382$, $p < .001$, KCC: $z = 6.207$, $p < .0001$, JUE: $z = 5.924$, $p < .0001$. Furthermore, KCC's and JUE's imageability effect points to the use of the lexical-semantic route and a further functional deficit of the direct lexical route for repetition. In contrast,

MCB, who was less impaired in nonword repetition than JUE or KCC, seemed to use a combination of sublexical and direct lexical or lexical-semantic processing routines in word repetition (see Table 3).

VISUAL WORD PROCESSING

For MCB and KCC, overall accuracy of visual lexical decision was within the normal range. However, both participants scored just below the normal range for low-imageability and low-frequency words, while all other subsets of words were processed normally. JUE's overall accuracy was impaired, but her responses were not significantly influenced by either imageability or frequency. The overall number of errors for JUE and the qualitative effect in MCB and KCC point to a mild functional deficit of the visual input lexicon in all participants.

Reading of words was mildly impaired in KCC and moderately impaired in JUE and MCB. All participants were significantly better at reading high-imageability than low-imageability words, Fisher exact (two-tailed): JUE: $p < .0001$; MCB: $p < .05$; KCC: $p = .01$. JUE and MCB produced semantic errors, whereas in KCC mainly no-responses occurred.

All participants were worse at reading nonwords than words—Fisher exact (two-tailed), MCB: $z = .5.207$, $p < .0001$; KCC: $z = 8.589$, $p < .0001$, JUE: $z = 4.363$, $p < .0001$—which points to a functional deficit of orthographic-phonological conversion procedures in all participants. Furthermore, lexicalisations formed the major category of errors for all participants. This, in combination with imageability effects in all participants and semantic paralexias in MCB and JUE, points to the use of the lexical-semantic route in reading (see Table 3).

Nevertheless, evidence for partially preserved orthographic-phonological conversion was present in JUE and MCB, who were partially able to transcode single letters into their corresponding phonemes. KCC was severely impaired on this task (see Table 2).

SEMANTIC PROCESSING OF WORDS AND PICTURES

Both spoken and written word-to-picture matching was within the normal range for MCB and KCC. JUE's spoken word-to-picture matching was preserved, whereas written word-to-picture matching was moderately impaired. At least part of her impaired performance seemed to be attributable to a pre-semantic disorder of her visual input lexicon (see above).

JUE and MCB were mildly impaired in auditory and written synonym judgements. KCC showed a marked impairment in auditory synonym judgements (written results not available). Semantic processing from pictures was just outside the normal range for all participants (Pyramids and Palm Trees Test, Howard & Patterson, 1992) (see Table 4).

NAMING

Spoken naming was studied initially using 224 black-and-white line drawings. Written naming was investigated using a subset of those stimuli ($N = 42$). Spoken naming was moderately to severely impaired, with semantic paraphasias and no-responses as the main error-types for all participants. In addition, some phonological errors were produced by each participant.

TABLE 3
Background assessments: Auditory and visual processing of words and nonwords

PALPA test no.	Task	n-items	MCB	KCC	JUE
5	Auditory lexical decision	160	146 (91.3)	135 (84.4)	141 (88.1)
	hi image/hi fre	20	20	17*	20
	hi image/lo fre	20	20	19*	20
	lo image/hi fre	20	18*	17*	20
	lo image/lo fre	20	20	13*	17*
	nonwords	80	68*	69	64*
9	Repetition, words	80	65 (81.3)	49 (61.3)	70 (87.5)
	hi image/hi fre	20	18*	16*	19
	hi image/lo fre	20	17*	13*	20
	lo image/hi fre	20	14*	12*	16*
	lo image/lo fre	20	15*	9*	15*
9	Repetition, nonwords	80	44* (55)	10* (12.5)	33* (41.2)
25	Visual lexical decision	120	114 (95)	114 (95)	103 (85.8)
	hi image/hi fre	15	15	15	15
	hi image/lo fre	15	14	14	13*
	lo image/hi fre	15	14	15	13*
	lo image/lo fre	15	13*	13*	11*
	nonwords	60	58	57	51
31	Reading words	80	45 (56.3)	64 (80)	36 (45)
	hi image/hi fre	20	15*	20	16*
	hi image/lo fre	20	12*	17*	14*
	lo image/hi fre	20	8*	15*	3*
	lo image/lo fre	20	10*	12*	5*
	Reading, nonwords (from PALPA 25)	60	7* (11.7)	3* (5)	0/32* (disc.)
	initial sound correct (lexicalisations excluded)		26/53 (49)	2/55 (3.6)	11/32 (34.4)

The table shows absolute number correct and percent correct in parentheses (subtests mainly taken from PALPA, Kay, Lesser, & Coltheart, 1992). Where available, norm data were considered, and a performance was scored as impaired when it was at least two standard deviations below the mean normal score (see Kay et al., 1992).
*Impaired performance.

Written naming was severely impaired in all participants. However, JUE and MCB were sometimes able to retrieve the initial letter of the target word, whereas KCC was severely impaired with mostly totally unrelated responses in written naming.

Underlying functional deficit

There was some mild impairment of semantic processing, particularly for KCC. However, while some degree of semantic impairment may contribute, it seems likely that the anomia in the participants largely resulted from a primarily post-semantic deficit in accessing lexical entries for production.

FACILITATION STUDY

Method

Stimuli. The complete item set consisted of 224 black-and-white line drawings with a mean name agreement of 95% (from 16 language-unimpaired adults). The target

TABLE 4
Background assessments: Semantic processing and picture naming

PALPA test no.	Task	n-items	MCB	KCC	JUE
47	Spoken Word-Picture-Matching	40	38/40 (95)	36/40 (90)	38 (95)
48	Written Word-Picture-Matching	40	38/40 (95)	38/40 (95)	32* (80)
49	Auditory synonym judgements	60	49* (81.7)	41* (68.3)	48* (80)
	high imageability	30	26	22	29
	low imageability	30	23	19	19
50	Written synonym Judgements	60	48* (80)	nt	46* (76.7)
	high imageability	30	26		25
	low imageability	30	22		21
54	Picture naming, written	40	nt	nt	2/20* (disc.)
	Pyramids and Palm Trees Test (Howard & Patterson, 1992, all picture version)	52	46* (88.5)	45* (86.5)	47* (90.4)
	Picture naming, spoken (Lorenz, unpublished)	224	100/224 (44.6)	70/224 (31.3)	114/175 (subtest) (65.1)
	Picture naming, written (Lorenz, unpublished)	42	14/42 (13.33)	0/5 (disc.)	nt

disc. = discontinued, nt = not tested.   The table shows absolute number correct and percent correct in parentheses. Where available, norm data were considered, and a performance was scored as impaired when it was at least two standard deviations below the mean normal score (see Kay et al., 1992).
*Impaired performance.

words had one to three syllables. The mean log frequency was 1.3 (*SD* 0.59, range 0.55–2.86; combined spoken and written lemma-frequency, Celex lexical database, Baayen, Piepenbrock, & van Rijn, 1995). The target words were classified as irregular, regular, or ambiguous according to regularity of orthography-phonology conversion (OPC regularity) for the initial letter. We classified words as *irregular* when the most frequent pronunciation of the first letter in isolation did not correspond to the first phoneme of that word (for example the first *letter*-phoneme conversion in KNIFE is /k/ but the initial phoneme is /n/). Stimuli were classified as *regular* when the phoneme of the initial letter always corresponded to the first phoneme of the word (for example BOTTLE, B→/b/). We classified words as *ambiguous* when the most frequent pronunciation of the initial letter of the word corresponded to the first phoneme of the word, but other correspondences existed for that letter (for example, CAT, C→/k/ but in ceiling, church, C does not correspond to /k/).

Assessments of picture naming. The target pictures were presented in the middle of the screen of a laptop. A time limit of 10 seconds was used in the pre-assessment and the two post-assessments (24 hours post and 1 week post), and a time limit of 6 seconds was used in the facilitation sessions. The first response was analysed. Minor phonological errors (substitution, deletion of one phoneme, singular/plural errors) were counted as correct (cf. Howard et al., 1985; Nickels & Howard, 1995). The Universal Data Acquisition Program (UDAP) was used for the controlled presentation of target pictures and cues (Zierdt, 1998–2005). All naming responses were audio-taped for later analysis.

Pre-assessment. Participants were required to attempt to name in randomised order the set of 224 pictures of objects, which comprised the complete set of treatment and control stimuli. In order to control for stability of naming performance prior to treatment, a pre-treatment baseline of spoken naming was established with MCB and KCC for half of the stimuli (Set B: $N = 112$). JUE also participated in two naming baseline assessments using a subset of stimuli ($N = 143$) prior to treatment.

Facilitation of spoken picture naming. The set of 224 stimuli were divided into matched subsets of stimuli: 112 items that received treatment and 112 controls that received no treatment. Of the treated items, half received phonological cues and half orthographic cues. In both the phonological and the orthographic condition, the initial segment of the target word was presented before the target picture. The letter cues remained on the screen for 600 ms, the duration of the phoneme cues varied between 100 and 450 ms, depending on type of phoneme (plosives around 100 ms, vowels around 450 ms). The target pictures were presented immediately after provision of the cues and remained on the screen for 6 seconds. If a picture could not be named within this time frame, no further help or feedback was given, and the next picture (preceded by its cue) was presented for naming. Similarly, in the control condition, each picture was presented for spoken naming with a time limit of 6 seconds, but no cue was given. No feedback was provided in any of the three conditions.

With MCB and KCC, two short facilitation phases were conducted, consisting of three consecutive sessions each. Half of the items were treated in the first phase and the other half were treated in the second phase. With JUE, only one facilitation phase was conducted using a subset of 175 object pictures. Within each facilitation phase the same items were presented repeatedly over three consecutive sessions in blocked sets. In each session, one set was treated using phonological cues (the first phoneme in the word), another set was treated using orthographic cues (the first letter in the word), and the final set consisted of uncued control pictures ("naming controls"). Furthermore, the order of presentation of conditions (orthographic cue, phonological cue, no cue) was rotated each session in order to minimise possible order effects. In addition to the naming control stimuli that were presented as often as the treated pictures, another set of untreated items was only presented once before and once after the whole facilitation phase ("unseen controls").

The four different sets (phoneme cue, letter cue, naming controls, unseen controls) were matched individually for each participant, considering pre-treatment accuracy of spoken picture naming as well as combined lemma frequency (Baayen et al., 1995), word length (number of phonemes), and animacy (T-test, two-tailed $p > .05$ all comparisons). The latter factors can be significant predictors of word retrieval in aphasic patients (Nickels & Howard, 1995). For KCC and MCB, who received two facilitation phases, matching of items in the four different conditions was done for set A and set B separately. Furthermore, the two facilitation sets and the naming controls each included the same number of irregular, ambiguous, and regular words. The unseen controls each included fewer irregular words than the other sets, other than this all four sets were closely matched according to the above factors. In addition, irregular, ambiguous, and regular subsets of items did not differ according to any of the above factors both within conditions and for the whole set—T-test (two-tailed): $p > .05$ all comparisons (see Table 5).

TABLE 5
Stimulus set

N224 (whole set)							
Set A (N112)				Set B (N112)			
Set A (N56): cued TREATMENT		Set A (N56): uncued CONTROL		Set B (N56): cued TREATMENT		Set B (N56): uncued CONTROL	
Sound- 1 (N28)	Letter- 1 (N28)	Naming control- 1 (N28)	Unseen control- 1 (N28)	Sound-2 (N28)	Letter- 2 (N28)	Naming control- 2 (N28)	Unseen control- 2 (N28)
irreg.: N7	irreg.: N7	irreg.: N7		irreg.: N7	irreg.: N7	irreg.: N7	
ambig.: N7	ambig.: N7	ambig.: N7		ambig.: N7	ambig.: N7	ambig.: N7	
reg.: N14	reg.: N14	reg.: N14		reg.: N14	reg.: N14	reg.: N14	

Post-assessments. All items were named again following treatment to determine any lasting effects of treatment. Effects of treatment were measured in the end of each training session (15–20 minutes after facilitation of picture naming) using both cued and uncued but seen pictures ("naming controls"). A further post-test was done 24 hours after the end of each training phase or three facilitation sessions. Here the whole item set was tested including the unseen control pictures that were not presented during the facilitation sessions. In addition, with MCB and KCC a follow-up test was conducted 1 week after the end of the first facilitation phase (Set A) using the same pictures as in the 24 hours post-test.

RESULTS

Figures 1–5 give proportions of correct responses in spoken naming over time. Both immediate and delayed naming is provided. Furthermore, the effects of phases 1 and 2 are presented separately for MCB and KCC. JUE received only one facilitation phase.

All participants showed a stable pattern in the pre-treatment baseline sessions— for MCB and KCC see Figures 2 and 4: BL_B0 vs BL_B1, for JUE see Figure 5: BL_0 vs BL_1, McNemar exact (two-tailed): $p > .05$ each. Furthermore, naming of set A and set B did not differ significantly for MCB or KCC prior to treatment (see Figures 1 and 3: BL_B0 vs. BL_A0: $p > .05$ each, Fisher exact (two-tailed)).

When not indicated differently, the exact version of the McNemar test (one-tailed) was used for the following analysis of cue effects in the different facilitation sessions, considering both immediate and delayed effects.

MCB and KCC

Both MCB and KCC showed more specific and stronger effects within the first than the second facilitation phase.[1]

Orthographic cues. Within the first phase, both participants profited from the initial letter cue, with significant benefits being present for both immediate and

---

[1] This cannot be attributable to the stimulus items in the two phases because KCC received almost 90% of MCB's set B items in the first phase and vice versa; other than that the different subsets within the phases were individually matched.

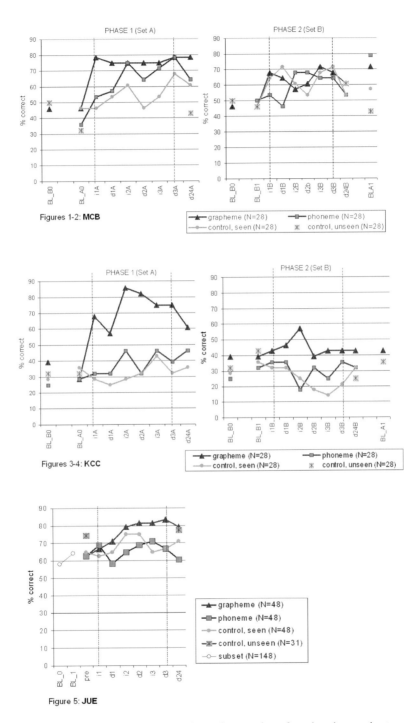

Figures 1–5. Proportion of correct responses in spoken naming of cued and uncued sets over time. BL = baseline; pre = pre-assessment; i1–i3 = immediate effects, sessions 1–3; d1–d3 = delayed effects, sessions 1–3; d24 = delayed effects, 24 hours after end of facilitation phase; A = Set A; B = Set B; BL_A1 = follow-up test 1 week after end of facilitation phase 1 (Set A).

delayed naming in each facilitation session (all at least $p < .01$). Furthermore, in both participants the orthographic cue effect was still present 1 day after the end of this facilitation phase (24 hours post-test: MCB: $p < .01$; KCC: $p < .05$). MCB showed a stable effect 1 week later, whereas KCC's accuracy had dropped back to baseline (1 week post-test: MCB: $p < .05$, KCC: $p > .05$). Furthermore, in KCC, the letter cue effects were stronger in session 2 than session 1, with up to 68% correct in session 1 and 85% correct in session 2. This difference reached significance for delayed effects (session 1 vs 2: immediate: $p > .05$; delayed: $p < .01$). After that, no further improvement was shown in KCC. In MCB, no further improvement was found for the orthographic condition after the first facilitation session.

Phoneme cues. In the first facilitation session the initial phoneme was ineffective in both participants. KCC did not profit from the initial phoneme in any of the following sessions either ($p > .05$ in all sessions). In MCB, the initial phoneme was ineffective in the first facilitation session ($p > .05$), but significant effects of the initial phoneme were present in the second and third session both for immediate and delayed naming (session 2: immediate: $p < .01$; delayed: $p < .05$; session 3: immediate: $p < .01$, delayed: $p < .001$). As for orthographic cues, phonological cue effects were still present 1 day and 1 week later in MCB (24 hours post-test: $p < .05$; 1 week post-test: $p < .001$).

Naming controls. MCB showed a significant improvement with the naming control set in the third facilitation session of phase 1 for delayed naming, but not for immediate naming (session 3: immediate $p > .05$, delayed $p < .05$). Other than that, no effects were present with the naming controls in any of the sessions for MCB. MCB's naming of unseen control pictures remained stable ($p > .05$). KCC did not show any change for seen or unseen control pictures in any of the sessions (both control sets $p > .05$ in all sessions).

For MCB, phase 2 produced fewer specific effects than phase 1. Significant benefits from the initial letter were present in the first and third session but not in the second session (session 1: immediate: $p < .05$, delayed: $p > .05$; session 2: $p > .05$ each; session 3: immediate: $p < .01$, delayed: $p < .05$). No effects were present 1 day after the end of this phase for the initial letter cue (24 hours post: $p > .05$). In contrast to phase 1, no significant effects of the initial phoneme cue were present at all within the second facilitation phase (all sessions: $p > .05$). Furthermore, MCB improved significantly for spoken naming of the naming control pictures within sessions 1 and 3 of the second phase (session 1: immediate $p > .05$, delayed: $p < .05$; session 2: immediate and delayed: $p > .05$ each, session 3: immediate: $p > .05$, delayed: $p < .05$). However, she did not improve with unseen control pictures (unseen control set: $p > .05$).

In contrast to phase 1, no significant benefit of letter cues was found for KCC in phase 2 (all sessions $p > .05$). While naming of the orthographic set remained stable, naming of uncued and phonologically cued pictures even deteriorated. Naming of the orthographic set was significantly better than naming of the phonological set and the control set in the second facilitation session. In the third session this difference remained stable for the control set, but there was no longer a significant difference between phonologically cued and orthographically cued pictures—Fisher exact (two-tailed), session 2: orthographic set vs phonological set: $p < .01$; orthographic set vs control set: $p < .05$; session 3: orthographic set vs phonological set: $p > .05$, orthographic set vs control set: $p < .05$.

JUE. JUE profited significantly from the initial letter in spoken naming. Significant benefits were present within the second and third facilitation session both for immediate and delayed naming, but not within the first session (session 1: $p > .05$ each, session 2: $p < .05$ each; session 3: $p < .01$ each). Furthermore, the orthographic cue effect was still present 1 day later (24 hours post-test: $p < .05$). No further post-assessment was conducted with JUE.

In contrast to the orthographic condition, the initial phoneme cue did not produce any effects, and naming of uncued control pictures remained stable as well (all sessions: initial phoneme cue, naming controls, unseen controls: $p > .05$ each).

SUMMARY OF OVERALL EFFECTS

Both KCC (see phase 1) and JUE specifically benefited from the initial letter and showed no effects of the initial phoneme on spoken naming accuracy. In addition, naming of uncued control pictures remained stable in both participants. Furthermore, the effects were more pronounced in session 2 than session 1 in both participants. The superiority of letter cues was replicated in phase 2 with KCC, although no significant benefit could be found here. However, naming of letter-cued pictures remained stable while naming of phonologically cued pictures or uncued pictures deteriorated.[2]

In contrast to the other participants, MCB profited from both letter and phoneme cues (phase 1). However, letter cues produced significant effects in session 1 (phase 1) whereas she only profited from the initial phoneme cue in the later sessions. With regard to stability of effects, letters and phonemes produced similar improvements for MCB, which were still present 1 week later. In addition, there was some evidence for an improvement with naming control pictures in MCB, despite the fact that these pictures were presented without any cues or feedback. However, since naming of control pictures fell back to baseline in the two post-assessments, both letter and phoneme cue effects can be interpreted as specific effects as the result of this type of information. The second facilitation phase produced fewer benefits for MCB, although letter cue effects were still present. In addition, once again, MCB improved in naming seen control pictures (naming controls) but not with unseen control pictures.

We have documented significant and specific effects, from cueing with the initial letter of the target word, on spoken naming in three participants. How were letter cues effective in our participants?

We discussed above that orthographic cues have been argued to be especially effective in participants who are able to sound out single letters or to read nonwords, which are tasks relying on the sublexical route for written material (e.g., Best et al., 2002; Nickels, 1992). However, all of our participants were impaired both in sounding out single letters and in reading nonwords. Nevertheless, for MCB and JUE there was some evidence that may point to partially preserved processing via the sublexical route (e.g., sounding out the initial letter in nonword reading). However, is

---

[2] KCC did report not sleeping very well during this time because of skin irritation. Probably this explains the absence of any improvement within phase 2.

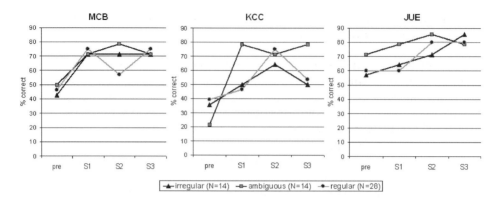

Figures 6–8. Naming of irregular (e.g., KNIFE), ambiguous (e.g., KING), and regular items (e.g., DOLL) in the pre-assessment and immediately after presentation of the letter cue (sessions 1–3). (JUE received only 20 items within the regular set)

that enough to be able to explain the letter cue effects in these participants using orthographic-phonological conversion procedures? A direct lexical mechanism and/ or a lexical-semantic mechanism seem to be possible alternative accounts. In order to investigate this we included words with initial letters that are *irregular* according to orthographic-phonological conversion (as described above). These are stimuli where the first letter of the word, when sounded out, does not correspond to the first phoneme of the same word said aloud. For example, the first letter in CHEF, C, would normally be pronounced "kuh" which does not correspond to the correct first phoneme "sh". Hence, if a patient has better picture naming when a letter cue is given, even when this letter does not correspond to the first phoneme of the word (e.g., C for CHEF), we can be sure that the letter cue is working directly (via the visual input lexicon) and not via conversion to the corresponding phoneme.

Figures 6–8 give proportion of correct responses for regular, irregular, and ambiguous target words in the letter cue condition. For MCB and KCC the data from phases 1 and 2 have been combined. Overall, OPC regularity did not seem to have a very strong impact on letter cue effects in our participants. The overall pattern of letter cue effects did not differ significantly between irregular and regular or ambiguous items for any of the participants—irregular vs regular, irregular vs ambiguous, ambiguous vs regular: $p > .05$ each, Wilcoxon two sample test (two-tailed).

DISCUSSION

We have documented specific effects of orthographic cues on spoken naming in three people with anomia. In all participants, both immediate and delayed benefits for naming were found after presentation of the initial letter of the target. Two of the participants showed pure orthographic cueing effects: they profited only from letter cues but not from phoneme cues (KCC and JUE). Similarly the third participant (MCB) profited from letter cues alone in the first facilitation session. However, in the following sessions both types of cues produced similar and long-lasting effects (1 week).

This led us to the conclusion that the effects of letter cues do not rely on the same processing mechanisms as phonological cues. In contrast to the arguments of Bruce and Howard (1988), letter cues can be effective even in participants who cannot profit from phoneme cues.

In addition, we found that not all cueing effects were apparent in the first facilitation session. For example, JUE profited significantly from letter cues in the second and third session, but there were no effects in the first session. Similarly, for MCB no phonological cue effect was present in the first session, but an effect did occur in the following sessions. Furthermore, in KCC the letter cue effect was significantly stronger in the second than the first session. These results make it clear that effects of a single application of a cue do not necessarily indicate whether this type of information might be an effective cue when applied over a longer period of time.

The results of Best et al. (2002), who examined the effects of a cue after a single facilitation session, contrast with our findings. They found that there was no significant difference between the efficacy of orthographic and phonological cues when their patients were analysed as a group. However, on the other hand they argued that phonological and orthographic cues rely on different mechanisms for their effects. Phonological cues were argued to work via the lexical system, and orthographic cues via the sublexical system (Best et al., 2002).

In two of our participants phonological cues were totally ineffective. One reason could be that the cues were presented by a computer program and without any mouth-shape information. In contrast, in many other studies phoneme cues have been presented by the experimenter. In this case, mouth-shape information is usually also provided and hence no pure phoneme cue effects are assessed. Probably the addition of mouth-shape information allows for stronger effects than the presentation of pure phoneme cues in our study. It is unlikely that impaired auditory analysis of single phonemes could account for the lack of efficacy of phonological cues for JUE and KCC: neither had a deficit on the auditory discrimination task. Furthermore, JUE was only mildly impaired in the repetition of single phonemes (without mouth-shape information), although KCC was moderately impaired. As discussed above, Best et al. (2002) argued for a lexical (but non-semantic) mechanism of effectiveness for phoneme cues. Could this lexical mechanism be impaired for JUE and KCC? They both showed impaired word repetition, although it was significantly better than repetition of nonwords, suggesting some use of a lexical route.

However, both participants' word repetition was influenced by imageability, which leads to the assumption that word repetition relied mainly on the lexical-semantic route. Interestingly MCB, who profited significantly from phonological cues, did not show a significant effect of imageability in word repetition. Perhaps then, for MCB, phonological cues are effective by a "direct" lexical route from phonological input lexical representations to the phonological output lexicon (which may or not be via lemmas) and not the lexical-semantic route. This direct lexical route seems to be impaired in JUE and KCC but was partially preserved in MCB, resulting in benefit from phonological cues for MCB but not for JUE and KCC. However, while MCB failed to have a significant imageability effect, her overall word repetition accuracy was similar to JUE, and somewhat better for nonwords. Could her superior nonword repetition (compared to JUE and KCC) indicate that a sublexical route might contribute to the efficacy of cues? This is not what Best et al.'s data suggest, and indeed the fact that JUE and MCB showed similar accuracy for repetition of single phonemes (but JUE did not show any benefit from phonological cues) also makes this account less plausible. Hence, we suggest that a lexical or lexical-semantic mechanism is most likely, but still need to explain why this route is not effective for JUE, who shows a similar degree of impairment. We will discuss this further below.

With regard to the underlying functional mechanisms of effectiveness of orthographic cues, different accounts have been pointed out in the literature. The most prevalent account is that letter cues are effective by reliance on the sublexical route for written material (orthographic-phonological conversion). According to this theory, the patient would create his or her own phonological cue by sounding out the initial letter of the target word (e.g., Bachy-Langedock & de Partz, 1989; Bastiaanse, Bosje, & Franssen, 1996; Bruce & Howard, 1988; Nickels, 1992). If self-generated phonological cues work in the same way as provided phonological cues, letter cues (=self-generated phonological cues) should only be effective in participants who profit from (provided) phonological cues. However, our data do not support this assumption (see above). Following this, it seems quite likely that either self-generated cues work differently from presented phoneme cues or letter cues become effective without mediation from the corresponding phoneme.

All of our participants were severely impaired in nonword reading, but for MCB and JUE there was some evidence for partial functioning of the sublexical OPC route (49% and 34% initial phonemes correct). However, there was no evidence for preserved sublexical processing in KCC (only 3.5% initial phonemes correct in nonword reading). In addition, letter cue effects were not strongly influenced by OPC regularity of the initial letter of our target words. A similar overall pattern of cue effects was observed with words starting with regular (e.g., DOLL, D → /d/) and irregular letters (e.g., KNIFE, K → /k/, but not /n/). Hence, we would suggest that at least part of the letter-cueing effects in our participants rely on direct lexical or lexical-semantic processes.

However, word reading was mildly to moderately impaired in our participants, with strong imageability effects in all participants. Semantic paralexias were produced by JUE and MCB but not by KCC, who produced mainly no-responses (but only with low-imageability words). It is quite obvious that all participants used the lexical-semantic route in word reading, accounting for imageability effects in reading. Following this logic, we should conclude that the underlying mechanism of effectiveness for letter cues is the lexical-semantic route.

We have concluded that both types of cues had their effects mainly by lexical rather than sub-lexical processing routines. However, for phoneme cues we suggest that the mechanism is ineffective for JUE and KCC, and yet for letter cues we have argued that this same mechanism is effective. Can we justify this seeming contradiction—the same mechanism being effective in one modality (written – letter cues) but not in the other (spoken – phonemic cues)?

Why were phoneme cues totally ineffective in JUE and KCC whereas letter cues produced strong effects? For KCC it may be a matter of degree of impairment. He shows greater impairments on auditory tasks than written tasks at several levels: auditory lexical decision is more impaired than visual lexical decision, and word repetition is more impaired than word reading (see Table 3). Hence, KCC has a greater impairment to lexical and semantic access from the auditory modality than from the written modality. It follows then that an auditorily presented phoneme cue will be less effective than a visually presented letter cue, even if the same underlying mechanisms are involved. For JUE this account cannot hold; if anything, she had better processing of auditory word forms than written word forms. However, we would argue that the nature of the cue itself may account for the difference. We presented our written cues for 600 ms, whereas the spoken cues lasted for shorter periods of time. Hence the longer presentation duration for written cues may result in stronger activation within the lexical system than spoken cues, and this may be the case even when the underlying functional processes are more impaired for the written than the spoken modality. A further contributing factor may be impaired auditory-verbal short-term memory (AVSTM; e.g., an impaired phonological input buffer), which would prevent refreshing of the activation of the phonological cue. Many aphasic individuals have co-occurring AVSTM impairments, one symptom of which is impaired nonword repetition (as shown by JUE). In contrast, visual memory is often less impaired. While not tested in our patients, such a dissociation would also predict greater effectiveness for letter cues compared to phonological cues.

In conclusion, letter cues have been relatively neglected in the clinical arena, with phonemic cues having precedence. Our data suggest that this is misguided and that clinicians should look to letter cues as a tool for facilitating word production, even in those individuals who show little response to phonemic cues, and regardless of sublexical transcoding abilities for print.

REFERENCES

Baayen, R. H., Piepenbrock, R., & van Rijn, H. (1995) *The Celex Lexical Database* [CD-ROM]. Philadelphia, PA, Linguistic data consortium.

Bachy-Langedock, N., & Partz, M.-P. (1989). Coordination of two reorganisation therapies in a deep dyslexic patient with oral naming disorder. In X. Seron & G. Deloche (Eds.), *Cognitive approaches in neuropsychological rehabilitation* (pp. 211–247). Hillsdale, NJ: Lawrence Erlbaum Associates, Inc.

Basso, A., Marangolo, P., Piras, F., & Galluzi, C. (2001). Acquisition of new "words" in normal participants: A suggestion for the treatment of anomia. *Brain and Language, 77,* 45–59.

Bastiaanse, R., Bosje, M., & Franssen, M. (1996). Deficit-oriented treatment of word-finding problems: Another replication. *Aphasiology, 10,* 363–383.

Best, W., Herbert, R., Hickin, J., Osborne, F., & Howard, D. (2002). Phonological and orthographic facilitation of word-retrieval in aphasia: Immediate and delayed effects. *Aphasiology, 16,* 151–168.

Bruce, C., & Howard, D. (1988). Why don't Broca's aphasics cue themselves? An investigation of phonemic cueing and tip of the tongue information. *Neuropsychologia, 26,* 253–264.

Hickin, J., Herbert, R., Best, W., & Howard, D. (2002). Phonological therapy for word finding difficulties: A re-evaluation. *Aphasiology, 16,* 981–999.

Howard, D. (2003). Single cases, group studies and case series in aphasia therapy. In I. Papathanasiou & R. De Bleser (Eds.), *The sciences of aphasia: From therapy to theory* (pp. 245–258). Oxford, UK: Elsevier Science Ltd.

Howard, D., & Harding, D. (1998). Self-cueing of word retrieval by a woman with aphasia: Why a letter board works. *Aphasiology, 12,* 399–420.

Howard, D., & Patterson, K. E. (1992). *Pyramids and Palm Trees.* Bury St. Edmunds, UK: Thames Valley Test Company.

Howard, D., Patterson, K. E., Franklin, S., Orchard-Lisle, V., & Morton, J. (1985). The facilitation of picture naming in aphasia. *Cognitive Neuropsychology, 2,* 49–80.

Kay, J., Lesser, R., & Coltheart, M. (1992). *Psycholinguistic assessment of language processes in aphasia (PALPA).* Hove, UK: Lawrence Erlbaum Associates Ltd.

Lorenz, A. (2004). *Die Behandlung von Wortabrufstörungen bei Aphasie: Eine methodenvergleichende Studie zum Bildbenennen.* Dissertation. 1-265, Universität Potsdam. (http://pub.ub.uni-potsdam.de/volltexte/2005/183/).

Monsell, S. (1987). On the relation between lexical input and output pathways for speech. In A. Allport, D. MacKay, W. Prinz, & E. Scheerer (Eds.), *Language perception and production: Relationships between listenings, speaking, reading and writing* (pp. 273–311). London: Academic Press.

Nickels, L. A. (1992). The autocue? Self-generated phonemic cues in the treatment of a disorder of reading and naming. *Cognitive Neuropsychology, 9,* 155–182.

Nickels, L. (2002). Therapy for naming disorders: Revisiting, revising, and reviewing. *Aphasiology, 16,* 935–979.

Nickels, L., & Howard, D. (1995). Aphasic naming: What matters? *Neuropsychologia, 33,* 1281–1303.

Patterson, K. E., Purell, C., & Morton, J. (1983). Facilitation of word retrieval in aphasia. In C. Code & D. J. Müller (Eds.), *Aphasia Therapy* (pp. 76–87). London: Edward Arnold.

Wambaugh, J. L., Linebaugh, C. W., Doyle, P. J., Martinez, A. L., Kalinyak-Fliszar, M., & Spencer, K. A. (2001). Effects of two cueing treatments on lexical retrieval in aphasic speakers with different levels of deficit. *Aphasiology, 15,* 933–950.

Zierdt, A. (1998–2005). *Universal Data Acquisition Program (UDAP) V3.22.* Clinical Neuropsychology Research Group (EKN), City Hospital Bogenhausen, Munich, Germany.

APHASIOLOGY, 2007, 21 (6/7/8), 687–701

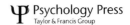

Longitudinal study of reading and writing rehabilitation using a bigraph–biphone correspondence approach

Kelly Bowes and Nadine Martin

Temple University, Philadelphia, PA, USA

Background: Treatments for sound-blending ability in phonological dyslexia that train single grapheme–phoneme correspondences have had mixed success. A more recent approach to re-establishing sound-blending abilities is to train correspondences of bigraph–biphone units (CV + VC = CVC) (Berndt, Haendiges, Mitchum & Wayland, 1996; Friedman & Lott, 2002). This approach has proved beneficial thus far, although the reasons for its success are not yet fully understood.

Aims: The purpose of this longitudinal investigation was to use the bigraph–biphone segment-blending approach to improve both reading and writing abilities in an individual with phonological dyslexia/dysgraphia. Re-establishing this ability laid the foundation for continued treatment with longer words and phrases.

Methods & Procedures: A case study design combining reading and writing treatment was used in three treatment protocols. Initially, treatment focused on improving the participant's awareness of bigraph–biphone correspondences and sound-blending abilities for one-syllable nonwords. The successful completion of this protocol was followed by two treatments to extend these abilities to reading and writing two-syllable words and eventually phrase-length material.

Outcomes & Results: Gains were made in all treatment protocols. The participant progressed from an inability to read one-syllable nonwords to reading and writing phrase-length material.

Conclusions: This study provides further evidence that using bigraph–biphone correspondences to train sound-blending abilities can improve both reading and writing abilities in cases of phonological dyslexia. Furthermore, the success of this treatment programme illustrates the benefit of a targeted treatment programme even 5 years post onset of aphasia, for reading and writing rehabilitation.

Acquired dyslexia and dysgraphia present unique challenges to both participants and clinicians. Recovery of reading and writing skills following brain injury can be critical for return to functional independence. This need highlights the importance of developing effective remediation strategies for adults with acquired reading and writing disorders. We report a longitudinal treatment study of an individual with acquired phonological dyslexia and dysgraphia. A cardinal feature of this syndrome

Address correspondence to: Kelly Bowes, Center for Cognitive Neuroscience, Department of Communication Sciences, Temple University, Weiss Hall Room 110, 1701 North 13th Street, Philadelphia, PA 19122, USA. E-mail: Kbowes@temple.edu

Many thanks to MQ for her enthusiasm and diligence during this project. We also thank Lianne DiMarco MA, SLP, Francine Kohen MS, CCC/SLP, James Reilly PhD, CCC/SLP, and Michelene Kalinyak-Fliszar MS, CCC/SLP for their assistance during this project. This study was supported by Dean's Research Incentive Award, 2003 (College of Health Professions, Temple University) and NIDCD Grant DC01924-11 awarded to Temple University (PI: Nadine Martin).

http://www.psypress.com/aphasiology DOI: 10.1080/02687030701192117

is the inability to read or write nonwords, reflecting an impairment of learned correspondences between graphemes and phonemes. Additionally, reading and writing is affected by the imageability of words (high better than low) and grammatical category (nouns and adjectives better than verbs and functors).

Models of reading and writing (e.g., Coltheart, Patterson, & Marshall, 1980) postulate lexical and sublexical routes of word processing. The lexical route processes words as whole units and enables reading of irregularly as well as regularly spelled words. This route is influenced by lexical and semantic factors. The sublexical or phonological route processes oral reading of written words via grapheme–phoneme correspondences. This route enables the reading of novel words via these direct correspondences. Impairment to the lexical route leads to a dependence on the sublexical route, resulting in an impaired ability to read or write irregularly spelled words (surface dyslexia/dysgraphia). Impairment to the sublexical route (phonological dyslexia/dysgraphia) leads to a dependence on the lexical route to read and write, increasing influence of lexical-semantic factors on word reading and impairment of nonword reading. A third syndrome, deep dyslexia/dysgraphia, shares the features of phonological dyslexia, with the addition of semantic errors. This disorder has been postulated to be a more severe form of phonological dyslexia/dysgraphia (Friedman, 1996; Glosser & Friedman, 1990).

Treatments of both phonological and deep dyslexia/dysgraphia begin with re-establishment of the ability to link graphemes with their corresponding phonemes. There have been several reports of treatments that succeed at this stage (e.g., dePartz, 1986; Laine & Niemi, 1990; Mitchum & Berndt, 1991; Nickels, 1992). The second stage of remediation involves re-establishing the ability to blend sounds together into syllables. The use of single grapheme–phoneme correspondences to train sound blending has yielded mixed results. The participant in dePartz's (1986) study learned to blend single grapheme–phoneme correspondences into words after considerable practice. Other attempts have not been as successful (e.g., Laine & Niemi, 1990). The participants in Mitchum and Berndt's (1991) and Nickel's (1992) studies learned to produce consonant-vowel (CV) and vowel-consonant (VC) blends, but not CVC combinations. Both Laine and Niemi (1990) and Mitchum and Berndt (1996) suggested that the limited short-term memory (STM) of their participants prevented them from maintaining the phonemes long enough to blend them together.

The difficulty in re-establishing sound-blending abilities was addressed in a study by Berndt et al. (1996). They tested 11 participants, 5 with aphasia and phonological dyslexia and 6 controls, in a variety of word and nonword reading tasks. In one experiment, they compared phoneme blending and CV-VC segment blending. All the participants with phonological dyslexia performed significantly better with the CV-VC segment blending.

Friedman and Lott (2002) adapted Berndt et al.'s (1996) bigraph–biphone correspondences approach to sound blending in a treatment study of two individuals, LR and KT, who each presented with moderate nonfluent aphasia and deep dyslexia. There were three training sets, each comprising consonant-vowel bigraphs (CVs), vowel-consonant bigraphs (VCs), and consonant-vowel-consonant words (CVCs) matched for part of speech and frequency. In each training set, CVs were trained first and were followed by VCs and CVCs. Treatment for the bigraphs involved pairing the target bigraph with a "relay" word that began with that bigraph. Words were trained by presenting the written word on flashcards and instructing the participant to repeat the CV-VC in "rapid succession" until it blended to sound like a word. Both participants reached criterion on all trained bigraphs and words. Improvements on trained bigraphs did not generalise to untrained bigraphs, but generalisation was observed from trained to untrained words comprised of the trained bigraphs.

Friedman and Lott (2002) note that this approach may be more successful than using single grapheme–phoneme correspondences because it is easier to blend syllables than sounds. But what makes it easier? One possibility is that blending syllables is more natural and closer to the actual pronunciation of a word (/pæ/ - /æt/) than blending single grapheme–phoneme correspondences, which can include a schwa following each consonant (/pə- /æ/- /tə). Limitations in short-term memory may also preclude maintaining activation of three phonemes long enough to blend them together. Other possible factors that have varied considerably across studies of treatments for phonological dyslexia are length of treatment time, type of aphasia, and severity of aphasia.

Here we report a study of the bigraph–biphone sound-blending approach applied to rehabilitation of the reading and writing abilities of a single participant, MQ, with acquired phonological dyslexia. We follow the approach of Friedman and Lott generally, but have extended it, in that we use nonwords in training rather than real words in order to discourage our participant from relying on lexical strategies to read. After mastering CV and VC blending in one-syllable nonwords, MQ progressed to reading and writing two-syllable words and eventually phrase-length material. In the General Discussion, we offer some possible reasons why this approach worked so well with MQ.

METHOD

Participant

MQ, a 45-year-old, right-handed female, experienced an acute left CVA in May 2000, involving the left frontal and parietal lobes and insular cortex. She had been employed as a sports writer with a local newspaper. After discharge from a rehabilitation hospital, MQ was enrolled in outpatient speech therapy for 8 months. MQ remains employed by the same newspaper, but her duties have been modified to accommodate her aphasia and restricted reading and writing abilities.

MQ enrolled in this study 2.8 years post-onset, at which time she presented with chronic output conduction aphasia. Measures of her language functioning (Table 1) indicated relatively intact semantic abilities and significantly impaired output phonological abilities. Her reading was best characterised as phonological dyslexia, and writing as phonological dysgraphia. The critical pattern in this syndrome is superior word reading compared to nonword reading. MQ exhibited impaired oral reading of words as well as nonwords, although her word reading was superior (Table 2).

Procedure

Design. A case study design with pretest, baseline, and post-test was used. Three treatment programmes aimed at improving MQ's ability to read and write nonwords, words, phrases, and sentences were administered over a 3-year period from 2003 to 2005.

TABLE 1
Measures of MQ's language processing

	Raw score	Percentage correct
Tests of semantic comprehension		
Boston Naming Test[1]	23/60	.38
Philadelphia Naming Test[2]	96/175	.55
Peabody Picture Vocabulary Test – Form L[3]		
Raw	144	
Standard Score	85	
Philadelphia Comprehension Battery[4]		
Lexical Comprehension	44/44	1.00
Synonymy Judgments Noun/Verb	29/30	.97
Synonymy Judgments Concrete/Abstract[4]	44/48	.92
Pyramids and Palm Trees Test[5]		
Picture	49/52	.94
Written	50/52	.96
Short Term Memory Span[6]		
Pointing Digits	3.3	
Pointing Words	3.0	
Repetition Digits	3.3	
Repetition Words	3.0	
Nonverbal	5.8	
Tests of phonological processing		
Rhyme Judgement[6]		
Word Pairs	53/64	.83
Nonword Pairs	58/64	.91
Philadelphia Repetition Test[2]	127/175	.73
Repetition – One Word[6]	51/60	.85
Repetition – One Pseudoword[6]	16/60	.27
Phoneme Discrimination (no interval)[6]		
Word	79/80	.99
Nonword	79/80	.99
Phoneme Discrimination (5 second filled interval)[6]		
Word	77/80	.96
Nonword	71/80	.89
Auditory Lexical Decision[6]		
Word	171/180	.95
Nonword	171/180	.95

[1]Kaplan, Goodglass & Weintraub (1983). [2]Dell, Martin & Schwartz (in press). [3]Dunn & Dunn (1981). [4]Saffran, Schwartz, Linebarger, Martin & Bochetto (1988). [5]Howard & Patterson (1992). [6]Martin, Schwartz & Kohen (2006).

Background language assessment. Semantic comprehension and phonological-processing abilities were tested using a battery of published tests and tests developed by our research group before treatment was initiated (Table 1). These measures indicate relatively preserved semantic processing, mild impairment of MQ's input phonological abilities, and more severe impairment of her output phonological processing abilities. In tasks such as reading, repetition, and naming, MQ's primary errors are phonological. For examples of MQ's naming and repetition errors, see Schwartz, Dell, Martin, Gahl, and Sobel (2006) and Dell, Martin, and Schwartz (in press). Span measures indicate impairment on verbal span tasks.

TABLE 2
Selected measures from the PALPA pre and post Treatment Protocol 1

	Pre-Treatment Protocol 1		Post-Treatment Protocol 1	
PALPA 22: Letter Naming & Sounding				
See Letter/Name Sound	.85		.96	
Hear Letter/Name Sound	.85		.92	
PALPA 23: Spoken Letter–Written Letter Matching				
	.73		.88	
PALPA 36: Nonwords	*Write*	*Read*		
3 Letter	0	.67		
4 Letter	.33	.67		
5 Letter	0	.50		
6 Letter	0	.67		
PALPA 29: Letter Length	*Write*	*Read*	*Write*	*Read*
3 Letter	1.0	1.0	1.0	1.0
4 Letter	1.0.	1.0	1.0	1.0
5 Letter	1.0	1.0	1.0	1.0
6 Letter	.50	1.0	.67	1.0
PALPA 30: Syllable Length	*Write*	*Read*	*Write*	*Read*
1 Syllable	.88	1.0	1.0	1.0
2 Syllable	.63	.50	.88	.88
3 Syllable	.75	.38	.38	.75
PALPA 31: Imageability and Frequency				
High Imageability	.75	.78	.78	.93
Low Imageability	.38	.33	.63	.55
High Frequency	.45	.48	.83	.75
Low Frequency	.53	.63	.58	.73
PALPA 32: Grammatical Class				
Nouns	.65	.50	.55	.65
Adjectives	.65	.75	.70	.80
Verbs	.65	.65	.68	.85
Functors	.50	.50	.60	.60
PALPA 35: Spelling–Sound Regularity				
Regular	.67	.70	.77	.87
Exception	.69	.57	.72	.76
PALPA 37: Sentences				
Reversible		.47		
Non-reversible		.63		

Background testing of reading and writing. Before treatment was initiated, MQ's reading and writing abilities were assessed using the *Psycholinguistic Assessment of Language Processing in Aphasia* (PALPA, Kay, Lesser, & Coltheart, 1992) (Table 2) and the *Reading Comprehension Battery for Aphasia* (RCBA, LaPointe & Horner, 1998). The results are summarised below.

Grapheme–phoneme knowledge. MQ had moderate difficulty producing a sound when the sound's corresponding letter was presented both visually and auditorily.

Oral reading and writing. Both of these abilities were impaired, but writing was more severely impaired. MQ demonstrated imageability effects but frequency and length effects were inconsistent. Oral sentence reading was poor. Three months prior to enrolling in this treatment programme, MQ's nonword reading, varied for letter length, was assessed (PALPA 36). As part of the background assessment for this study, we administered the comparable letter-length reading task (PALPA 29). Although the tests were not administered concurrently, neither was administered in acute stages of recovery. A comparison of performance on these two measures indicates a clear disparity between word (1.0) and nonword (.63) reading. The characteristics of MQ's reading and writing (imageability effects, length effects, lexical effects) are most consistent with that of phonological dyslexia and dysgraphia, which are part of a more general deficit in phonological processing that affects output (repetition, naming) more than input (phonological discrimination, rhyming).

Reading comprehension. MQ scored perfectly or near perfectly on all subtests of the Reading Comprehension Battery for Aphasia (RCBA; LaPointe & Horner, 1998) with exception to the morpho-syntax subtest (.60 correct). These results, indicating impaired oral reading of words and near perfect reading comprehension, further implicate the locus of impairment as output phonological processing.

TREATMENT PROTOCOLS AND RESULTS

Overview

Initially, treatment focused on improving MQ's awareness of grapheme–phoneme correspondences and sound-blending abilities for one-syllable nonwords. The successful completion of this protocol was followed by two treatments to extend these abilities to reading and writing two-syllable words and phrase-length material. For all three treatment protocols, a baseline was established before training began, all trained and control items were probed at the beginning of each session to track progress, items were trained until a criterion of 90% accuracy was reached over two consecutive sessions, and training of writing immediately followed training of reading. Writing treatment involved the same words that were trained in reading, but with a new baseline measure. During all treatment sessions, modelling was provided when needed, and practice on a trained item continued until MQ was accurate. We compared performance on initial and final baselines separately from a comparison of final baseline and post-test scores using McNemar and Binomial tests of change (the latter used when expected frequencies are less than 10; Siegel, 1956). In Treatment Protocols 2 and 3a, we compared performance on the pretest used to select items for training and control sets with final baseline. These statistical comparisons are noted in the results of each protocol. The initial baseline served as the pretest for Treatment Protocols 1 and 3b. Because MQ often made several attempts at a response, only scores for final responses are reported. Initially, training sessions were 1 hour, three times per week, and later twice per week due to scheduling conflicts. MQ was not involved in other treatment studies. The treatment descriptions and results are reported below.

Treatment 1: Rehabilitation of sound-blending abilities using bigraph–biphone correspondences

This was a replication and extension of Friedman and Lott (2002). MQ relied on a lexical reading strategy that often resulted in incorrect guesses when reading words aloud. We therefore began training with one-syllable nonwords to discourage use of this lexical strategy. Bigraph units (CV and VC) of the nonwords were linked to corresponding biphones and used to train sound-blending abilities. Two sets of stimuli were developed, one with CVC words and nonwords and the other with

CCVC and CVCC words and nonwords. Four vowels were used in each training set (eight altogether). Each set contained 30 nonwords for training and 30 control items (15 nonwords and 15 real words) matched for CV structure. Reading training involved the following steps:

1. Consonants and vowels in the training set were reviewed.
2. A flashcard with a CV or VC representation from a trained nonword was presented for oral reading (e.g., BE, EK). Limitless trials were allowed before MQ moved onto the next bigraph.
3. A new flashcard in which bigraphs of the nonword and the nonword as a whole appeared. MQ orally read each bigraph separately before blending them together to form the nonword.
4. CCVC items were trained in the same way but using trigraphs and bigraphs (e.g., GRI, IB).

   Writing training involved the following steps:

1. Consonants and vowels in the training set were reviewed.
2. Spoken biphones (e.g., /bɛ/ɛk/) from a trained nonword were presented for MQ to write. If a bigraph was incorrect after two attempts without a self-correction, the bigraph was explained and written for her. MQ was encouraged to repeat the bigraph as she wrote it.
3. The spoken nonword (e.g., /bɛk/) was presented for MQ to write. The first bigraph was written first, then the second, and finally the nonword as a whole. MQ was encouraged to orally produce the bigraphs and nonword as she was writing them.

   CCVC items were trained in the same way as CVC items, but using biphones and triphones.

Results: Treatment Protocol 1. Reading CVC nonwords. MQ reached criterion on the first CVC set before treatment was initiated. Following this remarkable improvement, we developed a second set of CVC nonwords with different vowels (see Figure 1a). A rising baseline stabilised after eight sessions (high score .73). Change from the first (.50) to last (.67) baseline tended towards significance (Binomial Test, $p < .09$). Once treatment was initiated, MQ's accuracy improved significantly to .97 after 8 treatment sessions (Binomial Test, $p < .02$) and control items improved from .67 to .93 (too few items for statistical test). Scores were maintained at an 8-month follow up.

Writing CVC nonwords. MQ found this task to be very difficult and after 14 sessions treatment was terminated on the first set of training items without reaching criterion. With the new set of CVC items, MQ achieved a stable baseline in five sessions (Figure 1b), with a high score of .93. Once treatment was initiated, MQ's accuracy improved from .83 at final baseline to .93 in six treatment sessions. Control items improved from .87 to 1.00. These changes were not statistically significant (Binomial Test, $p < .188$). At a 4.5-month follow-up, accuracy rate for trained items was .90.

Reading CVCC and CCVC nonwords. MQ achieved a stable baseline in six sessions (.77; change from first to final baseline not significant, Binomial Test, $p < .172$). She had a high baseline score of .90. Once treatment was initiated, MQ's accuracy

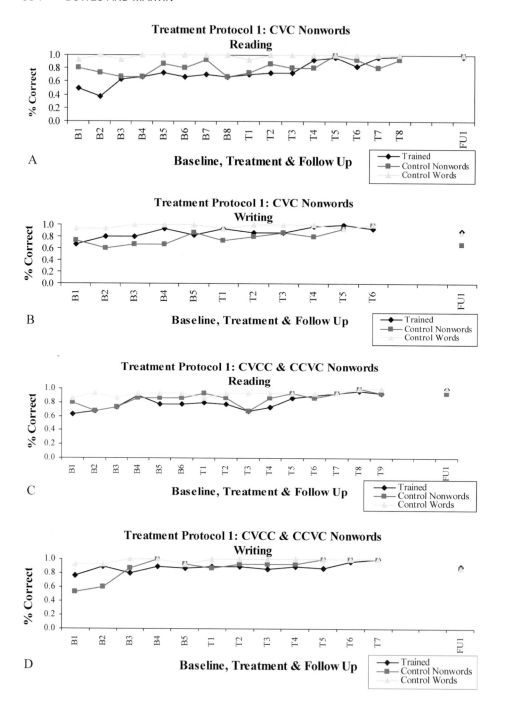

Figure 1. Treatment Protocol 1. Graphs of percent correct during baseline, treatment, and follow-up.

improved to .93 (a change that tended towards significance, Binomial Test, $p < .09$) in nine treatment sessions (Figure 1c). Control items improved from .87 to .93 (too few items for statistical comparison). At follow-up 5.5 months later, accuracy for trained items increased to 1.00.

Writing CVCC and CCVC nonwords. MQ achieved a stable baseline in five sessions (.87), with a high score of .90 (nonsignificant change from first to final baseline: Binomial Test, $p < .363$). Once treatment was initiated, MQ's accuracy improved to 1.00 (too few items for statistical comparison) in seven treatment sessions (Figure 1d). Control items improved from .93 to 1.00. At a 1-month follow-up, accuracy rate for trained items was .90. MQ also made improvements on the PALPA (Table 2).

Treatment 2: Extension of Treatment Protocol 1 to two-syllable words

This treatment protocol introduced two-syllable words with CVCVC, CVVCVC, and CVCCVC structures. A set of 180 concrete and abstract words varied for frequency (range 1–472, Francis & Kucera, 1982) was generated. A total of 80 words that MQ was unable to read or write consistently were chosen as trained and untrained items (40 each). However, due to the high scores of the untrained items, they could not be used for control comparison. Reading training involved the following steps:

1) Consonant clusters and vowels in the training set were reviewed.
2) A flash card was presented with three versions of the same word in descending order:

    (a)   the word divided into three bigraphs (e.g., CA – ME – EL);
    (b)   the word divided into CV - CVC (or CVV- CV-VC, CV-VC-CV-VC) form (e.g., CA – MEL);
    (c)   the word as a whole (e.g., CAMEL).

3) Each version of the word was shown alone with the other versions concealed from view. MQ read aloud each version progressing from bigraphs to syllables and then to the whole word.

   Writing training involved the following steps:

1. Spoken biphones were presented one at a time (e.g., /kæ/, /mɛ/, and /ɛl/) to write.
2. Spoken syllables were presented (e.g., /kæ/, /mɛl/) for MQ to write.
3. The spoken word was presented (e.g., "/kæmɛl/") for MQ to write.

Results: Treatment Protocol 2. Reading. From pretest to final baseline, MQ's accuracy on trained items improved from .33 to .43, with a high baseline score of .45. This change was not significant, $\chi^2(1) = 1.563$, $p < .30$. MQ's accuracy improved significantly from final baseline (.43) to .93 after six treatment sessions, $\chi^2(1) = 18.05$, $p < .001$ (Figure 2a). Scores for untrained items changed from .88 to .95. Accuracy at follow-up testing was .88 at 3 months and .95 at 13 months.

Writing. MQ's accuracy on items chosen for training was zero at the 180-item pretest. Reading treatment always preceded writing treatment and the same words were used in reading and writing protocols. It is interesting to note that MQ's baseline on writing these words increased from zero at pretesting to .73 correct (with a high baseline score of .83) by the time writing training was initiated. Thus, her ability to write these words improved considerably as a consequence of the reading

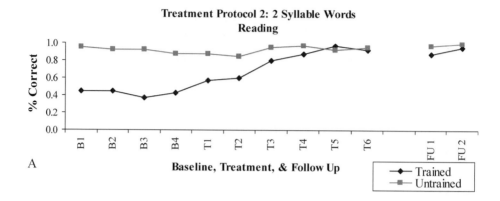

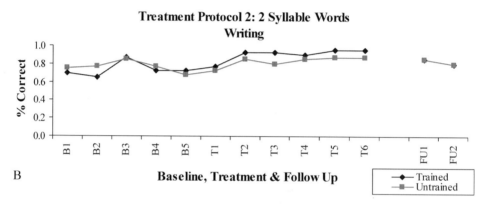

Figure 2. Treatment Protocol 2: Two-syllable words. Graphs of percent correct during baseline, treatment, and follow-up.

training. Once treatment began, MQ's accuracy increased further to .95 after six sessions (Figure 2b). Untrained items also improved from initial pretesting score of zero to .68 at baseline and to .88 correct at treatment's end. Improvements in accuracy were significant from pretest to final baseline, $\chi^2(1) = 27.03$. $p < .001$, and from final baseline to post-test, $\chi^2(1) = 5.818$, $p < .02$. Follow-up tests at 1 month and 13 months resulted in lower scores on trained items, but above final baseline (.85 and .80 respectively).

Treatment 3: Extension of Treatment Protocol 2 to noun-verb/verb-noun phrases and noun-verb/verb-noun plus prepositional phrases

Two-syllable nouns from the 180-item pretest in Treatment Protocol 2 that were inconsistently accurate and not used as trained or untrained items, were paired with verbs to make 48 noun-verb phrases (e.g., "the model struts") and verb-noun phrases (e.g., "prepare the lesson"). Verbs were not controlled for frequency. A baseline was established for the 48 items (25 trained, 23 untrained) before training began. Reading training involved the following steps:

1. Flashcards of the nouns and verbs were presented separately for reading.

2. Emphasis was placed on reading syllable by syllable and blending syllables.
3. Flashcards of the trained phrases were presented for reading.

Writing training involved writing each word of the phrase, emphasising a syllable-by-syllable strategy.

After reading and writing criteria were reached, the phrases were paired with prepositional phrases (e.g., "for the students") to make new, more difficult phrases (e.g., "prepare the lesson for the students"). MQ was familiar with part of the phrase (the noun and verb) and had to learn the new part (prepositions and new nouns). Training for these extended phrases involved the same steps as above.

Results for Treatment Protocol 3: Reading noun-verb and verb-noun phrases. For both reading and writing, it was necessary for MQ to produce the whole phrase accurately in order for it to be scored as correct.

From pretest to final baseline, accuracy improved from .36 to .52, with a high score of .68. This change was not significant (Binomial Test, $p < .70$). A stable baseline was achieved after five probes. MQ then reached criterion within four treatment sessions (Figure 3a). Once training began, her accuracy improved significantly from .52 at final baseline to 1.00 at the end of treatment, $\chi^2(1) = 10.08$, $p < .01$. Untrained items improved from .78 at pretest to .96 at final baseline to 1.00 at the end of treatment (too few items to test change). MQ maintained her accuracy on trained items at a 12-month follow-up (1.00).

Writing noun-verb and verb-noun phrases. MQ achieved a stable baseline on the noun-verb and verb-noun phrases after four sessions. Once treatment was initiated, she reached criterion within four treatment sessions (Figure 3b). Her accuracy was inconsistent from pretest (.48) to initial baseline (.88) to final baseline (.84), with a high baseline score of .92. This difference was significant, $\chi^2(1) = 5.818$, $p < .02$. Due to MQ's ability to improve simply through exposure, this baseline score is quite high (at pretest before reading treatment was initiated, accuracy for trained writing items was .48). Her performance improved to 1.00 by the end of treatment (too few items to test change). Untrained items stayed the same (.96). At an 11-month follow-up, accuracy on trained items decreased (.84), but remained at the final baseline score.

Reading noun-verb and verb-noun with prepositional phrases. A pretest was not administered because the stimuli were the same as in Treatment Protocol 3a but with prepositional phrases added. From initial to final baseline, MQ's accuracy improved from .52 to .56 (with a high score of .68). This difference was not significant. MQ reached criterion within five training sessions. From final baseline, her accuracy improved further to 1.00 at the end of treatment (Figure 3c), $\chi^2(1) = 9.09$, $p < .01$. Untrained items improved from .65 at baseline to .91 at the end of training (too few items to test change). At 9-month follow-up, accuracy diminished slightly (.88).

Writing noun-verb and verb-noun prepositional phrases. MQ's accuracy was inconsistent from initial (.72) to final baseline (.68). There were too few items to test the significance of this change. MQ reached criterion within three training sessions, and her accuracy improved from .68 at baseline to .96 by the end of treatment. This change was not significant (Binomial Test, $p < .172$). Untrained

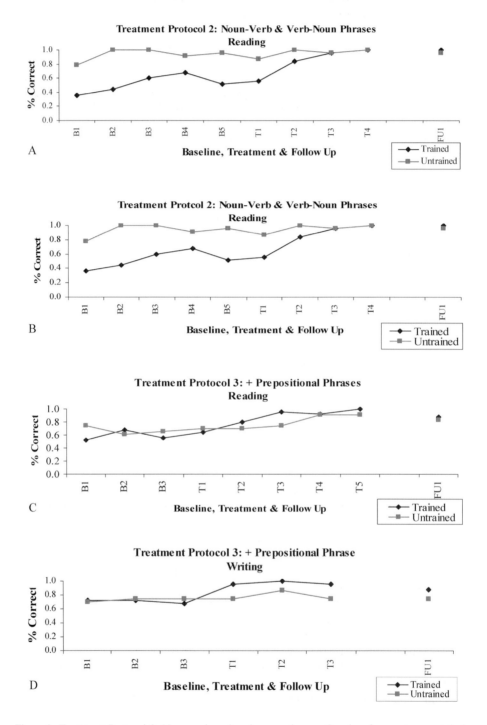

Figure 3. Treatment Protocol 2: Noun-verb and verb-noun phrases. Graphs of percent correct during baseline, treatment, and follow-up.

items remained steady throughout treatment. Accuracy rate for trained items was .88 at 8.5-months follow-up.

GENERAL DISCUSSION

Before treatment, MQ's grapheme–phoneme conversion abilities were impaired. She tended to use a lexical, whole-word approach to reading. This often resulted in incorrect guessing of a word based on partial phonological information. Using nonwords as stimuli necessitated the use the grapheme–phoneme conversion route to read. This approach was also effective for writing. Establishing this ability prepared MQ for reading and writing training of two-syllable words, phrases, and short sentences.

In all but one training set, MQ's improvements on trained items generalised to control and untrained items. Moreover, in Treatment Protocol 2 she also showed generalisation of improvements in reading to her ability to write these same words. Her writing accuracy from the pre-treatment test increased considerably following reading training, evidenced at the baseline measure preceding writing treatment. Although reading and writing are intimately related, it is somewhat remarkable to observe this generalisation from one to the other. This suggests that it would be efficacious to train the two abilities together, or in close succession as was done in this study. It would also be interesting to determine if training reading alone were to improve writing abilities. This could be tested in future studies.

As noted earlier, treatment approaches for sound blending that use single grapheme–phoneme correspondences to facilitate sound blending have not always been successful. However, the bigraph–biphone correspondence training has been successful with a few cases reported to date. It is important, therefore, to gain more evidence of the efficacy of this approach and to understand why it is effective. There are factors related to the procedure itself. It has been suggested that training bigraph–biphone correspondences is more natural for phoneme blending, and approximates the pronunciation of a word more closely because the pronunciation of individual phonemes is different from in the context of a syllable (Friedman & Lott, 2002). This is a reasonable conclusion that is supported by direct empirical evidence comparing grapheme–phoneme and bigraph–biphone conversion abilities (Berndt et al., 1996).

Another task-specific factor is the short-term memory demands of the grapheme–phoneme conversion process (Laine & Niemi, 1990). Verbal STM impairments are ubiquitous in aphasia, and the ability to maintain activation of semantic and phonological representations has been hypothesised to be the link between short-term memory impairments and aphasia (Martin & Saffran, 1997). If we assume that STM capacity is sensitive to the number of item units and those units can be defined differently, it is conceivable that maintaining activation of three phonemes in STM while linking them with three graphemes could be more difficult than holding two bigraph–biphone correspondences and blending them together. Moreover, during training with single grapheme–phoneme correspondences, the consonant graphemes are often pronounced as bigraphs (consonant + schwa) when being linked, adding to the phonological content to be maintained in STM. Thus, the hypothesis that STM limitations contribute to the difficulty in learning to blend sounds has merit, but should be investigated further with a direct comparison of numbers of graphemes and bigraphs being processed.

Other contributing variables that need to be investigated systematically in future studies of this treatment approach (as well as training blending with single grapheme–phoneme correspondences) are length of treatment, type of aphasia, and severity of aphasia. In the case studies reported to date there is considerable variation of each of these factors. It is conceivable that this treatment will work for one type of aphasia and not another. With the exception of Berndt et al.'s (1996) participants, other individuals who received treatment for sound blending were nonfluent and/or had poor auditory comprehension. MQ presented with conduction aphasia with good semantic processing and a relatively circumscribed phonological deficit. Martin, Fink, and Laine (2004) have shown that individuals with spared semantic processing benefit more from repetition priming than those with impaired access to semantics. Thus, even though this treatment for sound blending targets phonological processing, the integrity of semantic processing could be important to long-term benefits from the training. With respect to length of treatment, De Partz's participant, who learned sound blending with single grapheme–phoneme correspondences, was in treatment for a much longer period of time than Nickel's (1992) participant (who did not learn the sound blending). Future studies should address these factors systematically.

CONCLUSION

This longitudinal study supports the use of bigraph–biphone correspondence training (Berndt et al., 1996; Friedman & Lott, 2002) to improve sound-blending abilities. Using this approach resulted in MQ's progression from an inability to perform grapheme–phoneme correspondence tasks consistently to reading and writing phrase-length material. An important clinical implication of this study is that this treatment was effective with an individual with chronic aphasia (5 years post onset). Currently, MQ is enrolled in a treatment protocol that is building on her 3 years of intense training and extending it to workplace skills. Combining direct impairment-based with functionally based treatment should maximise the relevance of treatment to the everyday functional needs of this participant.

REFERENCES

Berndt, R. S., Haendiges, A. N., Mitchum, C. C., & Wayland, S. C. (1996). An investigation of nonlexical reading impairments. *Cognitive Neuropsychology, 13*(6), 763–801.

Coltheart, M., Patterson, K., & Marshall, J. C. (1980). *Deep dyslexia*. London: Routledge & Kegan Paul.

Dell, G. S., Martin, N., & Schwartz, M. F. (in press). A case-series test of the interactive two-step model of lexical access. Predicting word repetition from picture naming. *Journal of Memory and Language*.

dePartz, M. P. (1986). Re-education of a deep dyslexic participant: Rationale of the method and results. *Cognitive Neuropsychology, 3*(2), 149–177.

Dunn, L., & Dunn, L. (1981). *Peabody Picture Vocabulary Test – Revised*. Circle Pines, MN: American Guidance Service.

Francis, W., & Kucera, H. (1982). *Frequency analysis of English usage: Lexicon and grammar*. Boston: Houghton Mifflin.

Friedman, R. B. (1996). Recovery from deep alexia to phonological alexia: Points on a continuum. *Brain and Language, 52*, 114–128.

Friedman, R. B., & Lott, S. N. (2002). Successful blending in a phonological reading treatment for deep alexia. *Aphasiology, 16*, 355–372.

Glosser, G., & Friedman, R. B. (1990). The continuum of deep/phonological alexia. *Cortex, 26*, 343–359.

Howard, D., & Patterson, K. (1992). *The Pyramids and Palm Trees Test: A test of semantic access from words and pictures.* Bury St. Edmunds, UK: Thames Valley Test Company.

Kaplan, E., Goodglass, H., & Weintraub, S. (1983). *Boston Naming Test scoring booklet.* Philadelphia: Lea & Febiger.

Kay, J., Lesser, R., & Coltheart, M. (1992). PALPA. *Psycholinguistic Assessments of Language Processing in Aphasia.* Hove, UK: Lawrence Erlbaum Associates Ltd.

Laine, M., & Niemi, J. (1990). Can the oral reading skills be rehabilitated in deep dyslexia? In M. Hietanen, J. Vilkki, M. L. Niemi, & M. Korkman (Eds.), *Clinical neuropsychology: Excursions into the field in Finland* (pp. 80–85). Helsinki: Suomen Psykologinen Seura.

LaPointe, L., & Horner, J. (1998). *Reading Comprehension Battery for Aphasia (RCBA-2).* Austin, TX: Pro-Ed International Publishers.

Martin, N., Fink, R., & Laine, M. (2004). Treatment of word retrieval with contextual priming. *Aphasiology, 18,* 457–471.

Martin, N., & Saffran, E. M. (1997). Language and auditory-verbal short-term memory impairments: Evidence for common underlying processes. *Cognitive Neuropsychology, 14*(5), 641–682.

Martin, N., Schwartz, M. F., & Kohen, F. (2006). Assessment of the ability to process semantic and phonological aspects of words in aphasia: A multi measurement approach. *Aphasiology, 20,* 154–166.

Mitchum, C. C., & Berndt, R. S. (1991). Diagnosis and treatment of the non-lexical route in acquired dyslexia: An illustration of the cognitive neuropsychological approach. *Journal of Neurolinguistics, 6*(2), 103–137.

Nickels, L. (1992). The autocue? Self-generated phonemic cues in the treatment of a disorder of reading and naming. *Cognitive Neuropsychology, 9,* 155–182.

Saffran, E. M., Schwartz, M. F., Linebarger, M., Martin, N., & Bochetto, P. (1988) *The Philadelphia Comprehension Battery* [unpublished test battery].

Schwartz, M. F., Dell, G. S., Martin, N., Gahl, S., & Sobel, P. (2006). A case series test of the two-step interactive model of lexical access: Evidence from picture naming. *Journal of Memory and Language, 54,* 228–264.

Siegel, S. (1956). *Nonparametric statistics for the behavioral sciences.* Tokyo: McGraw-Hill.

APHASIOLOGY, 2007, 21 (6/7/8), 702–716

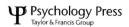

Talking across time: Using reported speech as a communicative resource in amnesia

Melissa C. Duff

University of Iowa College of Medicine, Iowa City, IA USA

Julie A. Hengst

University of Illinois at Urbana-Champaign, IL USA

Daniel Tranel

University of Iowa College of Medicine, Iowa City, IA USA

Neal J. Cohen

University of Illinois at Urbana-Champaign, IL USA

Background: Patients with amnesia may have more than pure memory deficits, as evidenced by reports of subtle linguistic impairments on formal laboratory tasks in the amnesic patient HM. However, little attention has been given to the impact of memory impairments on language use in regular, colloquial interactions. We analysed *reported speech* use by individuals with amnesia. Reported speech (RS), in which speakers represent thoughts/words from another time and/or place, requires management of two temporal frames, making it an interesting discourse practice in which to explore the impact of memory deficits on interactional aspects of communication.

Aims: This study: (1) documents frequency, type, and temporal contexts of reported speech used in discourse samples; (2) compares reported speech use by amnesic and comparison participants; (3) examines the interactional character of reported speech use in these discourse samples.

Methods and Procedures: Derived from a broader study of the discourse practices of individuals with amnesia, this study uses quantitative group comparisons and close discourse analysis to analyse reported speech episodes (RSEs) in interactional discourse samples between a clinician and each of 18 participants, 9 individuals with amnesia and 9 comparison participants (NC).

Outcomes and Results: Reported speech was used by all participants. However, significantly fewer RSEs were produced in amnesia sessions (273) than in NC sessions (554). No significant group differences were observed for type or temporal domain. In addition, for the participants with amnesia, post-amnesia past RSEs differed qualitatively from the other RSEs in the data.

Conclusions: These findings have important implications for understanding the interdependent relationship of memory and language, point to the value of examining

---

Address correspondence to: Melissa C. Duff PhD, Department of Neurology, University of Iowa, 200 Hawkins Drive RCP 2100, Iowa City, IA 52242, USA. E-mail: melissa-duff@uiowa.edu

We thank Michelle Nolan and Lisa Cardella for transcribing the sessions and assisting in data coding. This study was supported by Program Project Grant NINDS NS 19632, NIDCD grant 1F32DC008825, NIMH grant RO1 MH062500, and a Mary Jane Neer Research Grant of the College of Applied Health Sciences at the University of Illinois at Urbana-Champaign.

---

http://www.psypress.com/aphasiology   DOI: 10.1080/02687030701192265

interactional aspects of communication in the empirical study of brain–behaviour relationships, and reconceptualise interaction as a target in the remediation of functional communication following brain injury.

The neuropsychological and neuroanatomical description of the seminal case of HM, throughout the 50 years of ongoing study of this patient (see Corkin, 2002; Scoville & Milner, 1957), provided significant insight into the organisation of human memory and its instantiation in the brain. We have learned from HM, and from other cases of amnesia (see Cohen & Eichenbaum, 1993; Squire, 1987), that damage to the hippocampus and related medial temporal lobe regions, whether by surgical resection, as in HM, or following anoxia or other neurological insult, results in a profound but circumscribed amnesia. The specificity of the impairment is critical. The observed impairment has been described as being specific *to* the domain of memory, as well as specific *within* the domain of memory. Thus, impairments are seen in aspects of memory function, disproportionate to any deficits in general cognitive or intellectual ability including language, attention, and reasoning. Moreover, the impairment affects only certain aspects, or forms of memory. The striking dissociation between spared and impaired memory abilities observed in HM and in other cases of amnesia (e.g., Cohen & Squire, 1980; Tranel, Damasio, & Damasio, 2000) documented that memory is not a unitary function, but rather is manifested in multiple functionally distinct memory systems supported by anatomically distinct brain systems. Evidence has accumulated that the crux of anterograde declarative amnesia due to hippocampal damage is a deficit in the ability to form and retain new long-term declarative memories (Cohen, 1984; Cohen & Eichenbaum, 1993; Eichenbaum & Cohen, 2001; Squire, 1992), including acquiring new vocabulary and facts (semantic memory) and memory for time- and place-specific experiences that are personal or autobiographical in nature (episodic memory).

One consequence of the observed specificity of amnesia has been to encourage a view of memory as a cognitive capacity distinct from the various cognitive domains (language, spatial processing, etc.) that it serves, and to see the impairment in amnesia as exclusive to a specific aspect of memory functioning. However, some recent work looking at the possible effects of amnesia on other aspects of cognition raises questions about the scope of amnesia as well as about the role(s) of memory in various domains of cognitive functioning. Among the cognitive capacities traditionally considered preserved in amnesia, language is a topic of debate. MacKay and colleagues (e.g., MacKay, Burke, & Stewart, 1998) suggest a critical role for the hippocampal system in certain language functions. Recent studies point to subtle lexical, phrasal, and sentence-level language impairments in HM that were previously unnoticed or de-emphasised. These language impairments appear to be quite subtle, though, particularly when compared to HM's profound memory impairments or compared to the deleterious deficits in linguistic form observed in aphasia or in pragmatic functioning in right hemisphere syndrome.

Thus far, investigations of the impact of amnesia, or the role of the hippocampus, in language function have been directed at formal aspects of language rather than to real-world aspects of language-in-use. This may underestimate the significance of any possible language problems, as a number of authors have commented on the impact of memory impairments on the ability to function in and manage everyday activities (Tate, 2002; Wilson, 1999) and the effects of amnesia on functional communication (see Ogden & Corkin, 1991; Wilson & Wearing, 1995), even if those effects are not as severe as those seen in aphasia. In our own work with individuals with amnesia, we have been struck by subtle disturbances in their conversational patterns (e.g., disruptions in timing of speaker turns, lack of engagement and support for their conversational partners, lack of detail or vagueness in their discourse), leading us to suspect that interactional aspects of language-in-use may be more disrupted than the more formal testing might suggest.

THE CURRENT STUDY

To begin to explore the impact of memory impairments on language-in-use, as part of a broad examination of the discourse practices of individuals with amnesia (Duff, Hengst, Nolan, Tranel, & Cohen, 2005), we collected interactional discourse samples from individuals with amnesia as well as from a group of healthy comparison participants. Presented here is an initial analysis from the data set, focusing on the use of reported speech in these interactions.

Reported speech (RS) is a pervasive discourse practice in which speakers represent, or re-enact, words or thoughts from other times and/or places (see Hengst, Frame, Neuman-Stritzl, & Gannaway, 2005; McCarthy, 1998; Tannen, 1989). Traditionally, RS has been classified into two canonical forms: direct reports, or quotes, of speech (e.g., *John said, "I'll be there at six"*), and indirect reports, or paraphrases (e.g., *John said that he would be here by six*). In addition to these canonical forms, researchers have identified a variety of ways in which speakers routinely represent the words of others, such as using blended direct and indirect forms (e.g., Volosinov, 1986), non-explicit descriptions of talk (e.g., Hickman, 1993), and simply pointing to talk using indexical markers (e.g., Hengst et al., 2005).

Of particular interest to us here is the way that reported speech, across all of its forms, weaves together two temporal contexts within one utterance. The *reporting context* is the current time frame in which the speaker produces the report, while the *reported context* refers to the temporal frame in which the reported words were originally spoken. Discursively, speakers may specify the reported context quite precisely (e.g., *When I walked through the door on my first day of kindergarten the teacher said, "hi John"*) or vaguely (e.g., *During one of our family trips my sister asked me if she could borrow my jacket*), or leave it unspecified, as when reporting habitual comments (e.g., *Every time they think of it the kids ask, "now can we have a puppy?"*). In all cases, there is a requirement for maintaining, relating, and moving (mentally) between two separate time frames, which would seem to implicate memory along with language capabilities.

Within traditional structural linguistic perspectives, reported speech has been construed as a relatively rare and specialised form functioning simply as a factual representation of past events. Although reported speech forms certainly could support veridical representation of the past, extensive empirical sociolinguistic research on the use of reported speech in everyday interactions has found it to be a common and diverse discourse practice serving a wide range of creative and interpretive functions. Speakers use reported speech forms to represent others' thoughts (including animals and inanimate objects), what might have been said (but wasn't), and what will (should or might) be said in the future, as well as to animate the voices of make-believe or fictional characters. In addition, speakers strategically construct, or reconstruct, others' thoughts and words (factual or hypothetical) to serve their own purposes (Clark & Gerrig, 1990; Tannen, 1989). In fact, Tannen (1989) has argued in favour of the term *constructed dialogue*, over reported speech, on the basis that speakers seldom simply represent others' words verbatim, and even when they do, the represented words are re-constructed for new purposes in the reporting context, as speakers select what details to represent, what tones to put with words, and what impression to leave with the listener. Regardless of which term we use, this view of reported speech emphasises the cognitive and interactional flexibility and generativity that is required for its effective use.

The current examination of reported speech is, to our knowledge, the first study of reported speech use in amnesia. Reported speech represents an especially interesting discourse practice for studying the impact of memory impairments on interactional aspects of communication in the discourse of individuals with amnesia, particularly given the memory demands that would seem to be a requisite part of its successful use. Different perspectives lead to a range of different predictions of possible outcomes. Based on a classical view of amnesia as a deficit exclusively of memory (i.e., sparing language and other cognitive abilities), we might anticipate that individuals with amnesia would accurately produce a full range of reported speech forms (e.g., direct, indirect). However, to the extent that reported speech depends heavily on memory for previous events, and given the hallmark deficits in the ability to form and recall long-term declarative memories of places, people, and the temporal and interactional relations among them (i.e., items constituting an episodic event), we might anticipate that patterns of reported speech use would be disrupted. Indeed, traditional accounts of reported speech as simply a veridical report of a past speech event lead to the prediction that there would be an absence of reported speech referring to relatively recent events from the post-amnesia-onset past (i.e., from the period of anterograde amnesia), but with a preservation of reported speech referring to more remote events from the pre-amnesic past (from the remote past outside the period of retrograde amnesia). Interactional sociolinguistic perspectives, which focus on the discursive and creative representation of temporal events, might suggest more complex patterns of disruption, or conceivably no discernable disruption at all. Finally, sociolinguistic studies of communicative accommodation, in which the productions of one person in an interaction often shape the subsequent productions of others (as when interlocutors come to match rates of speech) (e.g., Giles, Coupland, & Coupland, 1991), lead to the prediction that any disruptions in reported speech productions by amnesic participants would affect clinician productions as well.

Analyses of the interactional discourse samples from individuals with amnesia and from healthy comparison participants, each communicating with the first author, permitted examination of: (1) the extent to which participants with amnesia and the clinician use reported speech in their interactional discourse sessions (i.e., number of reported speech episodes), the types of reported speech used, and the temporal domains represented in the events of the reported speech episodes; (2) comparisons between the reported speech use of participants with amnesia and neurologically intact participants, in terms of frequency of use and type of reported speech forms, and the temporal periods represented in their reports; and (3) the interactional nature of reported speech use in these sessions, i.e., how reported speech is collaboratively produced and taken up by the participants and the clinician, for both amnesic and comparison participants.

METHOD

Participants and data set analysed

The analysis of reported speech was completed on interactional data obtained during discourse sampling sessions conducted by the lead author with each of 18 participants, 9 individuals with amnesia and 9 comparison participants.[1] Of the nine participants with amnesia, seven had sustained bilateral damage restricted to the hippocampus from an anoxic/hypoxic event (e.g., cardiac arrest, status epilepticus)[2] and two had sustained more extensive bilateral brain damage including to the hippocampus, amygdala, and surrounding cortices from herpes simplex encephalitis (HSE). At the time of data collection, all nine participants were medically stable and in the chronic epoch of amnesia, with time-post-onset ranging from 1 to 25 years ($M = 9.33$; $SD = 7.1$). The Wechsler Memory Scale–III General Memory Index scores for each participant were at least 25 points lower than their scores on the Wechsler Adult Intelligence Scale–III, and the mean difference between Full Scale IQ and General Memory Index was 31.2 points. The average Delayed Memory Index was 65.3, almost 3 standard deviations below population means. Finally, the participants with amnesia were on average 50 years old (range 42–58) and had 14 years of education (range 9–16). The nine normal comparison participants (NC group) were all healthy non-brain-injured individuals. NC participants were matched pairwise on sex, handedness, age, and education to each participant with amnesia.

The data were collected using a mediated discourse-elicitation protocol designed to support ecologically valid interactional discourse sampling in a clinical setting by putting the clinician in the role of conversational partner (Hengst & Duff, 2007). The goal of the data collection sessions was to obtain approximately 30 minutes of conversational-based interaction between the clinician and target participant and, within this conversational framework, to move through a set of targeted discourse tasks. Consistent with discourse studies of adults with neurogenic disorders (see Cherney, Shadden, & Coelho, 1998), the targeted discourse tasks were: one 10-minute conversation; three story-telling prompts (frightening experience, historical event, family story); three picture descriptions (Cookie Theft, Normal Rockwell, World Trade Center); and three procedural descriptions (making a favourite sandwich, shopping in an American grocery store, changing a tyre). Throughout the session the clinician participated as an appropriate interactional partner for discourse activities (e.g., as an audience to participant's story telling). Thus, the sessions yielded both pre-selected (i.e., target tasks) and spontaneous (i.e., between-task) interactional discourse for analysis. All sessions were videotaped and transcribed to support situated discourse analysis.

---

[1] All participants were drawn from the Amnesia Research Laboratory at the Beckman Institute at the University of Illinois or the Patient Registry of the Division of Behavioral Neurology and Cognitive Neuroscience at the University of Iowa. Data collection and analysis was conducted under IRB approval from both institutions.

[2] For a detailed description of the neuroanatomical data for five of these participants see Allen, Tranel, Bruss, and Damasio, 2006.

Data analysis

Through repeated viewings of the videotapes, supported by use of the transcripts, we analysed reported speech use throughout the sessions, which included reported speech produced by the clinician and the participants during both target discourse tasks (e.g., picture description) and non-task interactions (e.g., small-talk between target tasks). The analysis was completed in four phases. First, using a broad definition of reported speech, research assistants identified all possible reported speech episodes (RSEs), yielding 2943 possible RSEs. In the second phase, these possible RSEs were reviewed by the first two authors and recoded in order to omit RSEs that were directly read (e.g., clinician reading instructions), non-explicit representations of other's speech (e.g., *We talked for hours*), clinician's prompts for talk (e.g., *I'd like for you to tell me about a frightening experience*), and immediate, unframed repetitions of each other's speech (e.g., *I don't want to. Yeah, I don't want to*). In addition, during this review, turn and speaker boundaries for each RSE were reviewed, and nine RSEs were reinterpreted as simply continuations of adjacent episodes. At the end of this second phase, 827 explicitly marked RSEs, or approximately 30% of those initially identified, were retained for further analysis. In the third phase, the lead author categorised each of the 827 RSEs as one of five reported speech types (described below) and identified each as either accurately and completely produced or as containing errors (e.g., false starts, grammatical errors) and/or being incomplete (e.g., abandoned or interrupted). Finally, in the fourth phase the lead author analysed the temporal domain represented by the reported context (see below) for each RSE.

Coding types of reported speech. For this analysis, we used five explicitly marked reported speech types (direct, indirect, indexed, projected, undecided) developed by Hengst et al. (2005). In *direct reported speech* the represented speech is presented as a quotation, as if reporting the exact words of the original speaker (e.g., *Get a call later ..."Roger somebody called. They can't get their car started"*). In *indirect reported speech* the represented speech is presented as a paraphrase of the original speaker's words (e.g., *One of them said she wants to hand out candy*). In *projected reported speech* it is understood that the represented speech has never actually been said—i.e., what might have been said, but wasn't; what will or should be said in the future; or what animals or objects might say if they could speak (e.g., *"I brought my wrong glasses" is what I should say*). In *indexed reported speech* the represented speech is not actually presented, either directly or indirectly, but is simply pointed to, or indexed, often with deictic pronouns or demonstratives (e.g., *That's what I was going to ask you*). Finally, the *undecided* category captures reported speech that cannot be easily categorised into one of the above types, such as blended forms, or episodes that contain multiple linguistic errors, were abandoned, or were interrupted (e.g., *I I wouldn't say I'm cause I have a couple of sisters that are a lot funnier when they tell a story*).

Coding temporal domain of reported context. To identify the temporal domains that participants were discursively managing within RSEs, we categorised the reported context into one of four temporal domains: *past, in-session, future,* and *unspecified.* The *past* domain included reported contexts from across the lifespan, ranging from childhood through recent past up to the beginning of the session. In order to code the reported context as past, the RSE or surrounding discourse needed to contain a reference to a specific past time or event (e.g., *When I went to the Breeder's Cup in 2000 …*). The *in-session* domain included reported contexts from the immediate past, specifically within the data collection session. This category included RSEs that had a within-session temporal reference (e.g., *And like I said earlier I'm interested …*), indexed reports of something said within the session (e.g., *That's not what I said*), and the hypothetical, or projected, reports that participants often used during target discourse tasks (e.g., giving voice to characters in the picture description: *And the girl said … saying, "shh be quiet"*). The *future domain* included reported contexts that were anticipated or forthcoming, typically presented as projected reports (e.g., *I'm gonna call him and tell him this is unacceptable*). The *unspecified* domain included reported contexts that were vague, ambiguous, or not specified. However, this also included RSEs produced within jokes (e.g., *One guy says, "I used to have a problem but now that I'm all better, its just that I know I'm perfect is my only problem"*) and representations of habitual thoughts or speech (e.g., *I always think that if I get some more time I'd like to take piano lessons*).

Reliability

Point-by-point inter-rater and intra-rater reliability of coding of the five types of reported speech and the temporal domains of each RSE was obtained on 10% of the data. Five consecutive RSEs for each of the 18 sessions were selected. The original researcher-coder and a researcher unfamiliar with the data independently recoded the data. Intra-rater and inter-rater reliability was 94% and 87% for RS type and 93% and 84% for temporal domain, respectively.

RESULTS

Frequency and type of reported speech

Across the data set, reported speech was available to, and used by, all participants and the clinician in all 18 sessions analysed, with a range of 1–78 episodes produced per person per session. However, on average only half as many RSEs were produced in the amnesia discourse sessions ($M = 30.3$; $SD = 16.9$) than in the NC sessions ($M = 61.5$; $SD = 30.1$), a difference that was significant, $t(16) = 2.713$, $p = .015$. This difference cannot be attributed to a more limited production of RSEs by the amnesic participants alone. During the amnesia discourse sessions, both the participants and the clinician produced fewer RSEs than during NC sessions. In NC sessions the clinician produced 28% of the total 554 RSEs (participant RSEs = 400; clinician RSEs = 154), and in amnesia sessions the clinician produced 32% of the total 273 RSEs (participant RSEs = 185, clinician RSEs = 88). Finally, across all sessions, the majority of RSEs were coded as completely and accurately produced, with an accuracy level of 88.9% in NC sessions (participant productions at 87.75%, clinician productions at 92.2 %) and an accuracy level of 84.6% for amnesia sessions (participants 83.2%, clinician 87.5%).

All five types of reported speech were used in these sessions. Across all 18 sessions, direct reported speech was produced most often, accounting for 43% (359/827) of total RSEs. Indirect and projected reported speech were produced less often, accounting for 18% (151/827) and 10% (84/827) of total RSEs, respectively.

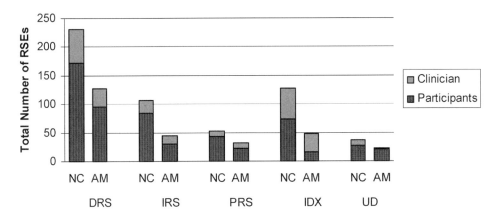

Figure 1. Total number of reported speech episodes (RSEs) by type and group. NC, normal comparison; AM, amnesia; DRS, direct reported speech; IRS, indirect reported speech; PRS, projected reported speech; IDX, indexed reported speech; UD, undecided.

Productions of indexed reported speech were surprisingly high, accounting for 21% (174/827) of total RSEs. However, the majority of indexed reports were produced by the clinician during her management of the target discourse tasks (e.g., *Do you want to add or change anything to that?*). Only 7% (59/827) of total RSEs were coded as undecided. Figure 1 displays the distribution of total RSEs by type and participant group.

Beyond overall differences in the total number of RSEs produced, we were interested in whether there were differences in the use of reported speech types between groups. Focusing on the productions of the NC participants and participants with amnesia, we calculated the proportion of RSEs per person and by type for each group. Using a two-tailed Wilcoxon matched pairs signed rank and a Bonferroni correction for multiple comparisons (alpha of 0.01) we found no significant group differences for type of reported speech: direct RS ($Z = -0.65$; $p < .51$), indirect RS ($Z = -2.075$; $p < .038$), projected RS ($Z = -1.12$; $p < .26$), indexed RS ($Z = -2.433$; $p < .015$), undecided RS ($Z = -1.66$; $p < .096$). The stringency of the Bonferroni correction increases the risk of Type 2 errors. It is worth noting that, consistent with visual inspection, statistically significant group differences would have been observed for indirect and indexed reported speech without the correction, suggesting that there may be group differences for these types of reported speech.

Temporal domains of the reported contexts

Analysis of the reported contexts of the 827 RSEs revealed that all four temporal domains, *past*, *in-session*, *future*, and *unspecified*, were represented, and that the distribution of temporal domains was similar between groups. Across all sessions, 55% (456/827) of the reported contexts were coded as past, 24% (197/827) were coded as in-session, and 19% (155/827) were coded as temporally unspecified. Only 2% (19/827) were coded as having a future reporting context. We examined whether the proportion of RSEs of each of the four temporal domains produced by participants only (without clinician productions) differed between groups using a two-tailed Wilcoxon matched pairs signed rank test and a Bonferroni correction for multiple comparisons (alpha of 0.0125). No significant group differences were observed: past ($Z = -1.7$; $p < .08$); in-session ($Z = -1.2$; $p < .21$); future ($Z = -1.4$; $p < .17$); and unspecified ($Z = -0.77$; $p < .44$).

The finding of no group difference in the distribution of temporal domains represented in the reported contexts was surprising. Our clinical impressions, as well as our preliminary review of the data, suggested that the participants with amnesia had difficulties communicating about past events, and we anticipated that this would be reflected in a smaller percentage of past reported contexts within RSEs produced during amnesic sessions. One possible explanation was that any difficulty in discursively managing past reported contexts might be limited to the recent past (i.e., post-onset of amnesia), with the remote past (i.e., pre-onset of amnesia) reported contexts undisturbed. Such a subcategory disruption might have been masked in our original analysis, which combined all past reported contexts into one category. To further investigate this possibility we analysed the 106 RSEs with past reported contexts that were produced by participants with amnesia, subcategorising each as having a reported context of pre- or post-amnesia for the target participant. This was surprisingly easy to do as participants with amnesia frequently referred to their memory impairments, often using the onset of amnesia as a way to discursively organise events (e.g., *before my brain injury*). In other cases, participants referenced salient events (e.g., childhood vacations) that, within the broader conversation, could be easily located in the participant's life. In the few cases in which the pre/post amnesia distinction was not clear, the specific temporal references were compared with information available in medical records.

This follow-up analysis revealed that, although past reported contexts of RSEs produced by amnesia participants included both recent and remote past temporal domains, the majority of reported contexts were coded as pre-amnesia. For all 106 RSEs, 59% (63/106) were coded as pre-amnesia and 41% (43/106) as post-amnesia. However, the two HSE participants, who had the most extensive brain damage, did not produce any RSEs with post-amnesia reported contexts. Indeed, these two participants together only produced six RSEs with past reported contexts, and all six of these were coded as pre-amnesia past. It was striking that not once during these sessions did either HSE participant produce a RSE with a reported context representing a temporal domain after the onset of their amnesia, a time period of 25 years for one participant.

It was also our impression that RSEs produced by amnesic participants with a pre-amnesia reported context were qualitatively different from those with a post-amnesia reported context. Those with pre-amnesia reported contexts often seemed indistinguishable from RSEs produced in NC sessions or by the clinician in amnesia sessions—they were animated (e.g., use of gestures, changes in voice quality), detailed, and covered a diverse range of topics (e.g., families, pets, work, schooling). In marked contrast, RSEs with post-amnesia reported contexts seemed less detailed, or specific, and more topically limited, with the most common topic being the impact of amnesia in their daily lives (e.g., *He'll say things like … "well do you remember to take a shower every night?"*; *They said I have long-term memory; I'd cover the same topic over and over and over and over and because I couldn't remember that I'd asked the same question five minutes ago; I couldn't really remember where he said he was gonna be*). In fact, when we reviewed the topics for all post-amnesia RSEs we found that 74% (32/43) focused on the participants' memory problems or amnesia, and many of these reports were repeated throughout the session.

The interactional character of reported speech in these sessions

The mediated discourse elicitation protocol, which works to establish the clinician as a conversational partner throughout the session, also allowed us to begin to document the interactional character of reported speech in this data set. Functionally, reported speech was diversely deployed within the sessions and in support of different functional goals. By assigning all utterances to an interactional discourse activity—either one of the four target discourse types (e.g., conversation) or the more general talk that occurred between target tasks—we documented which discourse activities supported the most reported speech production. Although reported speech was used throughout the session, interestingly, across both groups, the majority of RSEs (51%, or 333/827) occurred during the between-task talk. For RSEs that occurred during the target discourse activities, most were produced during the conversational and narrative tasks, 31% (254/827) and 23% (189/827) respectively, with few produced during picture and procedural description tasks, each at only 3% of the total RSEs (24/827 and 22/827 respectively). Across these discourse activities, reported speech episodes were used to give voice to fictional characters, to project possible discourse, and to provide details and animate voices of narratives.

In these sessions there was also evidence of more collaboratively produced RSEs—i.e., episodes in which the discursively constructed social and temporal frames established by one partner were taken up by the other partner in the production of reported speech. Two marked examples of collaborative productions were episodes in which both speakers jointly produced the represented speech, and episodes in which the RSE was set up, or framed, by the previous speaker. For example, in joint constructions, the represented speech that was initiated by one speaker, either the clinician (Cl) or the participant with amnesia (AP), was completed by the other one, as seen in the example below:

> AP: *And it's like well ... you know "I just-"*
> Cl: *"I don't want to."*

In examples of collaboratively framed episodes, the speaker depends on a framework set up by their conversational partner, as seen in the example below:

> Cl: *So I watch ... this person being killed and then I go to bed and I'm you know lying there going, "well."*
> AP: *"Did I hear something?"*

The most intriguing examples of these collaborations were multi-turn, hypothetical conversations jointly enacted by both partners. During these play-conversations the conversational partners would both slip into character voices (without verbal set-up) and respond to each other's utterances within the established play frame, either sharing the same, or speaking from different, character roles. In the transcript below, a participant with amnesia (AP) sets up a frame in which she, as a store clerk, doesn't know how to help a customer. Then both the AP and the clinician (Cl) enact the scenario by directly reporting what the store clerk might say to a customer:

> AP: *Especially if a customer comes and wants to buy something. I'm just like, "what is that?"*

Cl: *"Come pick it out."*
AP: *"Yeah. Do do you know what it looks like?"*
Cl: *"Show me what it looks like"*

All 827 RSEs were reviewed to identify examples of marked collaborative production and uptake of reported speech (i.e., jointly produced represented speech, collaboratively framed episodes, and/or play-conversations). This review documented marked collaboration in 14 of the 18 sessions. Perhaps not surprisingly, we documented more of these examples in NC sessions (17 examples documented across all nine sessions) than in amnesia sessions (9 examples documented across five sessions). It is also interesting to note that none of these marked collaborative RSEs were produced in the sessions with the two HSE participants.

DISCUSSION

The current findings accord with interactional sociolinguistic perspectives that conceptualise reported speech as a pervasive, robust, and creative discourse form. Here, reported speech was available to, and successfully used by, the clinician and all 18 participants, and of the 827 reported speech episodes identified for analysis, the vast majority (>80%) were produced accurately (i.e., without linguistic errors) and completely (i.e., not interrupted or abandoned). In addition, all types of reported speech analysed (e.g., direct, indirect, indexed) were identified. Of particular interest here, of course, was the comparison between amnesic and neurologically intact participants. There was no significant group difference in the types of reported speech produced by participants with amnesia and the comparison participants. But, despite such clear evidence that the amnesic participants had sufficiently preserved linguistic abilities to accurately produce a variety of reported speech forms, as a group they produced only half as many reported speech episodes during these sessions as the comparison participants.

If there were a simple relationship between episodic memory abilities and the discursive representations of past time frames of reported speech, we might suspect that the lower reported speech use by amnesic participants would be accounted for by a sharp reduction of reported speech episodes from the period of their anterograde and retrograde amnesia. However, this was not the case. Not only did participants with amnesia produce reported speech contexts representing all four temporal domains (i.e., past, in-session, future, unspecified), but also, proportionally, we found no significant difference in the distribution of temporal domains used between groups. In addition, despite their severe anterograde declarative memory deficit, the participants with amnesia were not limited to the remote (or pre-amnesia) past, but also used representations of recent (or post-amnesia-onset) past. However, discourse analysis of those reported speech events referring to relatively recent episodes from the post-amnesia-onset period did find indications of disruption. Impressionistically, these episodes seemed more schematic, less detailed, and more prone to breakdown. Moreover, the majority of them dealt with the highly salient, daily experience of the participants' memory problems and amnesia; there was no single topic that was as current and salient to serve as a comparison event in the NC participants' reported speech.

The interactional analysis of reported speech use in these sessions pointed to more similarities than differences for the amnesia and comparison participant groups.

Specifically, both groups displayed a similar pattern of reported speech use across discourse activities (i.e., conversation, picture description, procedural description, story generation, between-task talk), and reported speech episodes with marked collaboration (i.e., jointly produced and collaboratively framed episodes and play conversations) between the clinician and the participant. In addition, the clinician's production of reported speech tracked with the participants' productions, whether with the higher use of reported speech episodes of the comparison group, or the lower use of the amnesia group. Although the dynamics that led to this attunement await further study, these findings make it clear that production and use of reported speech in these sessions were shaped by emergent interactional phenomena.

Although we did not check the veracity of the reported speech episodes, the findings presented here are consistent with previous research demonstrating that individuals with amnesia can produce remote autobiographical memories (Tranel & Jones, 2006) and with as much detail as individuals without brain injuries (e.g., Bayley, Hopkins, & Squire, 2003). However, findings from the current study suggest that even when producing vivid remote memories, individuals with amnesia are less likely to use reported speech as a communicative resource when representing these memories in communicative interactions. This may be because, although the static display of remote memories becomes independent of the hippocampus over time, the hippocampal system plays a critical role in the flexible expression of memory in novel situations (Cohen & Eichenbaum, 1993; Eichenbaum & Cohen, 2001). Reported speech requires flexible access to the larger temporal record of events as well as the ability to flexibly and creatively generate unique combinations of the elements of the representation to be reconstructed (what details to represent, what details to omit) to meet specific interactional goals. This flexibility and creativity would seem essential to forming both past and future or anticipated representations. Thus, although sociolinguistic perspectives de-emphasise the importance of veridical declarative memories in reported speech use, hippocampal damage, in addition to disrupting reported speech use for episodes referring to the post-amnesia-onset period, may also impair the creative and interpretive uses of reported speech events from all time periods in communicative interactions.

An intriguing finding, not fully explored here, was that the reported speech use by two HSE participants was clearly more restricted. In the qualitative analysis presented here, the HSE participants stood out as the only two participants with amnesia who produced no episodes of reported speech referring to events in the post-amnesia-onset period and no episodes with marked collaboration. Although the data were not broken out above, these two participants produced a markedly lower number of RSEs overall (7.5 on average per session) than the other seven participants with amnesia (24.3 on average per session). Critically, these observed differences in frequency of reported speech use do not appear to be due to the severity of the declarative memory impairment; for example, a participant with anoxia, whose IQ–MQ (memory quotient) difference was greater than that of either of the two HSE participants, produced more than twice as many RSEs as any other participant with amnesia. Instead, the paucity of reported speech use by the HSE participants may be related to the fact that their brain damage extends beyond the hippocampus. A potentially related observation in other patients with extensive medial temporal lobe and limbic system damage is disruptions in, and particularly a lessening of, emotions and motivations (e.g., O'Conner, Cermak, & Seidman, 1995; Tate, 2002). Tate (2002) posits that these blunt or shallow emotional responses may not be limited to an individual's own altered life circumstances but may also extend to their interpersonal relationships. Tannen (1989) has argued that reported speech is a key discourse resource for the ongoing display and creation of interpersonal and interactional involvement among interlocutors. In this sense, it is interesting that the most striking disruptions in reported speech use were in the HSE participants, who had more extensive brain damage, and whose sessions were marked in multiple ways by a lack of interactional engagement. This finding suggests that the use of reported speech may also critically rely on other brain systems that support, more generally, reciprocal social-emotional communication (e.g., amygdala, ventromedial prefrontal cortex).

Understanding the relationship between memory and language and the neural substrates supporting everyday language use are core themes in neuroscience, neuropsychology, and speech pathology. In the current work, we did not observe deficits in basic linguistic mechanisms in amnesia; rather, individuals with amnesia used all forms of reported speech. Instead, the difference between amnesic and comparison participants was in the less frequent use of this form of discourse by those with amnesia. Given that reported speech seems to place great demands on maintaining, relating, and flexibly moving back and forth (mentally) between different time frames, the finding here, that reported speech is called upon less often in individuals with damage to precisely that memory system—declarative memory— thought to support such memory demands, makes good sense. Thus, even if amnesia is specific to an aspect of memory, it can exert its effects in other cognitive domains when the processing in those domains places large demands on memory. Language- in-use in actual interaction among participants involves more than basic linguistic mechanisms, invoking memory and presumably other cognitive capacities. Indeed, when we shift our investigation to understanding the nature of language-and- memory-in-use in communicative interactions, the distinctions between memory and language become less clear, and we would argue, less important.

Finally, findings from this study point to the value of research protocols designed to focus on social interaction and the systematic examination of interactional aspects of communication, suggesting that this is a promising approach in the empirical study of brain–behaviour relationships. Indeed, in previous work (Duff, Hengst, Tranel, & Cohen, 2006) we found this approach to be robust for promoting and documenting new semantic learning in severely amnesic individuals as they interacted with a familiar partner across a series of collaborative interactions. Drawing attention to the functional systems of social interaction reveals the complexity of communication in context, which seems to have greater ecological validity than typical laboratory tasks, and has direct clinical application for understanding the functional impact of cognitive-linguistic deficits in everyday interaction, and how language and memory impairments can be accommodated to support successful communication.

REFERENCES

Allen, J., Tranel, D., Bruss, J., & Damasio, H. (2006). Correlations between regional brain volumes and memory performance in anoxia. *Journal of Clinical and Experimental Neuropsychology*, *28*(4), 457–476.

Bayley, P., Hopkins, R., & Squire, L. (2003). Successful recollection of remote autobiographical memories by amnesic patients with medial temporal lobe lesions. *Neuron*, *37*, 135–144.

Cherney, L. R., Shadden, B. B., & Coelho, C. A. (Eds.). (1998). *Analysing discourse in communicatively impaired adults.* Gaithersburg, MD: Aspen Publishers.

Clark, H. H., & Gerrig, R. J. (1990). Quotations demonstrations. *Language, 66,* 764–805.

Cohen, N. J. (1984). Preserved learning capacity in amnesia: Evidence for multiple memory systems. In N. Butters & L. Squire (Eds.), *The neuropsychology of memory* (pp. 83–103). New York: Guilford Press.

Cohen, N. J., & Eichenbaum, H. (1993). *Memory, amnesia, and the hippocampal system.* Cambridge, MA: MIT Press.

Cohen, N. J., & Squire, L. (1980). Preserved learning and retention of a pattern analysing skill in amnesia: Dissociation of know how and know that. *Science, 210,* 207–210.

Corkin, S. (2002). What's new with the amnesic patient H.M.? *Nature Reviews Neuroscience, 3,* 153–160.

Duff, M. C., Hengst, J., Nolan, M., Tranel, D., & Cohen, N. J. (2005, November). *Language and memory: Analysing discourse of individuals with amnesia.* Presentation at the American Speech-Language-Hearing Association (ASHA), San Diego, CA.

Duff, M. C., Hengst, J., Tranel, D., & Cohen, N. J. (2006). Development of shared information in communication despite hippocampal amnesia. *Nature Neuroscience, 9*(1), 140–146.

Eichenbaum, H., & Cohen, N. J. (2001). *From conditioning to conscious recollection: Memory systems of the brain.* New York: Oxford University Press.

Giles, H., Coupland, J., & Coupland, N. (Eds.). (1991). *Contexts of accommodation: Development in applied sociolinguistics.* Cambridge, UK: Cambridge University Press.

Hengst, J., & Duff, M. C. (2007). Clinicians as communication partners: Developing a mediated discourse elicitation protocol. *Topics in Language Disorders, 27,* 36–47.

Hengst, J., Frame, S., Neuman-Stritzl, T., & Gannaway, R. (2005). Using others' words: Conversational use of reported speech by individuals with aphasia and their communication partners. *Journal of Speech, Language and Hearing Research, 48,* 137–156.

Hickman, M. (1993). The boundaries of reported speech in narrative discourse: Some developmental aspects. In J. A. Lucy (Ed.), *Reflexive language: Reported speech and metapragmatics* (pp. 91–126). New York: Cambridge University Press.

MacKay, D. G., Burke, D. M., & Stewart, R. (1998). H.M.'s language production deficits: Implications for relations between memory, semantic binding, and the hippocampal system. *Journal of Memory and Language, 38,* 28–69.

McCarthy, M. (1998). *Spoken language and applied linguistics.* Cambridge, UK: Cambridge University Press.

Myers, G. (1999). Functions of reported speech in group discussions. *Applied Linguistics, 20,* 376–401.

O'Conner, M., Cermak, L., & Seidman, L. (1995). Social and emotional characteristics of a profoundly amnesic postencephalitic patient. In R. Campbell & M. Conway (Eds.), *Broken memories: Case studies in memory impairment* (pp. 45–53). Oxford, UK: Blackwell Publishers.

Ogden, J. A., & Corkin, S. (1991). Memories of H.M. In W. C. Abraham, M. Corballis, & K. G. White (Eds.), *Memory mechanisms: A tribute to G.V. Goddard.* Hillsdale, NJ: Lawrence Erlbaum Associates, Inc.

Scoville, W. B., & Milner, B. (1957). Loss of recent memory after bilateral hippocampal lesions. *Journal of Neurology, Neurosurgery, and Psychiatry, 20,* 11–12.

Squire, L. R. (1987). *Memory and brain.* New York: Oxford University Press.

Squire, L. R. (1992). Memory and the hippocampus: A synthesis from findings with rats, monkeys, and humans. *Psychological Review, 99,* 195–231.

Tannen, D. (1989). *Talking voices: Repetition, dialogue, and imagery in conversational discourse.* Cambridge, MA: Harvard University Press.

Tate, R. (2002). Social and emotional consequences of amnesia. In A. D. Baddeley, M. D. Kopelman, & B. A. Wilson (Eds.). *The handbook of memory disorders* (2nd ed., pp. 17–56). Chichester, UK: John Wiley & Sons Ltd.

Tranel, D., Damasio, H., & Damasio, A. R. (2000). Amnesia caused by herpes simplex encephalitis, infarctions in basal forebrain, and anoxia/ischemia. In F. Boller & J. Grafman (Eds.). *Handbook of neuropsychology* (2nd ed., pp. 85–110). Amsterdam: Elsevier Science.

Tranel, D., & Jones, R. (2006). Knowing "what" and knowing "when". *Journal of Clinical and Experimental Neuropsychology, 28*(1), 43–66.

Wilson, B. A. (1999). *Case studies in neuropsychological rehabilitation.* New York: Oxford University Press.

Wilson, B. A., & Wearing, D. (1995). Prisoner of consciousness: A state of just awakening following herpes simplex encephalitis. In R. Campbell & M. A. Conway (Eds.), *Broken memories: Case studies in memory impairment* (pp. 14–30). Cambridge, MA: Blackwell.

Volosinov, V. N. (1986) *Marxism and the philosophy of language* (L. Matejka & I. R. Titunik, Trans.). Cambridge, MA: Harvard University Press.

APHASIOLOGY, 2007, 21 (6/7/8), 717–725

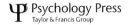

Gesture and aphasia: Helping hands?

Victoria L. Scharp, Connie A. Tompkins, and Jana M. Iverson

University of Pittsburgh, PA, USA

Background: The study of communicative gestures is one of considerable interest for aphasia, in relation to theory, diagnosis, and treatment. Significant limitations currently permeate the general (psycho)linguistic literature on gesture production, and attention to these limitations is essential for both continued investigation and clinical application of gesture for people with aphasia.
Aims: The aims of this paper are to discuss issues imperative to advancing the gesture production literature and to provide specific suggestions for applying the material herein to studies in gesture production for people with aphasia.
Main Contribution: Two primary perspectives in the gesture production literature are distinct in their proposals about the function of gesture, and about where gesture arises in the communication stream. These two perspectives will be discussed, along with three elements considered to be prerequisites for advancing the research on gesture production. These include: operational definitions, coding systems, and the temporal synchrony characteristics of gesture.
Conclusions: Addressing the specific elements discussed in this paper will provide essential information for both continued investigation and clinical application of gesture for people with aphasia.

The study of communicative gestures is of considerable interest for aphasia, in relation to theory, diagnosis, and treatment. For example, definitions and theories of aphasia differ in whether or not language impairment must cross all modalities of communication, including gesture. Some type or form of gesture is included in subtests of the Porch Index of Communicative Ability (PICA, Porch, 1967), scored in test batteries like the Communicative Abilities in Daily Living (CADL, Holland, 1980) and the pantomime recognition test (Duffy & Duffy, 1975, 1981), and modelled in the Promoting Aphasics Communicative Effectiveness (PACE) treatment programme (Davis & Wilcox, 1985). Also, aphasia researchers and clinicians consider gesture as both a means of communicative facilitation (e.g., Records, 1994) and compensation (e.g. Tompkins & Scharp, 2006).

Despite the broad potential relevance of gesture in aphasia, relatively little research has been done in this area. Thus the question remains as to how we can best advance the body of knowledge on gesture production in aphasia. Significant limitations currently permeate the general (psycho)linguistic literature on gesture production, and attention to these limitations is essential for both continued investigation and clinical application of gesture for people with aphasia.

Address correspondence to: Victoria L. Scharp, Communication Science and Disorders, University of Pittsburgh, 4033 Forbes Tower, Pittsburgh, PA 15206, USA. E-mail: scharpvl@hotmail.com

At the core of the limitations in the general gesture production literature is a theoretical difference among authors in the instantiation of the function of gesture during the communication process. More specifically, gesture is viewed either as a part of the communicative process that is driving language expression from its inception or as a supplemental aspect of communication enacted primarily during word finding. This paper discusses several fundamental differences between these two perspectives and pinpoints aspects of the current literature that require particular consideration including: an operational definition of gesture, description and implementation of coding systems for studying gesture production, and the nature of the relationship between temporal characteristics of gesture and speech. Finally, specific examples of necessary gesture production studies particularly for patients with aphasia will be provided.

CONCEPTUALISING GESTURE PRODUCTION

Existing models of gesture production reflect two major perspectives that differ on the central question: What is the function of gesture during communication? The proposed function of gesture for communication is in turn directly connected to its point of entry into the communication process. The two primary perspectives in the gesture production literature are distinct in their proposals about the function of gesture, and about where gesture arises in the communication stream. While individual elements of particular models of gesture production and comparisons between models are beyond the scope of this paper (for details of the models see de Ruiter, 2000; Krauss, Chen, & Gottesman, 2000; McNeill, 1992, 2005; Rose, 2006), this section outlines some general principles that underlie these two perspectives, as a springboard for discussing how these points of view motivate research questions and the execution of research in gesture production.

The first perspective on the function of gesture during communication is that gesture is an integral component at the conceptual level of expression. In his most recent book, McNeill (2005) proposes that gesture is integrated at the earliest stages of communication, and is part of the driving force of communication. According to McNeill, gestures are "conceived of as ingredients in an imagery–language dialectic that fuels speech and thought" (p. 3). The act of gesturing for communication is inseparable from the verbal message and rests at the *conceptual level*. Verbal communication and gesture are produced in parallel, and gesture is a potentially equal participant in the conceptual/planning stages. Communicative expression thus occurs via both verbal and spatial means, providing a temporally linked, non-redundant, multidimensional, content-rich message.

The Sketch model of gesture and speech production by de Ruiter (2000) is consistent with the perspective that gesture is enmeshed with verbal communication at the conceptual level. The Sketch model (designated by de Ruiter as a "speech" model because it is based on Levelt's 1989 model of speech production) purports that the primary function of gesture is for communication and that it emerges from the conceptualiser component of Levelt's model. The Sketch model and McNeill's perspective are also consistent with the Mutually Adaptive Modalities hypothesis (MAM, de Ruiter, 2006; Melinger & Levelt, 2004). The MAM states that if a speaker is unable to utilise one communication modality effectively (e.g., verbal communication in an excessively noisy place; gesture when face-to-face communication is not possible), the proportion of spatial information is skewed either towards gesture use or towards spatially loaded verbal expression respectively. While the Sketch model and MAM hypothesis are proposed to be able to accommodate the second major perspective outlined below, these principles clearly align with the view that gestures are conceptually driven.

The lexical retrieval hypothesis (Krauss et al., 2000) is the second major perspective on gesture production. In this view, gestures serve to assist in the retrieval of words from the mental lexicon. Krauss and colleagues' work focuses on "lexical gestures", which are defined as "spontaneous, complex, articulate hand-arm movements that seem related to the ideational content of the speech they accompany" (Morsella & Krauss, 2005, p. 415). Lexical gestures in this perspective are used predominantly as a supplemental mechanism to facilitate spoken language, and occur for the speaker's benefit (e.g., Butterworth & Beattie, 1978; Morrel-Samuels & Krauss, 1992). Krauss and colleagues (Krauss, Chen, & Chawla, 1996) in conjunction with Butterworth and Hadar (1989), posit that lexical gestures are engaged as a preverbal priming mechanism and are enacted most frequently during word finding, specifically when additional (spatial) information is needed to prime and access a word. This view of gesture production is particularly relevant to aphasia and normal ageing, given the widely reported word-finding difficulties that can accompany both.

Research cited in support of the word retrieval hypothesis includes studies that report an increase in "lexical" gestures during dysfluencies in language production (Butterworth & Beattie, 1978; Morrel-Samuels & Krauss, 1992) and studies utilising gesture restriction paradigms that yield an increase in dysfluent verbal productions (Rauscher, Krauss, & Chen, 1996; Rime & Schiaratura, 1991). The rationale for the hypothesis investigated in these studies is the link between "lexical" gestures and verbal fluency. As a speaker experiences a halting or stalled moment in their verbal communication, ostensibly due to a word-finding delay, lexical gestures increase; when a speaker is unable to use gestures, increases in pauses and dysfluencies occur.

The lexical retrieval hypothesis in its current instantiation cannot accommodate some of the fundamental observations that motivate the MAM hypothesis. However, a subset of communicative gestures beyond the lexical gestures of interest to Krauss and colleagues may fill this gap. As acknowledged by Krauss and Hadar (1999), this additional subset of gestures includes deictics, emblems, and pantomimes from Kendon/McNeill's continuum (Kendon, 1980; McNeill, 2005). The potential distinction between gesturing for communicative intent (gesturing for the listener) versus using gesture to enhance lexical retrieval (gesturing for self) again reflects the basic question of the function served by spontaneous movements of the hands and arms during communication.

When considering conceptual frameworks on gesture production, we are in agreement with a recent commentary by Rodriguez and Gonzalez Rothi (2006) that discusses the limitations of these models, and we underscore the need to view models as guiding tools that must continue to be developed, tested, and challenged. We also raise one further, specific consideration for both investigators and clinicians. The two perspectives on gesture production discussed above emphasise a key difference in the purpose and point of entry for gesture during communication, but they are not necessarily mutually exclusive. However, the proposed difference in the function of gesture during communication does impact the research emanating from each perspective. That is, the nature of the research questions, the methods used to elicit gesture, and the coding systems for setting boundaries of what is counted as a gesture are grounded in the perspective of the investigator, a fact that should be kept in mind when interpreting, comparing, and applying the results of various studies.

This conceptual framework debate has numerous implications for research on gesture production in aphasia, whether it be basic or clinical in nature. Four examples are provided here. First, aphasia research has not adequately considered the potentially important theoretical or clinical differences between gestures that are produced for the benefit of the (aphasic) speaker's communication partners, versus gestures that are produced for the aphasic person him/herself. Perhaps there are at least partially differentiable systems that support each of these gestural functions, and that can be differentially impaired or spared, or differentially trained or generalised. Investigating such questions in aphasia could also provide evidence about the theoretical (and anatomic) coherence or fractionability of the two conceptual frameworks. A second, more focused example refers to the types of gestures deemed relevant for study in each conceptual framework. It may be fundamental for advancing gesture research in aphasia to determine whether there are normative gestural profiles for various elements or types of gesture in various communicative contexts; e.g., with topics or communication partners that vary in familiarity. Third, the perspective on the function of gesture should help to determine the most relevant gesture elicitation methods. For example, the lexical retrieval perspective calls for a task designed to accentuate word-finding difficulties, while the stance that gestures emerge from a conceptual origin could be more fruitfully evaluated in a task that, for example, tapped gesture production incidental to the spatial working memory demands of the communication. Finally, the relevant profiles on which to classify adults with aphasia may vary depending on the conceptual framework. From the lexical retrieval perspective on gesture, it may turn out to be just as critical to establish aphasia participant profiles based on their gesture use as it is to classify and compare them on verbal expression. By contrast, if gesture is deemed to arise from the conceptual level of communication, verbal expressive characteristics may suffice for patient classification.

DEFINITIONS AND CODING SYSTEMS

A clear definition of the gestures of interest in any investigation or clinical application is a mandatory element for interpretation, but often this crucial aspect is left for the reader to surmise. It can be difficult to disentangle definitions from the coding systems used to outline what is coded as a gesture and if that gesture is considered "communicative". Additionally, the context in which a communicative gesture is produced impacts the analysis of the contribution of the gesture (i.e., naturalistic context, face-to-face communicative exchanges, spontaneous description, confrontation naming, etc.; Power & Code, 2006). Historically, operational definitions of gesture have been overlooked, and it is only recently that both definitions and models/frameworks of gesture production have been discussed in the same investigative circles (Rose, 2006).

Partly reflecting the typical lack of operational specificity, the gesture production literature is rife with terminological confusion. For example, the terms "emblems" (conventionalised symbolic gestures such as the okay sign; McNeill, 2005) and "iconics" (movements relating to the semantic content of the verbal expression; McNeill, 1992) are often interchanged in this literature. The term "gesticulation" used by Kendon (1980) to describe hand/arm movements of an illustrative nature, is now instantiated by McNeill (2005) as "motion that embodies a meaning relatable to the accompanying speech" (p. 5). Further complicating the picture, different terms and descriptions have been applied across perspectives and disciplines. For example, the "lexical-only" gesture perspective does not reference "beats" (McNeill, 1992, 2005) and "batons" (Efron, 1941), gestures that adhere to the prosodic/rhythmic features of language production and are integral for emphasis and communicative flow per McNeill.

Pantomimes are a unique gesture type that most authors agree encompasses movements of the hands, fingers, and arms without co-occurring verbal expression. Because these isolated and variable movements of the hands/arms (pantomimes can be executed in a variety of ways, unlike emblems which have a predictable static presentation; McNeill, 2005) are typically performed without verbal expression, the "point of entry" issue discussed in the prior section of this paper is irrelevant. Gesture researchers also tend to segregate self-touching or grooming movements of the hands and arms into a category distinct from gestures used during communication (Blonder, Burns, Bowers, Moore, & Heilman, 1995). These self-touching/ grooming gestures are not tied to verbal expression, which sets them apart from communicative gesture. Given that the field can agree on definitions for gestures that are predominantly executed independent from verbal expression, one might wonder why it is so difficult to define the co-verbal movements of the hands and arms.

We propose that the problem of inconsistent definitions rests to a large degree on the point of entry distinction discussed earlier. If there is a fundamental difference in the *function* of communicative gestures, then a range of definitions may be needed to encompass the relevant phenomena. Any single definition of communicative gesture would have to capture evolving perspectives on the function of gesture. In our view, in order to derive an inclusive but specific definition for "gesture", questions of the following sort need to be considered: Is it necessary to have a single definition that can cross all frameworks and populations, and that can encompass multiple gesture types? Are the gestures used in an adult/developed system fundamentally different in function from those that emerge during development or in an impaired system? Another definitional issue concerns whether gesture indeed falls into discrete categories, or whether it resides along a fluid continuum, as proposed by McNeill (2005), and how to capture apparent variations in gesture production in either case.

Rosenbek, LaPointe, and Wertz (1989) underscore both inclusionary and exclusionary aspects as critical components of definitions that are sufficiently comprehensive and specific, an emphasis with which we concur. While some may not consider an operational definition imperative, the lack of specifically and consistently defined terms in the gesture production literature challenges the integration of perspectives from multiple disciplines (e.g., neurology, cognition, and psycholinguistics), the continued development of conceptual frameworks and models, and the application of results from existing studies. Until the field is farther along in achieving definitional precision and consistency, individual researchers and clinicians would do a great service by specifically setting the boundary conditions of what they consider to be (and exclude from consideration) the gestures of interest in their work.

As a starting point, we sought out explicit definitions provided in the gesture and aphasia literature. An early example indicates that "gesture was conceived as a unit of expression which might consist of a number of individual movements … some of these gestural units could be grouped together into larger, more complex gestural phrases" (Cicone, Wapner, Foldi, Zurif, & Gardner, 1979, p. 329). A more recent definition from Cunningham and Ward (2003) stated that "gesture was defined very broadly as a purposeful, symbolic hand signal, purposeful pointing, or purposeful facial expression" (p. 691). Another example comes from Foundas et al. (1995), who write: "a single gesture was defined as a discrete movement of the arm and/or hand that resulted in one continuous motion followed by a visible pause in the action," (p. 207). While it is laudable that there are statements describing how gesture was defined in these studies, the three definitions overlap only slightly, in considering gesture to be some form of movement(s) of the hands/arms. The Cicone et al. definition also encompasses a series of movements that count as a singular gesture, and facial expression is included in the definition of Cunningham and Ward. This very slight overlap in explicit definitions leads to obvious difficulty in cross comparisons of studies of gesture in aphasia.

To begin to fill the definitional gap, we propose the following as a potential working definition of a communicative gesture: Communicative gesture includes spontaneous movements of the hands, arms, and fingers that are typically co-verbal and provide information that is consistent with the content of the verbal message, but can also provide additional information not contained in the verbal expression. Communicative gestures do not include self-touching, grooming gestures, or body-focused movements (Butterworth, Swallow, & Grimston, 1981). Additional features would need to be added to this definition depending on the type and context in which a gesture is to be studied. Such features could be captured in an explicit coding system, developed for that purpose.

A coding system is a template that guides authors in their analysis of gestures executed in an experimental context. Variation in coding systems also confounds the gesture production literature. The coding systems implemented to measure and study gesture are tightly knitted to the types of gestures being studied. While there are several templates for gesture coding systems (Krauss et al., 1996; McNeill, 1992) a single coding system (i.e., what "counts" as a specific type of communicative gesture) has yet to be agreed. This puts the reliability and validity of individual gesture studies in question, and makes virtually impossible the integration or meta-analysis of findings across gesture production studies.

Two examples will serve to illustrate the problem in coding system variability. In her study of cued recall for verbal targets, Frick-Horbury (2002) coded or classified elicited gestures into four categories: iconic, metaphoric, body-focused movements, and vague gestures. These four categories were used to guide analysis and interpretation of gesture use in that study. A quite different coding system was used by Alibali, Bassock, Solomon, Syc, and Goldin-Meadow (1999), who classified gestures into continuous representations (smooth, continuous motions of the hands/ arms), discrete representations (taps, points or beats), "both" representations (movements that incorporated both continuous and discrete representations), or "neither" representations. As with definitions, coding systems have also been applied differently by gesture point of entry, population, and communicative context. For example, studies motivated from the lexical retrieval perspective limit attention to a subset of "lexical" gestures, whereas work that reflects the view of McNeill and colleagues explores a range of gestures along a continuum (Kendon, 1980; McNeill, 2005). Coding is further complicated when any single gesture can involve several aspects of different gesture subtypes (see, e.g., McNeill, 2005).

In summary, along with the fundamental differences in perspectives on the function of gesture during communication, vague or idiosyncratic definitions and varying coding systems complicate the implementation and interpretation of gesture studies. These factors should be carefully considered by aphasiologists when investigating and considering treatment approaches that incorporate gesture for patients with aphasia.

TEMPORAL CHARACTERISTICS OF GESTURE

The timing features of gesture are of interest due to the predominantly co-verbal nature of communicative gestures (McNeill, 1992, 2005). Studying communicatively disordered populations, a common practice across aphasiology and related disciplines, may provide valuable insight into the intact gesture-language system for communication. For example, in one study Mayberry and Jaques (2000) observed that people who stutter halt their gesture stroke (while maintaining the hand-shape) until their dysfluency resolves, at which point the gesture stroke is continued or completed. Studies that incorporate hand/arm restriction paradigms also provide evidence on the synchronous nature of gesture and verbal communication (Rauscher et al., 1996; Rime & Schiaratura, 1991), emphasising a possible trade in the spatial content of the message between the verbal expression and gesture depending on whether movements are restricted (i.e., crossing the arms) akin to the MAM hypothesis discussed above.

The temporal characteristics of gesture are particularly relevant in a model proposed by Tuite (1993). In this model, gesture and speech are rooted in a "rhythmic" or "viscero-motor" component of communication. To illustrate the close relation of gestures to an internal "rhythmic pulse" (an unspecified term), Tuite superimposes a speaker's intonation peaks onto a movement display. Only limited data are provided as examples of this proposed phenomenon and, to our knowledge, no subsequent studies have been conducted to test this view. As such, Tuite's rhythmic hypothesis raises additional questions rather than offers conclusions.

However, the notion of a rhythmic pulse is an interesting one for research and practice on gesture production in aphasia and other communicatively impaired populations. One might investigate, for example, the concurrence between a rhythmic interruption and an unfilled pause during a word-finding attempt. Perhaps such a relationship could be quantified with respect to the halting of a gesture stoke, as described in studies of people who stutter (Mayberry & Jaques, 2000).

The temporal relationship between spoken language and spontaneous hand, arm, and finger movements during communication remains an understudied area in gesture production. The precise parameters of the gestural movement and the spoken utterance have typically been judged via a perceptual means, leaving much to interpretation and leaving inter-judge reliability almost absent from published studies in this domain. A replicable and valid method for studying this relationship is needed in typical populations prior to its application to disordered populations like those with aphasia. For example, studies that directly manipulate the variable(s) that are predicted to impact the temporal relationship between speech and gesture (i.e., prosodic stress, perturbation of movement, communicative context) are needed in order to gain any precision in measuring this elusive relationship. Once a fuller picture of the timing of the speech and gesture relationship is captured, perhaps more specific diagnostic and treatment approaches for people with aphasia can be shaped.

CONCLUSIONS

This paper presents a discussion of issues that, when appropriately considered, will enhance the conduct and interpretation of studies on gesture production in aphasia. There are clear limitations in the available body of gesture production literature in typical populations, ranging from vague and inconsistent definitions and coding systems to inadequate attention to temporal characteristics of gesture. Clinicians and investigators who wish to incorporate gesture into the diagnosis and treatment of a traditionally variable disordered population like those with aphasia will benefit from considering these issues.

As one step along a path to improving subsequent research efforts, we have provided a general working definition of communicative gesture, while emphasising that it will need to be tailored for specific purposes. We have also illustrated how the investigator's stance on theoretical perspectives for the function of gesture can affect other crucial study elements like the development of research questions, choice of gesture elicitation methods, and identification of an explicit coding scheme for identifying, analysing, and interpreting gesture. Furthermore, we have suggested a path for studies of the temporal synchrony between speech and gesture in which a precise relationship has yet to be established.

As a final comment, in order to gain further insight into the nature and function of gesture, it is vital to understand individual differences in gesture production. Knowledge about individual variability in typical populations will also provide a backdrop against which to assess and manage gesture use in a disordered population like those with aphasia.

In sum, a marriage is needed of sound theoretical orientation, operational definitions, and measurement approaches to yield valid and replicable studies of gesture production in aphasia. Only then will we make progress in disentangling whether, and how, incorporating gesture in aphasia diagnosis and treatment will provide a "helping hand".

REFERENCES

Alibali, M. W., Bassok, M., Solomon, K. O., Syc, S. E., & Goldin-Meadow, S. (1999). Illuminating mental representations through speech and gesture. *Psychological Science, 10*(4), 327–333.

Blonder, L. X., Burns, A. F., Bowers, D., Moore, R. W., & Heilman, K. M. (1995). Spontaneous gestures following right hemisphere infarct. *Neuropsychologia, 33*(2), 203–213.

Butterworth, B., & Beattie, G. (1978). Gesture and silence as indicators of planning speech. In R. Campbell & P. Smith (Eds.), *Recent advances in the psychology of language* (pp. 347–360). New York: Plenum.

Butterworth, B., & Hadar, U. (1989). Gesture, speech and computational stages: A reply to McNeill. *Psychological Review, 96*(1), 168–174.

Butterworth, B., Swallow, J., & Grimston, M. (1981). Gestures and lexical processes in jargonaphasia. In J. Brown (Ed.), *Jargonaphasia* (pp. 113–124). New York: Academic Press.

Cicone, M., Wapner, W., Foldi, N., Zurif, E., & Gardner, H. (1979). The relation between gesture and language in aphasic communication. *Brain and Language, 8*, 324–349.

Cunningham, R., & Ward, C. D. (2003). Evaluation of a training programme to facilitate conversation between people with aphasia and their partners. *Aphasiology, 17*(8), 687–707.

Davis, G. A., & Wilcox, M. J. (1985). *Adult aphasia rehabilitation: Applied pragmatics.* San Diego, CA: College Hill Press.

de Ruiter, J. (2000). The production of gesture and speech. In D. McNeill (Ed.), *Language and gesture* (pp. 284–311). Cambridge, UK: Cambridge University Press.

de Ruiter, J. (2006). Can gesticulation help aphasic people speak, or rather, communicate? *Advances in Speech-Language Pathology*, 8(2), 124–127.

Duffy, R. J., & Duffy, J. R. (1975). Pantomime recognition in aphasics. *Journal of Speech and Hearing Disorders*, 44, 156–168.

Duffy, R. J., & Duffy, J. R. (1981). Three studies of deficits in pantomimic expression and pantomimic recognition in aphasia. *Journal of Speech and Hearing Research*, 46, 70–84.

Efron, D. (1941). *Gesture and environment*. Morningside Heights, NY: King's Crown Press.

Foundas, A. L., Macauley, B. L., Raymer, A. M., Maher, L. M., Heilman, K. M., & Gonzalez Rothi, L. J. (1995). Gesture laterality in aphasic and apraxic stroke patients. *Brain and Cognition*, 29, 204–213.

Frick-Horbury, D. (2002). The use of hand gestures as self-generated cues for recall of verbally associated targets. *American Journal of Psychology*, 115(1), 1–20.

Holland, A. L. (1980). *Communicative abilities in daily living*. Baltimore, MD: University Park Press.

Kendon, A. (1980). Gesticulation and speech: Two aspects of the process of utterance. In M. R. Key (Ed.), *The relation between verbal and nonverbal communication* (pp. 207–227). The Hague: Mouton.

Krauss, R., Chen, Y., & Chawla, P. (1996). Nonverbal behavior and nonverbal communication: What do conversational hand gestures tell us? In M. Zanna (Ed.). *Advances in experimental social psychology* (Vol. 26, pp. 389–450). New York: Academic Press.

Krauss, R., Chen, Y., & Gottesman, R. (2000). Lexical gestures and lexical access: A process model. In D. McNeill (Ed.), *Language and gesture* (pp. 261–283). Cambridge, UK: Cambridge University Press.

Krauss, R., & Hadar, U. (1999). The role of speech-related arm/hand gestures in word retrieval. In R. Campbell & L. Messing (Eds.), *Gesture, speech, and sign* (pp. 63–116). Oxford, UK: Oxford University Press.

Levelt, W. (1989). *Speaking–from intention to articulation*. Cambridge, MA: MIT Press.

Mayberry, R. I., & Jaques, J. (2000). Gesture production during stuttered speech: Insights into the nature of gesture-speech integration. In D. McNeill (Ed.), *Language and thought* (pp. 199–214). Chicago, IL: Cambridge University Press.

McNeill, D. (1992). *Hand and mind: What gestures reveal about thought*. Chicago, IL: University of Chicago Press.

McNeill, D. (2005). *Gesture and thought*. Chicago, IL: University of Chicago Press.

Melinger, A., & Levelt, W. (2004). Gesture and the communicative intention of the speaker. *Gesture*, 4, 119–141.

Morrel-Samuels, P., & Krauss, R. M. (1992). Word familiarity predicts temporal asynchrony of hand gestures and speech. *Journal of Experimental Psychology*, 18(3), 615–622.

Morsella, E., & Krauss, R. M. (2005). Muscular activity in the arm during lexical retrieval: Implications for gesture-speech theories. *Journal of Psycholinguistic Research*, 34(4), 415–427.

Porch, B. E. (1967). *Porch index of communicative ability*. Palo Alto, CA: Consulting Psychologists Press.

Power, E., & Code, C. (2006). Waving not drowning: Utilising gesture in the treatment of aphasia. *Advances in Speech-Language Pathology*, 8(2), 149–152.

Rauscher, F. H., Krauss, R. M., & Chen, Y. (1996). Gesture, speech, and lexical access: The role of lexical movements in speech production. *Psychological Science*, 7(4), 226–231.

Records, N. (1994). A measure of the contribution of gesture to the perception of speech in listeners with aphasia. *Journal of Speech and Hearing Research*, 37, 1086–1099.

Rime, B., & Schiaratura, L. (1991). Gesture and speech. In R. Feldman & B. Rime (Eds.), *Fundamentals of nonverbal behaviour* (pp. 239–284). Cambridge, UK: Cambridge University Press.

Rodriguez, A. D., & Gonzalez Rothi, L. J. (2006). Even broken clocks are right twice a day: The utility of models in the clinical reasoning process. *Advances in Speech-Language Pathology*, 8(2), 120–123.

Rose, M. L. (2006). The utility of arm and hand gestures in the treatment of aphasia. *Advances in Speech-Language Pathology*, 8(2), 92–109.

Rosenbek, J. C., LaPointe, L. L., & Wertz, R. T. (1989). *Aphasia: A clinical approach*. Boston: Little, Brown & Co.

Tompkins, C. A., & Scharp, V. L. (2006). Communicative value of self cues in aphasia: A re-evaluation. *Aphasiology*, 20(7), 684–704.

Tuite, K. (1993). The production of gesture. *Semiotica*, 93(1/2), 83–105.

APHASIOLOGY, 2007, 21 (6/7/8), 726–738

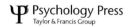

A cognitive and psycholinguistic investigation of neologisms

Arpita Bose and Lori Buchanan

University of Windsor, Ontario, Canada

Background: Jargon aphasia with neologisms (i.e., novel nonword utterances) is a challenging language disorder that lacks a definitive theoretical description as well as clear treatment recommendations (Marshall, 2006).

Aim: The aims of this two-part investigation were to determine the source of neologisms in an individual (FF) with jargon aphasia, to identify potential facilitatory semantic and/or phonological cueing effects in picture naming, and to determine whether the timing of the cues relative to the target picture mediated the cueing advantage.

Methods and Procedures: FF's underlying linguistic deficits were determined using several cognitive and linguistic tests. A series of computerised naming experiments using a modified version of the 175-item Philadelphia Naming Test (Roach, Schwartz, Martin, Grewal, & Brecher, 1996) manipulated the cue type (semantic versus phonological) and relatedness (related versus unrelated). In a follow-up experiment, the relative timing of phonological cues was manipulated to test the effect of timing on the cueing advantage. The accuracy of naming responses and error patterns were analysed.

Outcome and Results: FF's performance on the linguistic and cognitive test battery revealed a severe naming impairment with relatively spared word and nonword repetition, auditory comprehension of words and monitoring, and fairly well-preserved semantic abilities. This performance profile was used to evaluate various explanations for neologisms including a loss of phonological codes, monitoring failure, and impairments in semantic system. The primary locus of his deficit appears to involve the connection between semantics to phonology, specifically, when word production involves accessing the phonological forms following semantic access. FF showed a significant cueing advantage only for phonological cues in picture naming, particularly when the cue preceded or coincided with the onset of the target picture.

Conclusions: When integrated with previous findings, the results from this study suggest that the core deficit of this and at least some other individuals with jargon aphasia is in the connection from semantics to phonology. The facilitative advantage of phonological cues could potentially be exploited in future clinical and research studies to test the effectiveness of these cues for enhancing naming performance in individuals like FF.

Address correspondence to: Arpita Bose PhD, Department of Psychology, University of Windsor, 401 Sunset Avenue, Windsor, Ontario, N9A 5G8, Canada. E-mail: bosea@uwindsor.ca

We would like to express our deepest gratitude to FF and his wife for their interest and enthusiasm and their many hours of participation for this research. We also thank Dr Myrna Schwartz and Paula Sobel for sharing the digital pictures of the Philadelphia Naming Test, and we appreciate the help from Gillian Macdonald, Jenna Pawlow, and Kingsley Yang for their assistance in experimental development. This research was supported by the Toronto Rehabilitation Institute and Ontario Ministry of Health Post Doctoral Fellowship (AB), the Canada Research Chair Program, and the Social Sciences and Humanities Research Council of Canada MCRI program (LB).

http://www.psypress.com/aphasiology   DOI: 10.1080/02687030701192315

Jargon aphasia with neologism is a perplexing and challenging disorder. The language production in jargon aphasia is characterised by neologisms embedded in fluent well-articulated and long utterances with some underlying structures, such as good prosody and often with good syntactic form (for a review on characteristics of jargon aphasia see Marshall, 2006). Despite the well-articulated nature of their verbal production, word-finding difficulties, the presence of neologisms, and minimal content make the speech of jargon aphasic individuals difficult to understand (Buckingham, 1987). There is debate in the literature regarding the underlying source and nature of neologisms (e.g., Butterworth, 1992; Marshall, Robson, Pring, & Chiat, 1998; Moses, Nickels, & Sheard, 2004), and this lack of consensus may be behind the paucity of remediation recommendations for these individuals. The aim of this two-part investigation was to determine the source of neologisms in an individual with jargon aphasia (FF) and to identify potential facilitatory effects of semantic and/or phonological cues during picture naming. This study also examined whether the timing of these cues relative to these target picture had an impact on their effectiveness.

The literature describes various hypothesised sources of neologisms: poor awareness of speech errors and difficulty in self-monitoring (Ellis, Miller, & Sin, 1983; Marshall et al., 1998, but see Nickels & Howard, 1995); phonological distortion of the target and/or the error during phonological encoding (e.g., Kertesz & Benson, 1970); compensation of an initial failed attempt to retrieve the target word (e.g., "neologistic generator theory", Butterworth, 1992[1]); global weakening of connections within the lexical system (Schwartz, Saffran, Bloch, & Dell, 1994); localised impairment of connections between lexical and subword phonological segments (Hillis, Boatman, Hart, & Gordon, 1999); and impaired activation of phonological forms (Moses et al., 2004). One commonality among these diverse explanations is the assumption that neologisms reflect relatively circumscribed deficit in lexical retrieval within an otherwise normal lexical system. This assumption is supported by the fact that the errors are often target related (e.g., semantically related response) or the nonword contains elements of the target phonology (Marshall, 2006).

One reason for the limited theoretical consensus as described above may be the differences in definitions and classifications of neologisms across researchers (e.g., Christman, 1994; Moses et al., 2004). For the present study, we define a neologism as any nonword response, irrespective of its relationship with the target. We will first present FF's data from a variety of single-word processing tasks aimed at identifying spared or impaired cognitive and psycholinguistic processes. The data from these tasks also test some of the hypothesised causes of neologisms listed above, such as poor auditory monitoring skills, deficits in the semantic system, and/or deficit in accessing phonological forms to account for FF's neologisms.

The limited theoretical consensus regarding jargon aphasia is reflected in the lack of satisfying therapeutic interventions, and remediation of this disorder has proven to be very difficult (Marshall, 2001; Marshall et al., 1998). We performed a series of psycholinguistic experiments to determine which type of cueing (semantic versus phonological) might facilitate picture naming. These experiments were motivated by the common use of cueing procedures in the treatment of word production deficits in

---

[1] This lacks explanatory value to the extent that it simply moves the question back one level—the neologisms arise because the system made an error. This explanation is untestable because the cause of the error remains unspecified.

aphasia (e.g., Best, Herbert, Hickin, Osborne, & Howard, 2002; Le Dorze, Boulay, Gaudreau, & Brassard, 1994). The most typical phonological cue is the first phoneme of the target word (e.g., /cat/→ "k") and this type of cue is credited by some as facilitatory in word production and picture naming in aphasia (e.g., Best et al., 2002; Elman, Klatzky, Dronkers, & Wertz, 1992; Li & Williams, 1991, but see Croot, Patterson, & Hodges, 1999; Lambon-Ralph, Sage, & Roberts, 2000). A semantically related word (e.g., /fork/→ "spoon"), or a description of the target (e.g., /broom/ → "You sweep with it"), are often used as semantic cues (e.g., Li & Williams, 1991; Marshall et al., 1998). Unfortunately, the effect of semantic priming on picture-naming abilities in jargon aphasia is equivocal (Marshall et al., 1998; Robson et al. cited in Marshall, 2006), and the effectiveness of phonological cues has not been systematically investigated in these individuals. This study begins to fill these gaps in the clinical literature. We examined the effects of semantic as well as phonological cues in picture naming, and performed a follow-up experiment to determine if the timing of the facilitatory cue relative to the target picture had an effect on performance.

SECTION 1: SOURCE OF NEOLOGISMS

Participant

At the time of this study (autumn 2005), FF was a 75-year-old monolingual (English), retired high-school teacher with a college education. He suffered a single left cerebrovascular attack in August 2003. FF's medical history reports normal hearing and normal (corrected) visual acuity. FF exhibited right hemiparesis and continued to receive physiotherapy, which had led to substantial gain in his mobility of his arms and leg. Premorbidly he was right-handed but he now uses his left hand for activities of daily life. Detailed language assessments (e.g., Boston Diagnostic Aphasia Examination, BDAE, Goodglass, Kaplan, & Baressi, 2001, various subtests from Psycholinguistic Assessments of Language Processing in Aphasia, PALPA, Kay, Lesser, & Coltheart, 1992) supported a diagnosis of Wernicke's aphasia with severe neologisms. The following are examples of his conversational speech:

Examiner: Tell me about your work.
FF: *I used to drive.....I ...freda pridyburger.....then I was ...I did not work anywhere....i work but prior to that....was...uh...uh....taeba tigyban...pigyburger..i do not know.*

Picture description: Cookie theft (BDAE)
...like the cold air the water is breaking out of the sink and it's going under this floor...an um....going up the floor when uh birch go and ....and this kib.. is goboingbig is going pri on an ank...can't see what this dates got a lot of pigyham and poirb ib ib ts but over is yub ya.. she is got her job..and ...pigyburger...she got dentalated and one pigbigger ....and he pip en...

Story re-telling: Cinderella Narrative
.. and looks like the lugyburgers. It says oh we're gonna to pick a ligyburger that we want to get our liggyburgers. And so they, the..the king say or the so the men the uh the pigyburger say ah well here's the bigygurger and bloblah and all the rest of it and so they...they....they have a big big thing. And so the queen ago- or the old gigyburgers they all shodo betta sicki petegiburger and she hasn't she's couldn't..... tigybirger not go, and they go..

FF's spoken output was fluent and contained long and fairly grammatical sentences, with normal melodic line and phrase length but minimal content. His output was marked with neologisms, perseverations, and word-finding difficulty. BDAE testing showed naming difficulties and auditory comprehension difficulties that increased with sentence length and complexity. The predominant error types across naming tasks were neologisms and circumlocutory descriptions (e.g., /turkey/→"*figyburger*", /clock/ → "*kigyburger*"; /pineapple/ → "*bigyburger to eat*", /iron/ → "*you want to make your pigyburger nice*"). Information exchange during conversation was limited and required inference, questioning, and guessing on the part of the listener.

Materials and procedures

Various subtests from the PALPA (Kay et al., 1992), Philadelphia Naming Test (PNT, Roach et al., 1996), and Pyramids and Palm Trees Test (PPT, Howard & Patterson, 1992) were administered to determine FF's underlying language deficits and to test various hypotheses regarding the source of his neologisms.

Results and discussion

Table 1 shows FF's performance across the PALPA subtests, PNT, and PPT.

Output production tasks. FF's overall accuracy in naming PALPA 54 and PNT was 40% and 34%, respectively. He also showed a word frequency effect with greater accuracy for high-frequency words than for mid- and low-frequency words (Fisher Exact Test, $p = .04$). Neologisms were the most prevalent type of error followed by semantic errors and descriptions. Repetition was tested to examine whether FF would show similar difficulty in accessing and assembling phonological segments when the phonological forms were provided. FF performed very well on both word (96%) and nonword repetition (87%), with no demonstrated sensitivity to imageability or word frequency.

Testing across different modalities. The above two tasks revealed a clear dissociation between performance on naming and repetition. Such a dissociation would be difficult to explain within the context of global weakening of lexical connections (e.g., Schwartz et al., 1994). However, these tests differed in both requirements and items, and it could be argued that item differences were driving this dissociation. PALPA 53 provided the opportunity to rule out this argument by using the same items across both tasks (administered on different days). The pattern of performance (naming 40% < repetition 95%) combined with performance from PALPA 54, PNT, and repetition subtests (PALPA 8 and 9), suggested that the locus of FF's problem was not with production processes or with lack of access to phonological representation (e.g., Kertesz & Benson, 1970; Moses et al., 2004). FF's impairment was most evident when access to the phonological representations required for naming occurs via semantics. Such impairments could stem from an inability to access semantic representations or from a compromised connection between semantics and phonology. The following series of tests evaluates the former possibility.

Testing the semantic system. The spoken word picture matching (# 47), and auditory synonym judgement (# 49) along with PPT tests provided a broader picture

TABLE 1
Results of language assessments

Tests	Score (raw/total possible)	Percentage (%)
Output production tasks		
PALPA[1] # 54: Picture Naming × Frequency	24/60	40%
High-frequency words	15/20	75%
Mid-frequency words	5/20	25%
Low-frequency words	4/20	20%
Philadelphia Naming Test (Roach et al., 1996)	60/175	34%
PALPA # 9: Imageability (I) × Frequency (F) Repetition word	77/80	96%
High I–High F	20/20	100%
High I–Low F	19/20	95%
Low I–High F	19/20	95%
Low I–Low F	19/20	95%
PALPA # 8: Nonword Repetition	26/30	87%
1-syllable	9/10	90%
2-syllable	8/10	80%
3-syllable	9/10	90%
Performance across different modalities		
PALPA # 53		
Picture naming	16/40	40%
Repetition	38/40	95%
Auditory monitoring		
Monitoring of own response on PALPA 53 items on a different day	40/40	100%
PALPA 54: Word–nonword discrimination to picture stimuli	60/60	100%
Auditory comprehension		
PALPA # 2: Real-word minimal pair discrimination	66/72	92%
PALPA# 4: Minimal pair requiring picture selection	35/40	88%
Semantic system testing		
PPT[2]	46/52	89%
PALPA # 47: Spoken Word–Picture Matching	37/40	93%
PALPA # 49: Auditory Synonym Judgements	52/60	87%

[1]Psycholinguistic Assessments of Language Processing in Aphasia (Kay et al., 1992).   [2]Pyramids & Palm Trees Test (Howard & Patterson, 1989).

of FF's semantic abilities. FF's PPT performance of 89%, although marginally outside the normal range (>90%), suggested relatively intact semantic representations, and this suggestion was supported by his performance on PALPA 47 (93%) and 49 (87%).

Testing for monitoring difficulty. Marshall et al. (1998) suggest that neologisms reflect impairments of self-monitoring of speech that can be revealed through a careful evaluation of such abilities. Following Marshall et al., we presented FF with his own responses from the PALPA 53 naming subtest, and he was able to judge with 100% accuracy whether those responses were the correct names for the pictures. He was also able to distinguish word from nonword labels for the picture names for PALPA 54. Anecdotally, FF showed awareness of his errors with repeated attempts to self-correct, and he often rejected the neologisms by saying "*no that is not a pigyburger*", "*no no it is not a tigy.*" Additional support in favour of rejecting a monitoring-difficulty hypothesis came from FF's 92% performance on real-word minimal pair discrimination (#2) and 88% performance on minimal pair discrimination requiring picture selection (#4).

To summarise, FF's core deficit did not appear to be a loss of phonological codes, global weakening of connections, a loss of semantic representations, or monitoring failure. When word production involved accessing phonological forms by bypassing the semantic system, as in repetition, FF performed very well. When the semantic system was tested without phonological demands, as in PPT, his performance was also very good. This pattern implicates the connection between semantics and phonology as the underlying locus of FF's deficits (e.g., Hillis et al. 1999).

If the connection between semantics and phonology is compromised in FF, then increases in either phonological or semantic activation during picture naming may compensate for this and assist FF in picture naming. In the following experiments cueing was used as a potential source of increased activation. Experiment 1 examined the effects of semantic versus phonological cueing on picture naming. Experiment 2 then tested the effects of relative timing of these cue-target presentations.

SECTION 2: EFFECTIVENESS OF CUEING

Experiment 1: Effect of semantic versus phonological cueing in picture naming

Materials and procedures. A four-session computerised picture-naming experiment was developed using a modified 175-item Philadelphia Naming Test (Roach et al., 1996). These four testing sessions manipulated cue type (semantic versus phonological) and relatedness (related versus unrelated). The sessions were blocked by cue type: two sessions presented semantic cues and two sessions presented phonological cues. For each cue type, testing was conducted over two sessions such that the items that were preceded by related cues in one session were preceded by unrelated cues in the other session and vice versa. The verbal cues were generated by a native English-speaking female and recorded in a sound-treated room, and the pure tone was computer generated. A delay of 750 ms between cue and target was selected on the basis of a review of the aphasia literature—with delays that vary from a low of 350 ms to a high of 1400ms (Baum, 1997; Elman et al., 1991; Hagoort, 1997). We sought a middle ground that would allow sufficient processing time for the cue but would not unnecessarily extend the length of trails.

A trial consisted of the presentation of the recorded auditory cue, followed by 750 ms of silence, and then the target picture, which remained on the computer screen until a response was made. For the phonological cueing sessions, the auditory cue was either the first sound of the name of the picture (e.g., /ball/ → "b") in the related condition or 1 KHz pure tone in the unrelated condition. For the semantic cueing sessions, the auditory cue was a semantically related word to the target (e.g., /

candle/ → "wick") in the related condition or a semantically unrelated word in the unrelated condition (e.g., /candle/ → "grass"). The semantic cues were the first associates of the target items in the University of South Florida Word Association Norms (Nelson, McEvoy, & Schreiber, 1998). None of the semantic cues had the same initial phoneme as the target. The unrelated semantic cues were matched to the related cues for word frequency, syllable length, word class, and familiarity. The stimuli presentation was randomised within sessions, and relatedness and cue type were counterbalanced across sessions. There was a gap of at least 1 week between each of the four sessions. These sessions were recorded with a high-quality digital audio recorder and later transcribed for analysis.

Scoring and analysis. Despite instructions to limit naming attempts to a single word, FF produced many multiple responses. Although selecting one response when many were produced results in potentially useful information being discarded, we followed this standard practice, and for each trial the first complete non-fragmented naming attempt was classified into one of the following categories: (1) correct; (2) phonological error; (3) semantic error; (4) mixed error; (5) description; (6) neologism; (7) perseveration; (8) unrelated; and (9) no response (Croot et al., 1999; Roach et al., 1996; Schwartz, Wilshire, Gagnon, & Polansky, 2004). The Appendix provides descriptions of the error categories.

Reliability. All scoring was performed by the first author, and a trained research assistant performed the reliability checks for at least 40% of the sessions. The point-by-point inter-rater agreement was 98.3%, and disagreements were resolved by reviewing the scoring definitions and the transcripts.

Results. Figure 1's upper panel shows the performance across the semantic and phonological cueing conditions. In contrast to the semantic cues, phonological cueing resulted in an increase in correct responses in picture naming ($\chi^2 = 7.15$, $p < .01$). Figure 2's upper panel shows the error patterns across the cueing conditions, and indicates that the most common error types were neologisms, followed by semantic errors and descriptions. Statistical analyses were not performed given the small numbers associated with many of the error types. However, visual inspection of Figure 2 shows that semantic cueing appeared to increase the semantic errors and decrease the neologisms, whereas phonological cueing (top right panel) appeared to decrease semantic errors and descriptions. Because only the phonological cues resulted in improved picture naming, we focused on those cues in the development of the following experiment, which was designed to determine whether the timing of cue presentation relative to the target picture had an impact on the effectiveness of the cue.

Experiment 2: Effect of timing of the phonological cue on picture naming

This experiment began 4 weeks after the conclusion of Experiment 1, and was identical to the phonological cue condition of that experiment except for the modification of the timing of the phonological cue relative to the target in two cueing conditions: "with picture" and "after picture". In contrast to the phonological condition in Experiment 1 ("before picture"), where the cue was presented 750 ms

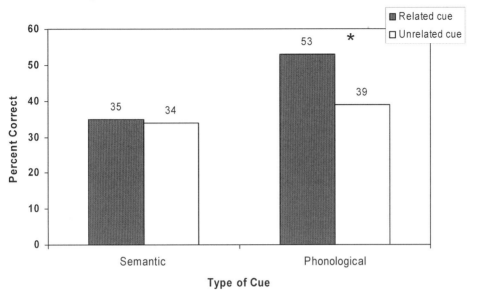

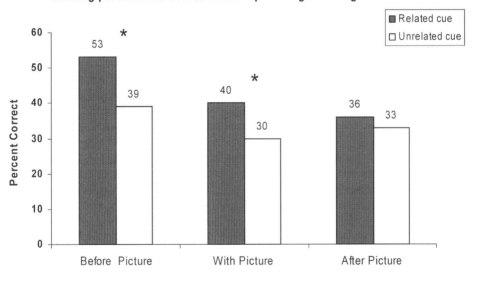

Figure 1. Percentage of correctly named items across different cueing conditions. * represents significant difference at alpha set at .05.

before the picture, in the "with picture" condition, the phonological cue and the picture were presented simultaneously, and in the "after picture" condition, the phonological cue was presented 750 ms after the picture appeared. This allowed us to determine when a phonological cue was most likely to assert an effect on

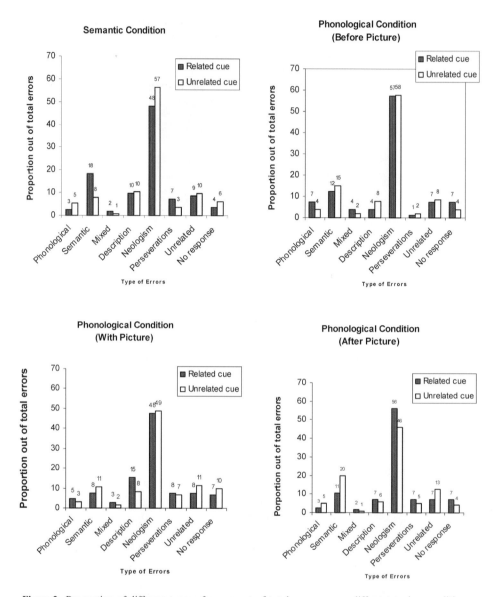

Figure 2. Proportion of different types of errors out of total errors across different cueing conditions.

picture-naming processes—either before semantic access, with semantic access, or after semantic access has been initiated. These conditions were presented over four testing sessions in a manner identical in all respects to Experiment 1.

Results. Phonological cues were effective in improving picture naming when they were provided before the picture as in Experiment 1, or with the picture ($\chi^2 = 5.16$, $p < .02$), but not after the onset of picture presentation ($\chi^2 = 0.29$, $p = .59$), as can be seen in the lower panel of Figure 1.

Figure 2's lower panel shows the error patterns for Experiment 2 with the same three prevalent error types as Experiment 1. In addition, similar to Experiment 1, small numbers associated with some error types precluded systematic statistical analysis and when considered together, the pattern of errors across cue type and cue condition appears much too varied to form a basis for strong claims. The large spread between neologisms across the two experiments, independent of relatedness condition, indicates that this variable may not be particularly sensitive to the cueing manipulation. We therefore restrict further discussion to accuracy data for the most part, and hope to establish a better understanding of error patterns through future work with FF.

Discussion: Experiments 1 and 2

Results of Experiment 1 showed that semantic cues were not as effective as phonological cues in improving picture-naming performance for FF. Failure to improve naming performance following semantic primes and lack of treatment gains following semantic therapy have been reported with other jargon-aphasic individuals, such as CM in Marshall et al. (1998) and JL in Martin and Laine (2000). This lack of impact may be because semantic activation is already present in the system as a consequence of picture processing, and any additional activation coming from the auditory presentation of a related word is insufficient to have an influence on the system. As suggested by Martin and Laine (2000), it may be that the cues increased spreading activation from the target word to semantically related lexical neighbours, giving rise to FF's increased semantic errors and decreased neologisms. However, without clearer error pattern data we are unable to strongly support this claim.

In contrast to the semantic cues, the phonological cues (Experiment 1) resulted in an increase in correct naming responses. A facilitatory effect of word-initial phonemic cue has been reported with aphasic individuals, particularly for patients whose production difficulties appear to be lexically mediated (Croot et al., 1999; Lambon-Ralph et al., 2000; Li & Williams, 1991). Similar to other such patients, FF made many semantic and descriptions errors, but fewer phonological errors (Croot et al., 1999; Lambon-Ralph et al., 2000; Wilshire & Saffran, 2005). Improved picture naming with phonemic cues is consistent with an explanation of the cueing advantage arising at a lexical selection stage whereby the cue increases activation of the target representation (e.g., Meyers & Schriefers, 1991) or activates a cohort of items beginning with the same phoneme ("phonological cohort effect", Best et al., 2002).

It is also possible that phonological cues work as constraints during lexical selection. Such an explanation is consistent with findings from Experiment 2, which show that the phonological cueing advantage was eliminated when FF received the phonological cue "after picture". In this condition, the phonological cue could not constrain a semantic system that had 750 ms available for the activation of a number of response alternatives. Elman et al. (1992) suggested that the timing of the cues for the posterior-aphasic patient is critical, as these patients can only be helped by prior cues. However, Elman et al.'s study included only one condition (cue prior to the picture), thus precluding any systematic comparison of the timing of cues on picture naming. To our knowledge, this study is the first to confirm Elman's claim through a systematic manipulation of the timing of the phonological cues and its effects on the accuracy of picture naming. Further research is under way to determine if cue timing will have similar effect on other types of aphasia.

SUMMARY, CONCLUSIONS, AND FUTURE DIRECTIONS

This article reports data from a study of an individual with jargon aphasia (FF) who produced severe neologisms in his verbal production. Results from a battery of cognitive and linguistic tests implicated the connection between the semantic and phonological systems as a potential locus of his deficit. A comparison of the effects of semantic versus phonological cueing showed a greater facilitatory effect for phonological cues than for semantic cues. The effectiveness of phonological cues was shown to be eliminated when target pictures were presented prior to the cue.

FF, like others with jargon aphasia (e.g., Marshall et al., 1998; Martin & Laine, 2000), did not demonstrate improved naming when provided with semantic cues. However, semantic cues may have strengthened the connection between related lexical items, as evidenced by increased semantic errors, but without stronger error pattern data we offer this as nothing more than an interesting speculation. Phonological cues provided prior to, or with, the picture possibly facilitated picture naming by acting as a constraining factor for the semantic system. Thus, FF's pattern of performance is consistent with theories that describe deficit in the connection between semantics and phonology as the likely source of neologisms in some jargon-aphasic individuals, similar to JBN in Hillis et al. (1999), CM in Marshall et al. (1998), and KVH in Moses et al. (2004). This finding generates the potential for future studies to incorporate the activation of the phonological system, specifically cues prior to or with the picture, for remediation of naming difficulties in people with neologisms. Our continued work with FF and other aphasic individuals will evaluate the generalisability of these findings.

This study contributes to the understanding of the underlying locus of neologism and provides evidence of a phonological cueing advantage in picture naming for an individual with severe neologism. Like many studies in this area of research, our study also presents additional questions and highlights a need for increased research on this very difficult form of aphasia. For example, a more detailed analysis of the phonological relationship of neologisms to their targets could form the basis for a more complete understanding of the disorder. A systematic comparison of the first versus later error responses in structured tasks like naming could shed light on error responses to naming failure. Finally, cueing experiments that systematically evaluate the effects of cue–target asynchrony would likely provide data of methodological, theoretical, and clinical relevance.

REFERENCES

Baum, S. (1997). Phonological, semantic and mediated priming in aphasia. *Brain & Language, 60*, 347–359.

Best, W., Herbert, R., Hickin, J., Osborne, F., & Howard, D. (2002). Phonological and orthographic facilitation of word-retrieval in aphasia: Immediate and delayed effects. *Aphasiology, 16*, 151–168.

Buckingham, H. W. (1987). Phonemic paraphasias and psycholinguistic production models for neologistic jargon. *Aphasiology, 1*, 381–400.

Butterworth, B. (1992). Disorders of phonological encoding. *Cognition, 42*, 261–286.

Christman, S. (1994). Target-related neologism formation in jargon aphasia. *Brain & Language, 46*, 109–128.

Croot, K., Patterson, K., & Hodges, J. R. (1999). Familial progressive aphasia: Insights into the nature and deterioration of single word processing. *Cognitive Neuropsychology, 16*, 705–747.

Ellis, A. W., Miller, D. M., & Sin, G. (1983). Wernicke's aphasia and normal language processing: A case study in cognitive neuropsychology. *Cognition, 15*, 111–144.

Elman, R. J., Klatzky, R. L., Dronkers, N. F., & Wertz, R. T. (1992). Phonologic priming and picture naming in aphasic and normal subjects. *Clinical Aphasiology, 21,* 255–262.

Goodglass, H., Kaplan, E., & Baressi (2001). *The assessment of aphasia and related disorders (Third edition).* Philadelphia, PA: Lea & Febiger.

Hagoort, P. (1997). Semantic priming in Broca's aphasics at a short SOA: No support for an automatic access deficit. *Brain & Language, 56,* 287–300.

Hillis, A., Boatman, D., Hart, J., & Gordon, B. (1999). Making sense out of jargon: A neurolinguistic and computational account of jargon aphasia. *Neurology, 53,* 1813–1824.

Howard, D., & Patterson, K. (1992). *Pyramids and palm trees test.* Bury St Edmunds, UK: Thames Valley Test Co.

Kay, J., Lesser, R., & Coltheart, M. (1992). *Psycholinguistic assessments of language processing in aphasia.* Hove, UK: Psychology Press.

Kertesz, A., & Benson, D. (1970). Neologistic jargon: A clinicopathological study. *Cortex, 6,* 362–386.

Lambon-Ralph, M. A., Sage, K., & Roberts, J. (2000). Classical anomia: A neuropsychological perspective on speech production. *Neuropsychologia, 38,* 186–202.

Le Dorze, G., Boulay, N., Gaudreau, J., & Brassard, C. (1994). The contrasting effects of a semantic versus a formal-semantic technique for the facilitation of naming in a case of anomia. *Aphasiology, 8,* 127–141.

Li, E. C., & Williams, S. E. (1991). An investigation of naming errors following semantic and phonemic cueing. *Neuropsychologia, 29,* 1083–1093.

Marshall, J. (2006). Jargon aphasia: What have we learned? *Aphasiology, 20,* 387–410.

Marshall, J., Robson, J., Pring, T., & Chiat, S. (1998). Why does monitoring fail in jargon aphasia? Comprehension judgement and therapy evidence. *Brain & Language, 63,* 79–107.

Marshall, R. (2001). Management of Wernicke's aphasia: A context-based approach. In R. Chapey (Ed.), *Language intervention strategies in aphasia and related neurogenic communication disorders.* Baltimore, MD: Lippincott Williams & Wilkins.

Martin, N., & Laine, M. (2000). Effects of contextual priming on impaired word retrieval. *Aphasiology, 14,* 53–70.

Meyers, A. S., & Schriefers, H. (1991). Phonological facilitation in picture–word interference experiments: Effect of stimulus onset asynchrony and types of interfering stimuli. *Journal of Experimental Psychology: Learning, Memory, & Cognition, 17,* 1146–1160.

Moses, M. S., Nickels, L. A., & Sheard, C. (2004). Disentangling the web: Neologistic perseverative errors in jargon aphasia. *Neurocase, 10,* 452–461.

Nelson, D. L., McEvoy, C. L., & Schreiber, T. A. (1998). *The University of South Florida word association, rhyme, and word fragment norms.* http://www.usf.edu/FreeAssociation/

Nickels, L., & Howard, D. (1995). Phonological errors in aphasic naming: Comprehension, monitoring and lexicality. *Cortex, 31,* 209–237.

Roach, A., Schwartz, M. F., Martin, N., Grewal, R. S., & Brecher, A. (1996). The Philadelphia Naming Test: Scoring and rationale. *Aphasiology, 24,* 121–133.

Schwartz, M., Saffran, E., Bloch, D., & Dell, G. (1994). Disordered speech production in aphasic and normal speakers. *Brain & Language, 47,* 52–88.

Schwartz, M., Wilshire, C., Gagnon, D., & Polansky, M. (2004). Origins of nonword phonological errors in aphasic picture naming. *Cognitive Neuropsychology, 21,* 159–186.

Wilshire, C. E., & Saffran, E. M. (2005). Contrasting effects of phonological priming in aphasic word production. *Cognition, 95,* 31–71.

APPENDIX: CRITERIA FOR CLASSIFYING THE NAMING RESPONSES

1. Correct: Phonologically accurate production of the target name or an acceptable alternative. Self-corrections, addition or deletion of plural morphemes (e.g., /grape/ → *grapes*), and addition of prepositional phrase (e.g., /can/ → *can of peas*) were accepted as correct responses.
2. Phonological error: Lexical error bearing phonological, but not semantic, resemblance to the target, minimally sharing the first phoneme and at least 50% or more phonemes with target (e.g., /anchor/ → *ankle*; /desk/ → *dress*).
3. Semantic error: Lexical error bearing semantic, but not phonological, resemblance to the target. Noun responses relating to the target as associative (e.g., /bench/ → *park*), synonyms (e.g., /toilet/ → *commode*), and/or categorical super-, sub-, and co-ordinate (e.g., /banana/ → *apple*) were included as semantic errors.
4. Mixed error: Lexical error bearing both semantic and phonological resemblance to the target (e.g., /crown/ → *king*).
5. Description: Responses that provided semantically related information to the target with no attempt to name. For example, description providing characterisation, explaining the function or purpose of the item to be named (e.g., /thermometer/ → *shove this in your throat*).
6. Neologism: Non-lexical/nonword errors (e.g., /monkey/ → *igyburger*; /glass/ → *kigyburger*).
7. Perseveration: Duplication of a response produced on any previous trial within the same session.
8. Unrelated: Lexical error not related to the target in any obvious way.
9. No response: Participant indicated verbally or non-verbally that he could not name the picture.

APHASIOLOGY, 2007, 21 (6/7/8), 739–749

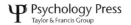

Towards a description of clinical communication impairment profiles following right-hemisphere damage

Hélène Côté

Institut universitaire de gériatrie de Montréal, Université de Montréal, and Hôpital de réadaptation Villa Medica, Montréal, Canada

Mélissa Payer

Institut universitaire de gériatrie de Montréal, and Université de Montréal, Canada

Francine Giroux

Institut universitaire de gériatrie de Montréal, Canada

Yves Joanette

Institut universitaire de gériatrie de Montréal, and Université de Montréal, Canada

Background: It is estimated that approximately 50% of individuals who incur right-hemisphere damage (RHD) have subsequent communication disorders. Lexical-semantic, discourse, prosodic, and pragmatic deficits have been reported following RHD, but the co-occurrence of these deficits within the same individual has not yet been systematically investigated. Therefore clinical profiles of communication impairments in individuals with RHD still have to be identified and described in order to appreciate their communication impairment and provide strategies for rehabilitation.
Aims: The goal of the present study was to explore the clinical profiles of communication impairments subsequent to a right hemisphere lesion.
Methods and Procedures: A total of 28 French-speaking individuals with a right-hemisphere lesion were evaluated using the *Protocole MEC* (Joanette, Ska, & Côté, 2004), a normalised battery allowing the assessment of communication deficits after RHD. A hierarchical cluster analysis was used to group participants according to similarities in their results on the 14 tasks.
Outcomes and Results: Four subgroups of RHD individuals were identified on the basis of the overall similarities of performance on the 14 tasks of the *Protocole MEC*. Participants in the first cluster showed impairments in all four language components evaluated, whereas the second cluster of participants was also impaired in prosodic, lexical-semantic, and pragmatic abilities, but was characterised by a relative preservation of discourse abilities. The third cluster of participants did not show any abnormal results. Finally, two individuals were mainly characterised by some lexical-semantic deficits.
Conclusions: The *Protocole MEC* used in conjunction with a cluster analysis provided a first step towards the identification of communication impairment profiles among the population of individuals with RHD. In the present study it was not possible to clearly identify the relationship between a given profile and factors such as lesion site, age, or

---

Address correspondence to: Hélène Côté, MOA Centre de recherche, IUGM 4565, chemin Queen-Mary, Montréal QC H3W 1W5, Canada. E-mail: helene.cote.1@umontreal.ca

---

© 2007 Psychology Press, an imprint of the Taylor & Francis Group, an informa business
http://www.psypress.com/aphasiology   DOI: 10.1080/02687030701192331

education. Incidence of communication impairments was estimated to be higher in a rehabilitation centre setting than the generally accepted 50% in the literature.

Almost 50 years have elapsed since Eisenson (1959) suggested that right-hemisphere brain damage (RHD) could lead to communication disorders. First vaguely referred to by Eisenson as *supra-ordinary alterations* or *loss of fine abilities*, these deficits have since been described more systematically, particularly over the past two decades. The non-exclusivity of the left hemisphere for language abilities is now widely endorsed, and the necessity of the integrity of the right hemisphere for a number of language components has been confirmed through the descriptions of communication impairments that can be observed in individuals with RHD (Code, 1987; Joanette, Goulet, & Hannequin, 1990; Myers, 1999; Tompkins, 1995). Thus, prosodic (Pell, 1999; Walker & Daigle, 2000), lexical-semantic (Gagnon, Goulet, Giroux, & Joanette, 2003; Joanette et al., 1990; Myers & Brookshire, 1995), discourse (Lojek-Osiejuk, 1996), and pragmatic (Chantraine, Joanette, & Ska, 1998; Gardner, Ling, Flamm, & Silverman, 1975; Vanhalle et al., 2000) deficits have been reported to occur in individuals following a right-hemisphere lesion.

Although such communication deficits have been described at length, there is growing evidence that they are not present in all individuals with RHD. No epidemiological studies have been undertaken on this topic, but some cues are available. Indeed, Joanette, Goulet, and Daoust (1991), as well as Benton and Bryan (1996), estimated that 50% of individuals with RHD are likely to present with communication disorders. Moreover, it is unclear if, when present, these communication deficits express themselves in the same way across individuals. Most studies on this question have considered components of communication separately, such as pragmatic or prosodic disorders. Surprisingly few attempts have directly addressed the question of the possible clinical profiles of communication deficits that might follow RHD. A clearer description of clinical profiles would allow a better appreciation of the communication impairments of an individual, and would also lead to the introduction of more adapted and relevant rehabilitation strategies for individuals with RHD in clinical settings. To our knowledge, only two studies examined this question directly.

In an attempt to explore the relationship between perceptual integration deficits and verbal expression after a right-hemisphere lesion, Myers (1979, 2005) partly addressed the question of clinical profiles of communication impairments in adults with RHD. Although only eight participants were included in this study, Myers (1979) reported the presence of some heterogeneity in the communication deficit profiles of the individuals with RHD evaluated, without being able to clearly identify distinctive profiles. One factor considered by Myers to limit the identification of clinical profiles of communication impairments in RHD individuals is the lack of a comprehensive published instrument to evaluate all components of RHD communication.

Joanette et al. (1991) made a first attempt at estimating the incidence of verbal communication deficits after RHD, and explored in preliminary terms the question of the clinical profiles of communication impairments. They analysed the performance of 33 participants with RHD who completed three different tasks: word naming, sentence completion, and story narration. Their results showed that, out of the 33 participants tested, four had overall performance similar to those of matched control participants, confirming that a lesion to the right side of the brain does not automatically impair communication abilities. Conversely, nine individuals with RHD were impaired on all tasks. However, the most interesting result was that the other 20 participants exhibited poorer performance on one or two tasks only, in such a way that some participants with RHD showed distinctive—and even contrasting—profiles of communication deficits that expressed themselves through double dissociations in some cases. The authors first concluded that not all individuals with RHD present with communication disorders, at least for the language components considered in their study. They also noted that, when communication impairments are present, the impaired abilities varied among participants, leading to heterogeneity of profiles. This first attempt had a number of limitations; one being that it was an a posteriori exploration, and another that it was based on the evaluation of only a limited number of communication components.

Blake, Duffy, Myers, and Tompkins addressed a similar question in 2002, searching for prevalence and patterns of right hemisphere cognitive and communicative deficits. To do so, they reviewed medical charts from 123 patients. Some correlations were reported (e.g., attention deficits were closely related to learning and memory deficits, hyporesponsivity was related to other cognitive deficits), but overall interpretation of the results was limited by the fact that no task was systematically used with all patients. Therefore, the analysis was solely based on health professionals' often subjective impression as to the presence or absence of communication and/or cognitive deficits.

Because the lack of a comprehensive assessment tool limits the exploration and description of clinical profiles associated with RHD, this issue will be briefly explored next. Very few batteries have been designed to specifically evaluate communication skills in individuals with RHD (e.g., Bryan, 1989, 1995; Halper, Cherney, Burns, & Mogil, 1996). Those that do exist appear to have both theoretical and methodological limits (Eck, Côté, Ska, & Joanette, 2001). Some of these batteries appear to lack coherence concerning what should be evaluated in order to address the communication impairments after RHD. Indeed, some of these clinical batteries tend to focus on non-communicative abilities, such as the evaluation of visual neglect. Of course, neglect may have an impact on the processing of written language, but it does not per se represent a communication deficit. Also, mainly inspired by the literature from the 1980s or earlier, these batteries did not benefit from the important theoretical advancements introduced in psycholinguistics and cognitive psychology over the last two decades.

In order to lessen the problem, our group recently developed such a clinical tool, now available in French (language- and culture-adapted versions are being currently prepared and normed in English, Spanish, Portuguese, and Italian). The *Protocole Montreal d'Évaluation de la Communication* (Joanette et al., 2004) allows the systematic evaluation of four components of verbal communication possibly affected following a right-hemisphere lesion. The *Protocole MEC* was standardised with 180 normal control participants representing three age groups (30–49, 50–64, 65–85) and two levels of education (HIGH and LOW by reference to each cohort's mean number of years of education). The *Protocole MEC* inter-rater reliability as well as its validity of content were shown to be good (Côté, Moix, & Giroux, 2004). Two aspects of the *Protocole MEC* are sources of obvious limitations. The first limitation results from the fact that the *Protocole MEC* does not provide exhaustive evaluation of the components of communication included; for instance, comprehension of humour and sarcasm is not evaluated, and only a limited number of tasks assess the semantic processing of words. The second limitation is shared by numerous clinical protocols; the *Protocole MEC* does not provide specific information as to the underlying sources of the verbal communication impairments. Nevertheless, and despite these limitations, the 14 tasks of the *Protocole MEC* appear to be the best compromise as a published and validated clinical tool that allows the evaluation of prosodic, lexical-semantic, discursive, and pragmatic abilities (see Table 1).

In summary, the clinical profiles of communication impairments that can be present in individuals with RHD are still largely unknown, despite some valuable but limited attempts to study them. The availability of a clinical battery allowing the evaluation of the main communication components likely to be impaired in individuals with RHD now permits us to revisit this longstanding question. The goal of the present study was to explore whether there are distinctive clinical profiles of communication impairments following RHD by using the *Protocole MEC* applied to consecutively admitted post-CVA patients with RHD recruited in specialised rehabilitation units. More specifically, it was intended to (a) estimate the proportion of individuals with RHD with communication impairments in rehabilitation settings, and (b) contribute to the description of clinical profiles of communication impairments subsequent to RHD.

METHOD

Participants

A total of 28 French-speaking volunteer participants (15 men and 13 women) were evaluated. Participants ranged in age from 26 to 90 years and had between 5 and 18 years of formal education. All but three participants were right-handers and had incurred a single vascular brain lesion ascertained by a CT or MRI scan, with no other neurological history. The remaining three had experienced a previous transient RH ischaemia. All were 3 to 14 weeks post-onset (with an average of 6 weeks post-onset). None had a history of psychiatric disease or drug and alcohol addiction. Recruited participants were unselected incoming patients admitted to the neurological unit of five different rehabilitation centres; they were thus not selected to participate in the study on the basis of the presence or absence of communication impairments.

Tasks

All 14 tasks of the *Protocole MEC* (Joanette et al., 2004) were used in the present study. See Table 1 for a brief description of each task.

Procedure

Each participant with RHD was evaluated by a trained speech and language pathologist (main evaluator) using the 14 tasks of the *Protocole MEC*. Evaluation was done in two or three 45–60-minute sessions in a quiet environment. All tasks were presented to each participant in the indicated sequence in the *Protocole MEC* in order to allow comparison between their results and the available norms. All participants' oral productions were audio-recorded and disagreements were resolved

TABLE 1
Description of the 14 tasks of the *Protocole MEC*

Language component	Task		Description
Prosody	Linguistic prosody	Comprehension	12 pre-recorded sentences (4 sentences of neutral content, each said with three different linguistic intonations). Participant identifies the intonation by pointing to a multiple choice of modality icons (previously ascertained as well recognised)
		Repetition	Same stimuli as previous. Participant repeats the sentences
	Emotional prosody	Comprehension	12 pre-recorded sentences (4 sentences of neutral content, each pronounced with three different emotional intonations). Participant identifies the intonation by pointing to a multiple choice of emotion icons (previously ascertained as well recognised)
		Repetition	Same stimuli as previous. Participant repeats the sentences
		Production	Nine short situational paragraphs inducing an emotion (three situations, three target sentences). Participant produces the target sentence orally with the appropriate intonation
Lexical-semantic	Verbal fluency	Unconstrained	Participant says as many words as possible in 2.5 minutes, without any criterion
		Semantic criterion	Participant says as many "clothes" names as possible in 2 minutes
		Orthographic criterion	Participant says as many words as possible starting by the letter "P" in 2 minutes
	Semantic judgement		24 pairs of words, 12 of them semantically related and 12 without semantic relationship. Participant indicates by YES or NO the presence of a semantic relationship and has to explain the nature of the semantic relationship
Discourse	Conversational discourse		10-minute conversation between participant and examiner on two different topics. 17-point observation grid filled in by the evaluator
	Narrative discourse – recall and questions		Five-paragraph narrative first recalled one paragraph at a time and then recalled globally, with 12 comprehension questions including inferences
Pragmatics	Metaphor interpretation		20 metaphors of which 10 are idioms (*frozen* or lexicalised) and 10 creative (*creative* or non-lexicalised) metaphors. Open question and multiple choices
	Indirect speech act interpretation		20 situations of which 10 end with a direct speech act, 10 end with an indirect speech act. Open question and multiple choices
Awareness of deficits	Questionnaire on deficits awareness		Seven yes/no questions

through consensus by two evaluators. Moreover, all results were reviewed by a single expert to ensure homogeneity in scoring and a strict comparison to the normative data. Reliability of results was not evaluated in the present study, but a previous study provided a good inter-rater reliability for the *Protocole MEC* (Côté et al., 2004). For each participant with RHD, a three-step *structured clinical impression* was also collected. First, the main evaluator filled out a 15-point screening questionnaire with a relative to collect information on pre-morbid communicative abilities of the individual with RHD and on any communicative changes noted by the relative since the stroke. Then a second trained speech and language pathologist had a 10-minute conversation with the participant with RHD, before completing a 17-point conversational discourse observation grid (part of the *Protocole MEC*), in order to obtain clinical impressions of possible deviant communicative behaviour, be they prosodic, lexical-semantic, discursive, or pragmatic. In the last step, both speech and language pathologists—the main evaluator having used the *Protocole MEC* and the second evaluator having used the conversational discourse observation grid— agreed on a "clinical impression", also taking into account the relative's perspective, as collected by the main evaluator. To do so, each judge made a decision (+/–) and then compared results with the other judges. A structured clinical impression was called positive when communication disorders were thought to be present by at least two of three judges—main evaluator, second evaluator, and relative. Conversely, the structured clinical impression was called negative when at least two of three judges considered the communication abilities to be preserved. The result of the structured clinical impression would later be used as a factor to describe the clusters.

RESULTS

Participants' communicative performance on each of the 14 tasks was first described in terms of the *Protocole MEC* standardised scoring procedure using the "*alert points*" (Côté et al., 2004). The *alert point* is the level of performance at which a behaviour is considered deviant for the task under examination (*cut-off*). It is the age- and education-adjusted performance and generally corresponds to the 10th percentile based on control participants' results obtained during the normalisation. The performance of all participants with RHD for all tasks was submitted to a hierarchical cluster analysis (Aldenderfer & Blashfield, 1985) to allow for the identification of subgroups of participants with RHD characterised by distinctive communication impairment profiles. However, before doing so, the results of each participant was transformed into z scores by reference to the normative data of the *Protocole MEC*. The z score permitted comparison of participants to each other, taking into account the normal impact of age and education. The hierarchical cluster analysis allowed the identification of three clusters. See Table 2 for a summary description of each cluster including participants' age, education, and cerebral region affected.

Following the identification of subgroups with a cluster analysis, a description of impaired communication abilities in each the subgroup was undertaken. In order to achieve this characterisation, the result for each task was considered impaired for a given subgroup under the following two conditions: (1) the overall mean z score of the cluster was below -1.5; and (2) more than 50% of the members of the cluster had a z score below -2 (see Table 3).

TABLE 2
Results of the hierarchical cluster analysis

Clusters (number of participants and gender)	Age (years)	Education (years)	Brain lesion (Number of participants in which a cerebral region was affected by the lesion)	
Cluster 1 (n = 5) 3♀ 2♂	26–61 (x = 44)	8–12 (x = 11)	Frontal 1 Temporal 0 Parietal 1 Sub-cortical 4	
Cluster 2 (n = 10) 3♀ 7♂	46–79 (x = 64)	6–16 (x = 11)	Frontal 3 Temporal 3 Parietal 5 Sub-cortical 5	
Cluster 3 (n = 11) 6♀ 5♂	50–90 (x = 73)	5–16 (x = 9)	Frontal 0 Temporal 2 Parietal 3 Sub-cortical 8	
Group 4 (n = 2) 1♀ 1♂	74–85 (x = 80)	9–16 (x = 13)	Frontal 0 Temporal 2 Parietal 0 Sub-cortical 0	

Each RHD participant represents a line on the left-sided ordinate axis of the figure; tinted areas indicate each of the four clusters.

Table 3 allows the identification of the communication profiles of each subgroup of participants with RHD. A qualitative analysis of all individual results—clinical notes—allowed a finer description of the impairments.

TABLE 3
Clusters mean z score for each task of the Protocole MEC

Variables	Cluster 1 (n = 5)	Cluster2 (n = 10)	Cluster 3 (n = 11)	Group 4 (n = 2)
Linguistic prosody – Comp	−1.10	**−2.02**	−0.33	0.33
Linguistic prosody – Rep	−1.84	**−4.35**	0.27	0.70
Emotional prosody – Comp	−2.34	−1.63	−0.29	−0.79
Emotional prosody – Rep	−1.02	−1.97	−0.88	−0.85
Emotional prosody – Prod	−1.09	−1.40	−0.72	−1.31
Verbal fluency unconstrained	−1.87	−1.82	−0.78	−1.24
Verbal fluency – semantic	−1.24	−1.67	−1.01	−0.48
Verbal fluency – orthographic	−1.84	−1.55	−0.44	−2.12
Semantic judgement	−0.64	**−2.70**	−0.04	**−17.14**
Conversation discourse	**−9.78**	**−3.53**	−1.26	−4.49
Narrative discourse – Recall	**−1.89**	−0.11	0.26	0.35
Narrative disc. – Questions	**−1.97**	−0.41	0.33	−0.67
Metaphors	**−2.61**	−1.72	−0.87	−3.89
Indirect speech acts	−1.40	−1.25	−1.19	**−2.77**

Bold results indicate tasks for which the group z score was ⩽ −1,5 AND for which 50%+1 of the participants obtained a z score ⩽ −2.

- Participants in the first cluster showed impairments in all four language components evaluated by the *Protocole MEC*. A qualitative analysis of these participants' results showed reduced verbal fluency, poor story recall, reduced comprehension of non-literal language, major difficulty in adapting their speech to their communication partner, and prosodic impairments. One of these five participants was evaluated as anosognosic.
- The second cluster of participants was characterised by a relative preservation of discourse abilities. Participants in that cluster also showed a reduced verbal fluency and difficulty in adapting their speech to the interlocutor, although less so than members of cluster 1. Out of 10 participants, 5 were anosognosic.
- Participants in cluster 3 showed globally normal communication abilities by reference to the *Protocole MEC* normative data. For five of these patients, both speech and language pathologists as well as a relative considered the participant to have normal communicational abilities (negative clinical impression). The six other participants of this cluster were suspected by the clinicians to have some degree of communication impairment. Each of these participants had at least one score below the norm at the *Protocole MEC*, but no task was impaired for all members of the group, and all mean Z scores were within normal range. Of the 11 participants, 2 did not notice any change in their communication behaviour although they scored below the norm on some measures.
- Two other participants fell outside the three clusters. They both presented severe deficits at the semantic judgement task and deficits in the indirect speech acts interpretation. Clinical notes for these two participants included difficulty in processing word semantics, reduced comprehension of indirect speech acts, slight prosodic impairments, conversational "malaise", and absence of emotional facial expression. Both participants were aware of changes in their communication abilities.

The descriptive analysis of the localisation of the brain lesion for every participant in each cluster did not allow the identification of a specific lesion site strongly associated with a specific cluster. However, the following observations were made. Three-quarters of the participants presenting a frontal lesion are in cluster #2, but we also see a variety of lesion sites affected in that same cluster. Cluster #3, presenting with normal results, seemed to be characterised by a high incidence of subcortical lesion. Age and education were fairly evenly distributed among the four subgroups, except that older and less-educated participants were over-represented in the third subgroup in which participants with RHD were most similar to normal participants. Participants of both genders were also evenly distributed in all clusters apart from a slight over-representation of women in the second cluster. No factor other than the right-hemisphere lesion itself thus appears to be responsible for the formation of the subgroups, despite the fact that the number of observations reported here probably does not allow for the identification of a given lesion site with a given communication impairment profile.

DISCUSSION

The use of the *Protocole MEC* in conjunction with a cluster analysis applied to the performance of individuals with RHD on 14 tasks including prosodic, lexical-semantic, discourse, and pragmatic abilities allowed the exploration of the possible profiles of communication impairments following a right-hemisphere lesion. Results showed the presence of heterogeneous profiles of communication impairments; however, this heterogeneity was not random—individuals with a right-hemisphere lesion actually share a number of communication impairments.

The presence of the three clusters and two outliers suggests two important points about the impact of a right-hemisphere lesion on verbal communication abilities. First, results confirm that a right-hemisphere lesion does not result in communication disorders in all individuals. Out of the 28 participants with RHD, a subgroup of 11 was identified by the cluster analysis as presenting with communication abilities globally comparable to that of age- and education-matched normal control participants, as none of their group average performances was below the alert point indicated in the *Protocole MEC*. However, 6 of these 11 participants with RHD were thought by expert clinicians to present some degree of communication impairment via positive structured clinical impression, but these were not apparent in the quantitative results obtained using the *Protocole MEC*. The other five participants of this group had a negative structured clinical impression, which means that these participants had both a clinical and a *Protocole MEC*-based indication that their right-hemisphere lesion was not a source of interference with their communication abilities. This number (5 out of 28, or approximately 18%) leads one to believe that the 50% incidence of communication disorders after RHD often stated in the literature (e.g. Joanette et al., 1991) is not descriptive of individuals in rehabilitation settings. Indeed, it suggests that the incidence of communication impairments in an unselected population of individuals requiring rehabilitation is more than 80%. This figure, which would have to be confirmed over a larger sample number of participants in rehabilitation clinical settings, probably expresses the fact that the less-impaired individuals with RHD do not require rehabilitation and are thus not referred to rehabilitation settings. However, this means that the incidence of communication impairments in RHD individuals who receive attention in a rehabilitation setting is very high. The systematic evaluation of possible communication impairments over a larger sample of individuals is necessary to gather more data on the actual incidence of communication impairments after RHD. Now that assessment tools are available, it would be of major interest for the field, as for public health planners, to use the instruments to estimate the incidence of communication disorders following RHD.

The second important point revealed by the presence of subgroups in the cluster analysis is that, when present, the combination of communication impairments can vary from one individual to another, although not in a totally random fashion, as is the case in aphasia after left-hemisphere stroke. The present exploratory study did not allow identification of factors possibly accounting for the observed subgroups, and collaborative studies done with a national sample would be needed in order to explore the impact of various factors such as lesion site and extent, age, education, and pre-morbid communication profiles. Although the limitations of the present study preclude an answer, lesion site and extension may represent a determinant factor in the profiles reported. If lesion site and extent in the right hemisphere are confirmed to correlate to communication profiles, there would be further evidence for specific contributions of the right hemisphere for communication. (Joanette & Goulet, 1994). On the contrary, if the different profiles of communication impairments were shown to be independent of site and extent of the lesion, this would argue for the non-specific contribution of the right hemisphere to communication abilities, as the heterogeneity would be due to other factors. Consequently, the question of the different profiles of communication impairments and their relationship with one another helps to reveal whether the contribution of the functional neural networks of the right hemisphere to components of communication is specific or not. A surprising finding was that participants in cluster 3—with relatively preserved language abilities—had predominantly subcortical lesions, therefore leading to the possible interpretation that subcortical structures are not essential for the treatment of language abilities under investigation in the present study. However, such an interpretation is mostly improbable considering the important recent literature pointing to the role of subcortical structures for language, especially for the processing of prosodic abilities (e.g., Van Lancker Sidtis, Pachana, Cummings, & Sidtis, 2006). More observations are needed in order to explore further this question.

The main limitation of the present study is surely the small number of participants evaluated, restricting the generalisation of results to the population of RHD. It will therefore be essential to reproduce a similar study with a larger number of participants.

Despite its limitations, this study represents a further attempt to describe clinical profiles of communication deficits following RHD. It now clearly appears that the occurrence of a right-hemisphere lesion is not responsible for communication impairments in all individuals, neither does it always express itself through the exact same profiles of disorders when impairments are present. The impact of such knowledge, hopefully enriched with more studies to come in the future, will be major in clinical settings, mainly for the development of rehabilitation strategies. These strategies would have to be adapted for each clinical profile. More studies concerning the incidence and the nature of the communication impairment profiles of individuals suffering from a right-hemisphere lesion will eventually guide clinicians in planning and adapting their interventions with this still under-served population.

REFERENCES

Aldenderfer, M. S., & Blashfield, R. K. (1985). *Cluster analysis*. Beverly Hills, CA: Sage Publications.

Benton, E., & Bryan, K. (1996). Right cerebral hemisphere damage: Incidence of language problems. *International Journal of Rehabilitation Research, 19*(1), 47–54.

Blake, M. L., Duffy, J. R., Myers, P. S., & Tompkins, C. A. (2002). Prevalence and patterns of right hemisphere cognitive/communicative deficits: Retrospective data from an inpatient rehabilitation unit. *Aphasiology, 16*, 537–547.

Bryan, K. L. (1989). *The Right Hemisphere Language Battery*. Kibworth, UK: Far Communications.

Bryan, K. L. (1995). *The Right Hemisphere Language Battery* (2nd ed.). London: Whurr Publishers Ltd.

Chantraine, Y., Joanette, Y., & Ska, B. (1998). Conversational abilities in patients with right hemisphere damage. In M. Paradis (Ed.), *Pragmatics in neurogenic communication disorders* (pp. 21–32). Tarrytown, NY: Pergamon Press.

Code, C. (1987). *Language aphasia and the right hemisphere*. Chichester, UK: Wiley.

Côté, H., Moix, V., & Giroux, F. (2004). Évaluation des troubles de la communication des cérébrolésés droits. *Rééducation Orthophonique, 219*, 107–122.

Eck, K., Côté, H., Ska, B., & Joanette, Y. (2001). *Analyse critique des protocoles d'évaluation des troubles de la communication des cérébrolésés droits*. Paper presented at the VII Congresso Latinoamericano de Neuropsicologia, São Paulo, Brazil, 30 October–3 November.

Eisenson, J. (1959). Language dysfunctions associated with right brain damage. *American Speech and Hearing Association, 1*, 107.

Gagnon, L., Goulet, P., Giroux, F., & Joanette, Y. (2003). Processing of metaphoric and non-metaphoric alternative meanings of words after right- and left-hemisphere lesion. *Brain and Language, 87*(2), 217–226.

Gardner, H., Ling, P. K., Flamm, L., & Silverman, J. (1975). Comprehension and appreciation of humor in brain-damaged patients. *Brain, 98,* 399–412.

Halper, A. S., Cherney, L. R., Burns, M. S., & Mogil, S. I. (1996). *RIC Evaluation of communication problems in right hemisphere dysfunction-revised (RICE-R).* Rockville, MD: Aspen.

Joanette, Y., & Goulet, P. (1994). Right hemisphere and verbal communication: Conceptual, methodological, and clinical issues. *Clinical Aphasiology, 22,* 1–23.

Joanette, Y., Goulet, P., & Daoust, H. (1991). Incidence et profils des troubles de la communication verbale chez les cérébrolésés droits. *Revue de Neuropsychologie, 1*(1), 3–27.

Joanette, Y., Goulet, P., Hannequin, D., with the collaboration of J. Boeglin (1990). *Right hemisphere and verbal communication.* New York: Springer-Verlag.

Joanette, Y., Ska, B., & Côté, H. (2004). *Protocole Montréal d'évaluation de la communication (MEC).* Isbergues: Ortho Édition.

Lojek-Osiejuk, E. (1996). Knowledge of scripts reflected in discourse of aphasics and right-brain-damaged patients. *Brain and Language, 53,* 58–80.

Myers, P. S. (1979). Profiles of communication deficits in patients with right cerebral hemisphere damage: Implications for diagnosis and treatment. In R. H. Brookshire (Ed.), *Clinical Aphasiology Conference Proceedings* (pp. 38–46). Minneapolis, MN: BRK Publishers.

Myers, P. S. (1999). *Right hemisphere damage: Disorders of communication and cognition.* San Diego, CA: Singular Publishing Group.

Myers, P. S. (2005). Profiles of communication deficits in patients with right cerebral hemisphere damage: Implications for diagnosis and treatment. *Aphasiology, 19*(12), 1147–1160.

Myers, P. S., & Brookshire, R. H. (1995). Effect of noun type on naming performance of right-hemisphere-damaged and non-brain-damaged adults. *Clinical Aphasiology, 23,* 195–206.

Pell, M. D. (1999). Fundamental frequency encoding of linguistic and emotional prosody by right-hemisphere-damaged speakers. *Brain and Language, 69*(2), 161–192.

Tompkins, C. A. (1995). *Right hemisphere communication disorders: Theory and management.* San Diego, CA: Singular Publishing Group.

Van Lancker Sidtis, D., Pachana, N., Cummings, J. L., & Sidtis, J. J. (2006). Dysprosodic speech following basal ganglia insult: Toward a conceptual framework for the study of the cerebral representation of prosody. *Brain and Language, 97*(2), 135–153.

Vanhalle, C., Lemieux, S., Joubert, S., Goulet, P., Ska, B., & Joanette, Y. (2000). Processing of speech acts by right hemisphere brain damaged patients: An ecological approach. *Aphasiology, 12*(11), 1127–1141.

Walker, J. P., & Daigle, T. (2000). Hemispheric specialization in processing prosodic structures: Revisited. *Brain and Language, 74*(3), 321–323.

APHASIOLOGY, 2007, 21 (6/7/8), 750–762

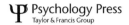

Problem-solving abilities of participants with and without diffuse neurologic involvement

Robert C. Marshall

University of Kentucky, Lexington, KY, USA

Susan R. McGurk

Dartmouth Medical School, Dartmouth, NH, USA

Colleen M. Karow

University of Tennessee, Knoxville, TN, USA

Tamar J. Kairy

Hofstra University, Hempstead, NJ, USA

Background: Impaired problem solving is a frequent consequence of brain trauma and other conditions that result in diffuse neurologic involvement. Information about how individuals with diffuse neurologic involvement solve problems is important to the development of strategies designed to help them achieve the highest degree of independent living despite neuropsychological compromise, and may aid clinical decision making in general.

Aims: To examine and compare problem-solving abilities of participants with and without diffuse neurologic involvement.

Methods & Procedures: We used the Rapid Assessment of Problem Solving test (RAPS; Marshall, Karow, Morelli, Iden, & Dixon, 2003a), a modification of Mosher and Hornsby's (1966) 20 Question task, to examine the problem-solving abilities of two groups of neurologically intact (NI) participants and three groups of participants with diffuse neurologic involvement (DNI). The RAPS is a clinical test of problem-solving abilities in which the client asks yes/no questions to identify a "target picture" in a 32-item array. The DNI groups included individuals with recent and chronic acquired traumatic brain injuries, and a third group of participants with severe mental illness. It was hypothesised that participants with DNI would perform less well on the RAPS than the NI participants, and that these differences would be reflected in lower scores on the RAPS and differences in the frequency with which certain types of questions were used to solve problems.

Outcomes & Results: Findings revealed significant differences between NI groups and two of the three DNI groups on objective scores, types of questions asked, and the strategies used to solve problems on the RAPS. The NI participants used a more systematic, organised approach to solving problems, whereas participants with DNI were less organised, inconsistent, and sometimes inflexible in their use of problem-solving strategies.

Address correspondence to: Robert C. Marshall PhD, Room 120F, CTW Building, University of Kentucky, 900 S. Limestone, Lexington, KY 40536-0002, USA. E-mail: rcmarsh@uky.edu

© 2007 Psychology Press, an imprint of the Taylor & Francis Group, an informa business

http://www.psypress.com/aphasiology

DOI: 10.1080/02687030601154076

Conclusions: Findings suggest the problem-solving abilities of participants with and without DNI are distinguishable in terms of selected components of Scholnick and Friedman's (1993) developmental theory of planning. These include a decision to plan, strategy choice and execution, and monitoring effects of prior actions.

Problem solving is one of several executive functions that permit individuals to engage in complex, novel, goal-directed activity (Lezak, Howieson, & Loring, 2004). Behavioural manifestations of impaired problem solving are well documented in persons with diffuse neurological involvement due to trauma (Goldstein & Levin, 1991; Kennedy & Coelho, 2005; Rath et al., 2004), dementia (Cummings & Benson, 1983; Willis et al., 1998), and mental illness (Chen, Chen, Cheung, Chen, & Cheung, 2004; Gold & Harvey, 1993). Information about how a patient solves problems is important in planning interventions and in clinical decision making. If one's ability to solve problems remains intact, the individual may be able to function independently despite impairment in other cognitive functions (Lezak et al. 2004).

Although it is has been determined that neurological damage and disease reduce one's ability to solve problems, no studies have compared problem-solving abilities of different brain-injured groups. One reason for the lack of comparative studies is that neurologically compromised individuals reflect a wide range of problem-solving limitations. This makes it difficult to assess this executive function in a cross-group study with any single measure, particularly standardised tests such as the Wisconsin Card Sorting Test (WCST; Grant & Berg, 1948) and Porteus Maze Test (PMT; Porteus, 1965) that are sometimes too complex for some individuals. A second reason for the lack of comparative studies is that some people may not perform at their best on tests of problem solving unless they perceive a relationship between the test and past experiences. With respect to the aforementioned two problems, one measure that appears well suited to examine and compare problem solving within and across brain-injured groups is the Rapid Assessment of Problem Solving test (RAPS; Marshall et al., 2003a). The RAPS is a recently developed, novel, clinical measure resembling Mosher and Hornsby's 20 Question task (20Q; Mosher & Hornsby, 1966). Patients are motivated to perform on the RAPS because its "game-like" format is familiar to them. Research shows the RAPS is sensitive to problem-solving deficits of patients with traumatic brain injuries (Marshall, Karow, Morelli, Iden, & Dixon, 2003b), severe mental illness (Marshall, McGurk, Karow, Kairy, & Flashman, 2006), and older neurologically intact participants (Marshall, Dixon, Iden, Karow, & Morelli, 1999). The test has also been used to measure changes in problem-solving abilities following intervention (Marshall, Capilouto, & McBride, 2007; Marshall et al., 2004).

The aim of this cross-group study was to compare the problem solving of two groups of neurologically intact (NI) participants and three groups of participants with diffuse neurological involvement (DNI). Two NI groups, older and younger, were used because earlier studies with the 20Q task (Denney, 1985; Denney & Denney, 1973; Denney & Palmer, 1981) and recent investigations with the RAPS (Marshall et al., 2003a, 2006) have yielded conflicting results about age effects on the type of problem-solving task offered by the RAPS. The DNI groups included recent and long-term survivors of a TBI and a group of individuals with schizophrenia (SWS). We included two TBI groups because no information exists with respect to the problem-solving abilities of recent and long-term survivors of a TBI.

The SWS group was included to expand the database for the RAPS and to provide additional comparative information on problem solving by TBI and subjects with schizophrenia (Chen et al., 2004). It was hypothesised that DNI groups would perform less well than the NI groups on the RAPS. Specifically, it was predicted that they would (a) have lower scores on the test, (b) use different types of questions to solve its problems, and (c) employ less efficient problem-solving strategies. No predictions were made with regard to whether or not the DNI groups would perform differently from one another.

METHOD

Participants

Each of our five groups had 20 adults. Information on age and education for the groups is provided in Table 1. Young NI participants were below age 50 and older NI participants were over age 65. All NI participants performed normally on a cognitive screening test, the Short Portable Mental Status Questionnaire (SPSMQ; Pfeiffer, 1975). Their responses to a questionnaire revealed that none had ever had a TBI or stroke, or been treated for psychiatric illness. Acute TBI participants were less than 1 year post-injury ($M = 3.45$ months; $SD = 2.45$), still receiving rehabilitation services, and not living independently. On the Rancho Lost Amigos Scale of Cognitive Function (Hagan & Malkmus, 1979) one of these participants was considered to be functioning at level 5 (confused-non-agitated), eight at level 6 (confused appropriate), seven at level 7 (automatic-appropriate), and four at level 8 (purposeful-appropriate). Chronic TBI participants were all more than 2 years post-injury ($M = 4.78$ years; $SD = 2.7$), not receiving rehabilitation, and lived independently. On the 36-item Raven Coloured Progressive Matrices (CPM; Raven, Court, & Raven, 1984), their scores ranged from 19 to 35 ($M = 30.0$; $SD = 5.64$). The SWS participants were outpatients in community-based vocational rehabilitation programme for patients with severe mental illness. Of these, 17 had a DSM-IV diagnosis of schizophrenia and 3 had a diagnosis of schizoaffective disorder (an intermediate, less severe form of schizophrenia). On the reading subtest of the revised Wide Range Achievement Test (WRAT-R; Jastek & Wilkinson, 1984) these participants' scores ranged from 64 to 103 ($M = 84.45$; $SD = 9.61$).

TABLE 1
Demographic information on participants with and without diffuse neurological involvement

	Young NI	Older NI	Acute TBI	Chronic TBI	SWS
Age					
Mean	34.1	71.4	37.8	35.3	39.3
SD	8.4	5.6	15.1	10.4	12.5
Education					
Mean	13.1	15.2	12.8	13.1	12.1
SD	1.8	2.8	2.7	2.4	1.9

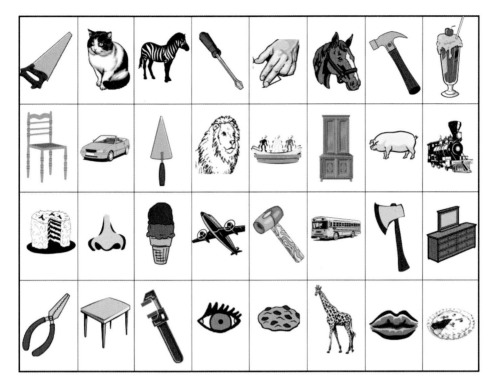

Figure 1. Example of problem-solving abilities board.

Materials

The RAPS includes three problems. Each involves asking yes/no questions to identify a target picture in an array (see Figure 1 for example). The nine-picture arrays of the RAPS have 32 pictures, half coloured, half black and white, belonging to familiar categories (e.g., transportation). The categories represented differ from array-to-array. Each array has one category of eight, two of six, and three of four pictures.

Administration

To begin the test, the examiner puts an array in front of the client and gives these instructions:

> We are going to play a question-asking game. I am thinking of one of these pictures. Your job is to find out which picture it is by asking me questions that I can answer yes or no. Try to do this by using as few questions as possible. When you are ready, ask the first question.

After each acceptable question the examiner answers "Yes" or "No", writes down the question, and crosses out the eliminated pictures. Acceptable questions include *constraints* and *guesses*. Constraints (e.g., Is it a form of transportation?) eliminate more than one picture regardless of whether they are answered yes or no. Guesses (e.g., Is it the car?) solve the problem with a yes and eliminate one picture with a no.

Unacceptable questions are those that cannot be answered yes or no (What is your favourite animal?), or are unrelated to the goal of the problem-solving task (e.g., Do you like animals?). Here, the examiner instructs the client to ask a question that can be answered yes or no, or to try a different question. If the client only guesses, the examiner defaults to a yes answer after 10 consecutive guesses. This solves the problem and terminates the task. However, if any constraint questions are asked before this point, the question-asking process continues until the target picture is identified.

Scoring

Four objective scores are used on the RAPS: mean number of questions, percent constraint questions, mean planning score, and mean efficiency score.

The *mean number of questions* is determined by summing and averaging the number of questions needed to solve each problem. A problem is considered solved after the client's questions have reduced the number of pictures to two or three, or the target picture is named. When two or three pictures remain, the client is allowed to ask additional questions to obtain closure, but these are not included in the question count because the only option available in this situation is to guess.

The *percentage of constraint questions* is determined by dividing the number of constraint questions by all questions (constraints/constraints + guesses) for the test.

Planning scores ranging from 1 to 6 are assigned the first question of each problem based on the number pictures targeted: 1 = one picture; 2 = two or three pictures; 3 = four or five pictures; 4 = six or seven pictures; 5 = eight pictures; 6 = nine or more pictures. The planning score is based on the assumption that a first question that eliminates approximately half of the pictures from consideration will facilitate solving of the problem. Scores are averaged to obtain a *mean planning score* for the test.

A *mean efficiency score* is computed for each problem. These are based on the reduction model used for the RAPS, which stipulates that the most efficient way of solving the problems is to ask questions that reduce the number of pictures from 32 to 16, 16 to 8, and so forth. This involves averaging efficiency scores for the first four questions of each problem. To compute an efficiency score of a question, the number of pictures targeted or eliminated (whichever was less) is divided by the number of pictures "in play" and multiplied by 2. Using Figure 1 as an example, consider that the target picture is *bus* and the first question "Is it an animal?" The question would be answered "No". Since this question both targets and eliminates six pictures, there is no smaller numerator and its efficiency score is .375 (6/32 × 2). Had the first question been "Is it transportation?" or "Is it the bus?" it would have been answered "Yes", and received lower efficiency scores of .25 (4/32 × 2) and .0625 (1/32 × 2) respectively, because the smaller numerators would be used. Mean efficiency scores for each problem are averaged to derive a *mean efficiency score* for the test.

Classification of questions

All questions are classified by type. Table 2 shows that constraint questions are classified as *novel, category-limited*, or *narrowing questions* and guesses as *frank guesses* or *pseudo-constraints* (questions phrased as constraints that are really guesses).

TABLE 2
Classification of questions on the RAPS

Constraints	Examples	Pictures targeted	Efficiency score
Novel			
Novel questions target pictures from more than one category, usually have an efficiency score of greater than .50, and have a greater impact on the problem-solving abilities effort that other questions	Is it a tool or an animal?	Cat, zebra, horse, lion, pig, giraffe, saw, screwdriver, trowel, mallet, axe, pliers, wrench	$14/32 \times 2 = .90$
Category-Limited			
Category-limited questions target all or some of the	Is it a tool?	Saw, screwdriver, trowel, mallet, axe, pliers, wrench	$8/32 \times 2 = .50$
pictures in one semantic category	Is it a jungle animal?	Zebra, lion, giraffe	$3/32 \times 2 = .187$
Narrowing			
A constraint question asked after the client learns the category of the target picture. For example, after getting a "yes" answer to the question "Is it a dessert?"	Is it cold?	Soda, sundae, ice cream cone	$3/6 \times 2 = 1.00$
Guess			
Frank guess	Is it the pig?	Pig	$1/32 \times 2 = .0625$
Pseudo-constraint	Is it the long-neck animal?	Giraffe	$1/32 \times 2 = .0625$

All examples are based on first questions for the picture array in Figure 1.

Procedure

Participants were tested once by familiar examiners in quiet, distraction-free rooms. Scoring and classification of the questions were done at a later time by the same examiner. A second examiner, blinded to the scores and classifications of the first, re-scored and re-classified 25% of the scores and questions respectively to assess reliability. Point-to-point agreement for the two examiners was greater than 90% for all scores and classifications.

RESULTS

Scores

Each group solved 60 problems. Young NI, older NI, Chronic TBI, Acute TBI, and SWS groups asked a total of 262, 268, 286, 378, and 405 questions respectively. Table 3 gives the group means and standard deviations for the scores of the RAPS. Separate one-way ANOVAs revealed significant differences between the group means for number of questions, $F(4, 95) = 12.26$, $p < .001$, percent constraint questions, $F(4, 95) = 22.10$, $p < .001$, planning, $F(4, 95 = 10.42$, $p < .001$, and efficiency scores, $F(4, 95) = 15.28$, $p < .001$. Dunnett T-3 tests used to make multiple comparisons among the means (Hochberg & Tamhane, 1987) showed that, except for the planning score, (a) means for the SWS and Acute TBI groups did not differ,

TABLE 3

Mean number of questions, percent constraint questions, planning, and efficiency scores

	Group					Significance
No. questions						
Mean	4.57 [1]	4.70 [2]	4.83 [3]	6.25 [4]	7.01 [5]	$F = 12.26$; $p < .001$
SD	.91	1.01	1.21	1.65	1.93	
% constraints						
Mean	.907 [1]	.833 [3]	.801 [2]	.494 [4]	.363 [5]	$F = 22.10$; $p < .001$
SD	.089	.231	.203	.242	.309	
Planning						
Mean	4.57 [1]	4.57 [2]	3.96 [3]	3.13 [4]	2.80 [5]	$F = 10.42$; $p < .001$
SD	.859	1.02	.611	1.29	1.59	
Efficiency						
Mean	.594 [1]	.558 [2]	.514 [3]	.352 [4]	.299 [5]	$F = 15.28$; $p < .001$
SD	.122	.170	.103	.144	.191	

For younger [1] and older [2]NI groups, Chronic-TBI [3], SMI [4], and Acute-TBI [5]groups. Any two means not underscored by the same line are significantly different at the .05 level or beyond.

but were significantly different from the two NI and Chronic TBI groups, (b) means for younger and older NI groups and the Chronic TBI group did not differ, and (c) the mean planning score for the Acute TBI group was significantly lower than all other groups.

Types of questions

Separate one-way ANOVAs were also used to examine differences in the types of questions asked. Table 4 shows that all groups asked novel questions less frequently than other questions. Younger and older NI groups asked more novel questions than the DNI groups, but the ANOVA for novel questions was not significant, $F(4, 95) = 1.94$, $p = .110$. Table 4 also shows that, except for the Acute TBI group, all groups asked predominantly category-limited questions. ANOVA results revealed group differences in the number of category-limited questions, $F(4, 95) = 3.39$, $p = .012$. Multiple comparison tests showed that the Acute TBI group asked significantly fewer category-limited questions than the Chronic TBI group, but there were no differences between any of the other groups. The largest group differences occurred for narrowing questions, $F(4, 94) = 13.66$, $p < .001$, and guesses, $F(4, 95) = 18.78$, $p < .001$. Multiple comparison tests indicated that the Acute TBI and SWS groups asked significantly fewer narrowing questions and did significantly more guessing than all other groups.

Other analyses

Table 5 provides information on the types of questions asked by the groups for the first six questions of the problem-solving task and types of questions asked early (question 1 or 2), midway (questions 3 and 4), and later (questions 5 and 6) in the

TABLE 4

Means and standard deviations for number of novel, category-limited, and narrowing questions, and guesses

	Group					F
Novel						
Mean	1.90 [2]	1.70 [1]	1.30 [5]	.859 [4]	.850 [3]	$F = 1.94$; $p = .012$ *ns*
SD	1.49	2.26	1.02	1.75	1.09	
Category-limited						
Mean	8.70 [3]	7.70 [2]	7.50 [1]	6.60 [4]	5.00 [5]	$F = 3.39$; $p < .05$
SD	2.59	3.54	2.54	3.47	4.01	
Narrowing						
Mean	3.00 [1]	2.20 [2]	2.05 [3]	.450 [5]	.600 [4]	$F = 13.66$; $p < .001$
SD	.887	1.14	1.17	1.67	1.08	
Guesses						
Mean	1.50 [1]	2.90 [3]	2.95 [2]	10.85 [4]	13.90 [5]	$F = 18.78$; $p < .001$
SD	1.40	3.63	3.73	7.38	9.05	

For younger [1] and older [2]NI groups, Chronic-TBI [3], SMI [4], and Acute-TBI [5]groups. Any two means not underscored by the same line are significantly different at the .05 level or beyond.

question-asking sequences. While these data were not analysed statistically, they do provide an indication of when or if groups used certain strategies in solving problems of the RAPS. Table 5 shows that (a) all groups asked most of their novel questions early and that more novel questions were asked by the NI groups, (b) younger and older NI groups predominantly asked category-limited questions on the first four questions, whereas the Chronic TBI group asked category-limited questions throughout the sequence, (c) NI groups asked narrowing questions on middle and later questions, Chronic TBI participants did not ask narrowing questions until later, and Acute TBI and SWS groups never reflected a "spike" in the use of narrowing questions, and (d) all groups guessed on later questions, but Acute TBI and SWS groups guessed throughout the problem-solving effort and almost exclusively on later questions.

DISCUSSION

Selected components of Scholnick and Friedman's (1993) developmental theory of planning are useful in discussing differences in problem solving by participants with and without DNI. These include, (a) decision to plan, (b) strategy choice, (c) strategy execution, and (d) monitoring the effects of prior actions.

Decision to plan

According to Scholnick and Friedman (1993), decision to plan involves making a judgment to analyse rather than to act. A decision to act rather than to plan would be seen in early guessing. Groups that performed poorest on the RAPS (Acute TBI and SWS groups) made more decisions to act. Table 5 shows that that Acute TBI

TABLE 5
Questions and guesses

Group	Early	Midway	Late
Younger			
Novel	25.5	3.5	0
Category-limited	62.5	53.0	23.5
Narrowing	9.5	33.0	44
Guesses	2.5	10.5	45.5
Older			
Novel	24.5	8.5	1.5
Category-limited	68.0	46.5	15.5
Narrowing	1.0	26.0	30.5
Guesses	3.0	18.5	51.5
Chronic TBI			
Novel	11.0	2.0	0
Category-limited	75.5	66.5	46.5
Narrowing	4.0	16.0	34.0
Guesses	7.5	21.5	34.0
Acute TBI			
Novel	15.0	4.5	1.0
Category-limited	35.5	27.5	14.5
Narrowing	1.5	4.0	2.5
Guesses	48.0	66.0	82.0
SMI			
Novel	12.5	1.0	0
Category-limited	49.5	44.0	15.5
Narrowing	1.5	3.0	2.5
Guesses	36.5	53.5	81.0

Percentages of novel, category-limited, and narrowing questions, and percentages of guesses asked in early (question 1 or 2), midway (questions 3 or 4) or late (questions 5 or 6) in the problem-solving abilities effort for younger and older NI groups, and Chronic TBI, Acute TBI, and SMI groups.

and SWS groups guessed 43% and 32% of the time respectively on question 1, whereas first-question guessing was rare by other groups. The Acute TBI and SWS groups also guessed rampantly throughout the problem-solving sequence (see Table 4). Early and frequent guessing by these participants may be due to impulsivity or possibly inability to do the type of planning and conceptual reasoning necessary to solve problems on the RAPS efficiently.

Strategy choice

Strategy choice relates to development of a plan of action to solve the problem. Post-hoc examination of the 300 solved problems indicated that participants chose two effective (category-driven and novel) and one ineffective (guessing) strategy. The *category-driven* strategy consisted of asking category-limited questions until the target picture category was identified and a narrowing question was needed. The *novel* strategy involved asking one or two novel questions in the first four questions, and ultimately solving the problem with a category-limited, a narrowing question, or sometimes a guess. The *guessing* strategy consisted of solving the problem solely by guessing. There were also times when problems were solved with no apparent strategy. This usually involved mixing constraints and guesses.

Post-hoc analysis reflected a hierarchical ordering of the groups in terms of strategy choices paralleling their overall performance on the RAPS and, in some respects, mirroring their cognitive status. The NI groups used the two effective strategies, category-driven (56%) and novel (44%), about equally, and never used the guessing strategy. The Chronic TBI group used the category-driven strategy almost exclusively (75% of the time) and rarely used the other strategies. The Acute TBI and SWS groups predominantly used a guessing strategy, and in some cases had no discernable strategy. Not choosing a strategy (e.g., mixing constraints and guesses) may indicate that some of these participants were aware that a strategy was needed, but were unable to use any one strategy consistently.

Strategy execution

To execute an effective problem-solving strategy, the client needs to use classification skills, recognise differences in picture category size, and ask narrowing questions. These meta-cognitive abilities are associated with asking constraint questions that coincide with the goal of solving the problem with as few questions as possible.

Classification skills (e.g., recognising that pictures belong to semantic categories, retrieving category labels) are important to the execution of the category-based and novel strategies. NI and Chronic TBI groups clearly showed the ability to use classification skills as evidenced by their high percentages of category-limited questions (see Table 4). However, that the Acute TBI group, and to a lesser extent the SWS group, asked fewer of these questions (See Table 4) suggests that some of their guessing was due to poor classification skills. Interestingly, a post-hoc analysis of guesses by the Acute TBI and SWS groups revealed that 33% and 19% of their guesses were clustered. Clustered guesses consisted of two or more consecutive frank guesses targeting pictures from the same category (e.g., Is it the zebra, the lion, the pig?), and were only seen for these two groups. This suggests that some of these participants may have recognised that pictures belong to categories, but were unable to retrieve the category labels to ask a category-limited questions.

Recognition of category size (four, six, or eight pictures) is also important to strategy execution since problem-solving efficiency is increased by asking questions that target larger rather than smaller picture categories, particularly on early questions. Post-hoc analyses revealed younger and older NI groups, SWS and Acute TBI groups asked 63%, 66%, 71%, and 78% of their eight-item questions early (first or second question), but that the Chronic TBI group only asked 49% of these questions at this time. Thus, while these participants used the category-driven strategy 75% of the time, they paid less attention to category size than the other groups. This suggests that they fail to make use of information about category size to maximise problem-solving efficiency.

Switching to a narrowing question when needed is also important to the execution of category-limited and novel strategies. One of the more obvious differences between participants with and without DNI was when and how frequently they asked narrowing questions. Table 5 shows that (a) the NI groups increased their use of narrowing questions on questions 3 and 4, (b) the Chronic TBI group did not increase their use of narrowing questions until questions 5 and 6, and (c) Acute TBI and SWS group scores never reflected an increase in narrowing questions. Significant differences in narrowing questions (see Table 4) between participants with and without DNI suggest that these questions may be too difficult for some participants with DNI, disrupt strategy execution, and reduce problem-solving efficiency. This is further supported by the fact that post-hoc analyses revealed that 93% of the guesses by the NI groups also represented failures to ask narrowing questions.

Monitoring the effects of prior actions

Self-monitoring behaviour was seen in differences in types of guesses made (frank guesses and pseudo-constraint questions) and the use of self-corrections by the groups.

Younger and older NI participants guessed a total of 90 times whereas participants with DNI guessed 557 times. Collectively, 81% of the guesses from the NI participants, but only 33%, 17%, and 26% by the Chronic TBI, Acute TBI, and SWS groups respectively were pseudo-constraints. Mosher and Hornsby (1966) suggested pseudo-constraints were an elegant form of guessing that suggested an awareness that guessing was a poor strategy and served as a "face-saving" device. Disparities in frank guesses and pseudo-constraints between the NI and DNI groups suggest that the latter may realise there are alternatives to guessing whereas participants with DNI do not. Also, the guesses (pseudo-constraints) from the NI groups were almost always associated with failures to ask narrowing questions. After many of these guesses, NI participants often self-corrected to a narrowing question on the next question to complete solving of the problem. These types of self-corrections were never seen for the participants with DNI. Usually, DNI participants, after failing to ask a narrowing question, continued to guess until the problem was solved.

Further research and clinical implications

Results of the study revealed no differences between younger and older NI participants on the scores of the RAPS and the types of questions used, but significant differences between the NI groups and two of three DNI groups (Acute TBI and SWS). Surprisingly, our third group of DNI participants (Chronic TBI) did not differ significantly from the NI groups. This result is not congruent with findings of a previous study (Marshall et al., 2003) that found differences between chronic community-dwelling TBI and NI participants on the RAPS. While the Chronic TBI and NI groups did not differ on statistical measures, performance of the Chronic TBI group differed qualitatively from the NI groups with regard to strategy choice, use of information about category size, and when they asked narrowing questions.

Several issues should be addressed in future research with the RAPS. One is to obtain information documenting tissue loss, site of lesion, and cerebral blood flow of DNI participants. Similarly, individuals with focal lesions also have problem-solving deficits (Glosser & Goodglass, 1990; LaPointe, Holtzapple, Pohlman, Katz, & Blackwood, 1995; Marshall, Harvey, Freed, & Phillips, 1996) and future studies with the RAPS should include these types of patients. Only limited information was available about the cognitive functioning of the DNI participants. Moreover, different methods were used to estimate levels of cognitive functioning for the Acute TBI (Rancho Los Amigos ratings), Chronic TBI (CPM), and SMI (WRAT-R) groups. Findings suggest there is a relationship between performance on the RAPS and level of cognitive functioning, but without using similar measures to assess all groups this cannot be determined. It would also have been advantageous to have information regarding latency to asking of the first question, which varied between individuals and possibly groups. Latency to asking the first question may reflect a number of processes important to problem-solving abilities including planning and information-processing speed. Since "decision to plan" (choosing to analyse rather than act) is an important component of problem-solving abilities (Scholnick & Friedman, 1993), future studies will evaluate the relationship of latency to asking the first questions to other neurocognitive processes, as well as problem solving on the RAPS. Finally, it is possible that more could be learned about problem-solving abilities of participants with DNI by asking poor problem solvers why they ask certain questions. For example, one individual guessed "Is it the tree?" on the first question. Later the examiner asked why the person asked this question and was told, "Oh, I know it's close to Christmas, and I just thought you might be thinking of a Christmas tree."

At this point in its development, the RAPS functions similarly to the word fluency test (Brookshire, 2003). Specifically, it is a test that is sensitive to brain damage, but as yet has not demonstrated the specificity needed to differentiate problem-solving abilities of different brain-injured groups. In this regard, the RAPS is similar to many other tests of executive functioning (Keil & Kaszniak, 2002). The RAPS does not replace standardised tests of problem solving, but may be useful in clinical settings where time is limited and the need for information about problem-solving abilities still exists. The test does fulfil some requirements of an executive function measure by allowing the individual tested some leeway to solve a problem on his/her own without direction from the examiner (Baddeley, 1992; Lezak et al., 2004). Currently, we are examining the use of the RAPS in assessing problem-solving abilities in persons with dementia and mild cognitive impairment, determining the relationship of RAPS performance to performance on a comprehensive neuropsychological battery in persons with severe mental illness, measuring changes in RAPS performance following behavioural and pharmacological interventions, and expanding our normative data.

REFERENCES

Baddeley, A. D. (1992). Working memory. *Science, 225*, 556–559.

Brookshire, R. H. (2003) *Introduction to neurogenic communication disorders* (6th ed.). St Louis, MO: Mosby.

Chen, R. C., Chen, E. Y., Cheung, E. F., Chen, R. Y., & Cheung, H. K. (2004). Problem-solving ability in chronic schizophrenia. A comparison study of patients with traumatic brain injury. *European Archives of Psychiatry and Clinical Neuroscience, 254*, 236–241.

Cummings, J., & Benson, D. F. (1983). *Dementia: A clinical approach*. Boston, MA: Butterworth.

Denney, N. W. (1985). A review of life span research with the twenty questions task: A study of problem-solving ability. *International Journal of Aging and Human Development, 21*, 161–173.

Denney, D. R., & Denney, N. W. (1973). The use of classification and problem-solving: A comparison of middle and old age. *Developmental Psychology, 9*, 275–278.

Denney, N. W., & Palmer, A. M. (1981). Adult age differences in traditional and practical problem-solving measures. *Journal of Gerontology, 37*, 323–328.

Glossser, G., & Goodglass, H. (1990). Disorders in executive control functions among aphasic and other brain-damaged patients. *Journal of Clinical and Experimental Neuropsychology, 12*, 485–501.

Gold, J. M., & Harvey, P. D. (1993). Cognitive deficits in schizophrenia. *Psychiatric Clinics of North America, 16*, 295–312.

Goldstein, F., & Levin, H. (1991). Question-asking strategies after severe closed head injury. *Brain and Cognition, 17*, 23–30.

Grant, D. A., & Berg, E. A. (1948). A behavioural analysis of degree of reinforcement and cease of shifting to a new response in a Weigl-type card-sorting problem. *Journal of Experimental Psychology, 38*, 404–411.

Hagan, C., & Malkmus, D. (1979). *Interaction strategies for language disorders secondary to head trauma.* Paper presented at the annual convention of the American Speech-Language Hearing Association, Atlanta, GA, USA.

Hochberg, Y., & Tamhane, A. C. (1987). *Multiple comparison procedures.* New York: Wiley.

Jastek, J. S., & Wilkinson, G. S. (1984). *Wide Range Achievement Test–Revised.* Wilmington, DE: Jastek Assessment Systems.

Keil, K., & Kaszniak, A. W. (2002). Examining executive function in individuals with brain injury: A review. *Aphasiology, 16*, 305–336.

Kennedy, M. R., & Coelho, C. (2005). Self-regulation after traumatic brain injury: A framework for intervention of memory and problem solving. *Seminars in Speech and Language, 26*(4), 242–255.

LaPointe, L. L., Holtzapple, P. A., Pohlman, K., Katz, R. C., & Blackwood, D. (1995). The Melinark Task: Reasoning and effects of training on concept acquisition in subjects with aphasia. *Journal of Medical Speech-Language Pathology, 3*(2), 95–107.

Lezak, M., Howieson, D., & Loring, J. (2004) *Neuropsychological assessment* (3rd ed.). New York: Oxford University Press.

Marshall, R. C., Capilouto, G. J., & McBride, J. M. (2007). Treatment of problem solving in Alzheimer's disease: A short report. *Aphasiology, 21*, 235–247.

Marshall, R. C., Dixon, J., Iden, K., Karow, C., & Morelli, C. (1999, November). *Problem-solving abilities efficiency of elderly participants: Effects of strategy-modeling training.* Paper presented at the convention of the American-Speech-Language-Hearing Association, San Francisco, CA, USA.

Marshall, R. C., Harvey, S., Freed, D. B., & Phillips, D. S. (1996). Question-asking strategies of aphasic and non-brain-damaged subjects. *Clinical Aphasiology, 24*, 181–191.

Marshall, R. C., Karow, C. M., Morelli, C. A., Iden, K., & Dixon, J. (2003a). A clinical measure for the assessment of problem-solving abilities in brain-injured adults. *American Journal of Speech-Language Pathology, 12*, 333–347.

Marshall, R. C., Karow, C. M., Morelli, C. A., Iden, K., & Dixon, J. (2003b). Problem solving by traumatically brain injured and neurologically intact participants on an adaptation of the twenty questions test. *Brain Injury, 17*, 589–608.

Marshall, R. C., Karow, C. M., Morelli, C. A., Iden, K., Dixon, J., & Cranfill, T. (2004). Effects of interactive strategy modelling training on problem solving by persons with traumatic brain injury. *Aphasiology, 18*, 659–674.

Marshall, R. C., McGurk, S. R., Karow, C. M., Kairy, T. J., & Flashman, L. A. (2006). Performance of participants with and without severe mental illness on a clinical test of problem-solving abilities. *Schizophrenia Research, 81*, 331–344.

Mosher, F. A., & Hornsby, J. R. (1966). On asking questions. In J. S. Bruner, R. B. Olver, & P. M. Greenfield (Eds.), *Studies in cognitive growth* (pp. 86–102). New York: Wiley.

Pfieffer, E. (1975). SPMSQ: Short Portable Mental Status Questionnaire. *Journal of the American Geriatric Society, 23*, 433–441.

Porteus, S. D. (1965). *Porteus Maze Test: Fifty years' application.* Palo Alto, CA: Pacific Books.

Rath, J. F., Langenbahn, D. M., Simon, D., Sherr, R. L., Fletcher, J., & Diller, L. (2004). The construct of problem solving in higher level neuropsychological assessment and rehabilitation. *Archives of Clinical Neuropsychology, 19*, 613–635.

Rath, J. F., Simon, D., Langenbahn, D. M., Sherr, R. L., & Diller, L. (2000). Measurement of problem-solving deficits in adults with acquired brain damage. *Journal of Head Trauma Rehabilitation, 15*, 724–733.

Raven, J. C., Court, J., & Raven, J. (1984). *Coloured Progressive Matrices.* London: H. K. Lewis.

Scholnick, E. K., & Friedman, S. L. (1993). Planning in context: Developmental and situational characteristics. *International Journal of Behavioural Development, 16*, 145–167.

Willis, S. L., Allen-Burge, R., Dolan, M. M., Bertrand, R. M., Yesavage, J., & Taylor, J. L. (1998). Everyday problem solving among individuals with Alzheimer's disease. *Gerontologist, 38*, 569–577.

APHASIOLOGY, 2007, 21 (6/7/8), 763–774

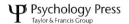

Making stories: Evaluative language and the aphasia experience

Elizabeth Armstrong

Macquarie University, Sydney, NSW, Australia

Hanna Ulatowska

University of Texas at Dallas, TX, USA

Background: Language used for expressing feelings and opinions—so-called evaluative language—is essential to the expression of the individual's identity. Illness narratives involving evaluative language are known to be important vehicles for coping with identity change during chronic illness, as well as reflecting on and sharing the experience. However, relatively little is known about the aphasic person's ability to engage in such narratives—in particular, the effects of their language difficulties on this endeavour.
Aims: This study discusses different types of evaluative language and ways in which they are relatively impaired or preserved in aphasia, focusing on stroke narrative.
Methods & Procedures: Examples from the stroke stories of three aphasic speakers are used as illustrations of their evaluative abilities. The stories were analysed according to evaluative language categories defined by Labov (1972) and Martin (2003). The function of each of these categories is described in terms of its contribution to the emotive nature of the discourse.
Outcomes & Results: The aphasic speakers were successful in using evaluative language and used similar devices to non-brain-damaged speakers. However, the realisation of the devices was simplified at both lexical and syntactic levels and in terms of quantity.
Conclusions: Emotive/evaluative language promises a different perspective on language usage across speakers of differing levels of severity for both assessment and treatment purposes. We will discuss implications of the use of emotive recounts in the clinical situation for facilitating language and working through identity issues.

Language used for expressing opinions and feelings—so-called evaluative language—is essential to the expression of the individual's identity. An individual's attitudes, judgements, and values are typically apparent in everyday discourse and are central to that individual's expression of who they are. In verbalising experiences from our own perspectives, we actually shape that experience and our reflections about it, and hence determine its significance in our lives. It has been suggested, for example, that illness narratives, usually highly emotive in nature, can function as coping mechanisms as speakers work through life-changing events (e.g., Alaszewski, 2006; Faircloth, Boylstein, Rittman, Young, & Gubrium, 2004). It is also in the

---

Address correspondence to: Dr Elizabeth Armstrong, Department of Linguistics, Macquarie University, North Ryde, NSW 2019, Australia. E-mail: barmstrong@ling.mq.edu.au

http://www.psypress.com/aphasiology   DOI: 10.1080/02687030701192364

sharing of a story that we engage other people in interaction. While the sharing of simple facts engages a listener to some extent, it is the speaker's "take" on the "facts" that stimulates real interest in the listener, and involves the listener in the speaker's world. Labov suggests that evaluation indicates "the point of the narrative, its raison d'etre: why it was told, and what the narrator is getting at" (1972, p. 366). Ochs and Capps (2001) refer to this in terms of the "tellability" factor. Martin (2003) suggests that evaluation provides "sites" in the discourse around which negotiation might take place. Hence, it is the fact that a speaker takes a particular stance in his/ her discourse that encourages the listener to respond in some way—either to agree or disagree, for example. Evaluative language, then, serves to directly engage the listener in a way that a relatively neutral presentation of facts does not.

The role of evaluative language in social interaction has been of interest to linguists concerned with the role of language in social life for a number of years (e.g., Labov, 1972; Martin, 1995; Stubbs, 1986). Its importance in narrative has been highlighted by applications of analysis to areas such as children's narrative development in the field of education (Taylor, 1986), developmental psycholinguistics (McCabe & Peterson, 1991), media studies (Van Dijk, 1988), as well as language use in particular ethnic sub-groups (Labov, 1972). To date, however, research into aphasic language has largely focused on the individual conveying relatively concrete, factual information, e.g., picture descriptions, story re-tell, procedural discourse. Little attention has been paid to the way the speaker conveys his/her particular stance or perspective on this information, engaging the listener in his/her experience. As aphasic speakers are restricted in terms of lexical and syntactic skills, it could be anticipated that they will have difficulty in this aspect of language, particularly as evaluative language tends to involve more "abstract" and less imageable words than factual language. The implications of this for the establishment and maintenance of interpersonal relationships is significant.

Emotive topics producing evaluative language have been used in some narrative studies of aphasic language, tapping both negative and positive experiences. However, the purposes of analyses to date have primarily been to investigate aphasic speakers' abilities to organise and maintain coherence across their discourse (Ulatowska & Olness, 2001; Ulatowska, Olness, Hill, Roberts, & Keebler, 2000), and to investigate hemispheric effects on pragmatic "appropriateness" (Borod et al., 1996; Borod et al., 2000) rather than to explore the lexical or grammatical resources used to convey the specific emotive content of the narratives. However, the fact that speakers with left hemisphere damage have been reported to produce "better" discourse when discussing emotional than non-emotional topics, and "better" discourse on positive emotional topics than negative ones (Borod et al., 2000), suggests that the element of emotion may be a facilitating and hence significant factor for speakers with aphasia. Hence, it appears that the use of evaluative language may well provide another avenue for improving communication.

Of the few studies that have commented on evaluative language in aphasia, Armstrong (2001, 2005) suggests that some aphasic speakers do have difficulty in the use of evaluative verbs and clauses. Ulatowska and colleagues' studies of the discourse of African Americans using recounts of negative experiences (Ulatowska & Olness, 2001; Ulatowska et al., 2000, 2004), while not focusing on evaluative language specifically, found that African American aphasic speakers overall used similar evaluative devices compared to their non-brain-damaged counterparts. However, they used simplified realisation, i.e., decreased lexical range and syntax, and their distribution of devices was different—e.g., repetition for emphasis in aphasic language was more contiguous, where non-brain-damaged speakers tend to reiterate at strategic points.

As noted above, the study of emotive illness narratives has recently become an increasingly important area of investigation in the understanding of chronic illnesses. To date, however, studies have largely explored the experiences of individuals suffering from cancer or those with other physical disabilities. Little is known about the person with aphasia's experience. It is acknowledged that people with aphasia are especially vulnerable to issues of identity change (Kagan & Duchan, 2004; LaPointe, 2001; Moss, Parr, Byng, & Petheram, 2004; Parr, Byng, Gilpin, & Ireland, 1997; Shadden, 2005). However, it is also important to acknowledge the fact that they are potentially restricted in the process of working through these issues via language, as other individuals would. This has implications for both the individual's mental state, and their interpersonal status in terms of involving other people in their world. Hence, it is important to understand their expressive abilities in this regard. The illness narrative—or in the person with aphasia's case, the stroke story—is an important social statement of the speaker's, and also a potentially rich source of evaluative language. Understanding more about evaluative language in general, and how it is used specifically in this context, may provide further insight into the aphasia experience—of benefit not only to the person involved, but also their families, significant others, carers, and health professionals.

The current study represents preliminary findings from an ongoing study specifically examining evaluative language in stroke stories across a range of individuals with aphasia from different ethnic backgrounds and across a variety of ages and severity. The purpose of the study is to examine whether aphasic speakers use evaluative language in their stroke stories, and if so, which particular devices they use, with what frequency, and whether any qualitative differences exist from the kinds of evaluative language used by non-brain-damaged speakers. The paper represents a platform for discussion of the whole area, raising issues related to evaluative language, rather than comprehensive case studies.

METHOD

The data

Out of a larger population of 25 speakers who produced stroke stories for an ongoing study, we selected 3 speakers for illustrative purposes in this paper in order to demonstrate the potential of this kind of analysis. Because many variables are involved in the production of evaluative language, the speakers represent a variety in order to demonstrate some of these variables. For example, we have selected both oral and written stroke stories (both important potential sources for gathering examples of evaluative language; Alaszewski, 2006), and have selected participants of varying severities and ethnic backgrounds.

Participants SL and CP provided oral recounts, elicited in response to direction to produce a personal narrative of a frightening experience. Participant MD's text was part of a diary written a year post stroke, covering the most significant events of his life. SL was a 55-year-old African American female, with mild aphasia, who was 5 years post stroke. CP was a 68-year-old African American female, with moderate aphasia, who was 3 months post stroke. MD was a 60-year-old Caucasian American male, with moderately severe aphasia.

The analyses

Hunston and Thompson (2003) suggest that evaluative devices are used to perform the following three functions within a discourse: (i) to express the speaker's or writer's feelings, and in doing so to reflect the value system of that person; (ii) to construct and maintain relations between the speaker or writer and hearer or reader; and (iii) to organise the discourse. Devices will be discussed below as they relate to these functions, although it must be noted that many devices can perform these functions concurrently.

The following evaluative devices were identified, as defined by Labov (1972), and Martin (2003): the use of repetition for emphasis, direct speech, metaphoric language, and use of emotive words and phrases. The first three have previously been investigated in terms of their contribution to coherence and "tellability" in African American aphasia discourse (Ulatowska & Olness, 2003; Ulatowska, Olness, Samson, Keebler, & Goins, 2004) and are related more to overall organisation of evaluative discourse. Emotive words and phrases have not been investigated specifically but constitute the contribution to evaluation at the level of specific wording. While these will be defined, elaborated upon, and illustrated below, it is important to note that these categories are not mutually exclusive, e.g., repetition can be embedded within reported speech.

Repetition involves reiteration or close paraphrase of words, phrases, clauses, or clause complexes, and can be contiguous or can occur at intervals in the discourse. According to Labov (1972), repetition has evaluative function in both intensifying a particular action, and potentially suspending the action of the narrative. It is a very powerful evaluative device but of course must be distinguished from perseveration, which is frequently observed in aphasic language. While such a distinction is potentially problematic, two primary "rules" can be applied. First, it is important to ascertain whether or not the repetition serves a function of emphasis. Second, repetition co-occurring with obvious word-finding difficulty is more likely to be perseveration.

Direct speech involves the narrator either reporting the speech of characters in the narrative speaking directly to each other, or the narrator reporting on his/her own speech to him/herself or to another person. Labov (1972) considers direct speech a complex form of evaluation in that it "translates our personal narrative into dramatic form" (p. 396). It brings the story to life and involves the listener, contributing to the "tellability" of the story (Ochs & Capps, 2001; Ulatowska et al., 2004). It has also been found to be related to high listener ratings of narrative quality when compared with narratives containing less direct speech (Ulatowska et al., 2004).

Metaphoric language refers to figurative terms and expressions "which bring two distinct domains (or concepts) into correspondence with each other" (Kovecses, 2000, p. 4) and involve a degree of abstraction. For example, in the expression "I was burning with anger", the speaker is bringing the concept of *burning* to bear on the level of intensity involved in his anger.

Particular *words and phrases* can also realise different kinds of evaluation (Labov, 1972; Martin, 2003). Such evaluation is most often expressed through adjectives (e.g., *terrible, scarey*), but can also be expressed through verbs (e.g., *hate, love*), nouns (e.g., *bastard, devil*), adverbs (e.g., *happily, gently, cruelly*), or phrases often involving intensifiers (e.g., *very scared, awfully rich, remarkably sane*). It is important to point out that words carry different values and connotations across age groups and cultures, to name but two of the variables involved. What is considered evaluative by one speaker may simply be considered factual by another. For example "cripple" may or may not be seen as evaluative, depending on the age and culture of the speaker. However, given some degree of subjectivity, and within a shared culture, it is through the use of the above devices that the individual shares personal information and engages the listener/reader, and in so doing, creates and maintains a mutual bond. It is the sharing of perspective, rather than facts alone, that is important in the establishment and maintenance of interpersonal relationships.

RESULTS

Repetition

Numerous examples of repetition were noted throughout the samples of the three speakers. An example of repetition emphasising emotions occurs in the discourse of participant SL when she was describing her efforts to overcome her initial physical difficulties after the stroke had just happened:

> *I talked to my arm, I talked to my arm and I said please let me get up. I got to get up and no please to it. I got to get up and so I got into a position to where I got my arm behind me and under me and I pushed and pushed*

(SL)

Repetition in this example gives cohesion to the discourse in the face of linguistic disruption, emphasising what SL felt was important at the time and reflecting her emotional engagement with the situation.

Another example is the following from participant CP:

> *In my right hand it really tried to scare me because I couldn't write. And that was one time I was really scared. And I was scared then to first when they told me I had to have my heart surgery and that really scared me.*

(CP)

These repetitions occurred in relatively uninterrupted stretches of discourse, with little distance between repetitive words and phrases. Such repetition differs somewhat from more complex forms of repetition where the speaker will reiterate particular points of emphasis or interest at different points throughout the discourse. However, it could also be that repetition might be the easiest form of evaluative language for aphasic speakers, given their restricted lexical repertoire.

It must also be pointed out that repetition and direct speech (to be discussed below) are said to be characteristic of a "high involvement style" of discourse (Tannen, 1989) used by certain groups of African Americans in particular (Ulatowska & Olness, 2003; Ulatowska et al., 2000). Hence, both cultural and personal style differences in use of these devices can be expected.

Direct speech

Direct speech was used by two of the participants, SL and CP. They both engaged the listener in their story in an immediate way through the use of direct speech, re-creating the event for the listener as if it was happening again. Consider the following examples (reported speech in bold):

> *That was in my mind. I said **I'm handicapped, but I will not be** but at that moment I was that picture, I said, **No**. If it was the devil showing me the way that I was going to be **he is a liar. He is a liar, he is a liar. Because I'm not down yet**.*
>
>   (SL)

> *And they said **we better call somebody***
> *And they called my pastor*
> *And he said*
> ***It kinda look like she done had a stroke***
>
>   (CP)

Such examples constitute what Labov calls embedded evaluation, where the evaluation is part of the story itself. This contrasts with external evaluation, where the narrator actually interrupts the story, and inserts some form of evaluation directed at the listener, or states explicitly to the listener what the point is.

Metaphoric language

While there were few instances of the direct type of metaphor exemplified in the definition above, SL drew on numerous images, using much metaphoric language to convey her feelings. In the setting stage of her narrative, she recounted the following:

> *And all I have to do is get up off this couch. And it felt like, it felt like it was one of those naked Ninja. This is just a parable but what is he called Ninja wrestle, a big old fat Ninja was pushing down on my and all of his weight with his hands. I was trying to push him up, to get up, I had to get up off the couch and I said, "I got to get up, I got to get up."*
>
>   (SL)

SL also used imagery to create a real sense of her emotional state at the time:

> *At that time, in my mind, I could see the picture of the old lady. When I say old, I mean a hundred, a hundred and two or a hundred and five and she was sitting in a wheelchair........ And there was a nurse prancing prancing around in front of her and made a a attempt to feed this lady in her mouth and I pictured that as being me. And I said no no God this can't be me.....*
>
>   (SL)

Neither CP nor MD used metaphorical language.

Evaluative words/phrases

In the above examples, the adjectives *scared* and *handicapped* were used, and the intensifier *really* amplified the speaker's feeling of being scared. The word *liar* in SL's example above also reflected the intensity of her feelings. Similarly in the following extract, CP uses evaluative lexical items (in bold) embedded within the action and dialogue:

*And ah, I got up, I tried to get up. But I fell back down and then my daughter em said what's **wrong** with you momma. I said, I don't know what's **wrong**. And they said sit down before you fall again. I said, **shoot** it's something **wrong** with me. And they looked at me and said it sho' is.*

(CP)

However, while the aphasic individuals used these evaluative words, there was a restricted range of usage, with the main lexical items related to fear "scared, scariery, afraid".

It is of interest, however, that even in the presence of clauses that are not syntactically or semantically "correct," evaluation can obviously be present. Consider the following extract from the narrative of MD:

*I know I was gonna be **sick** some day. I know it. Maybe it was for dreams I did have....Anyway **I did do cripple**. Yeah **I did sick** it was my head. Ha. I guess I had it for sixty years but I had some fun...It is to laugh. I have **I am still for fun**...It is to laugh. I have **I am still for fun** because I am still alive....*

(MD)

In this example, lexicogrammatical breakdown is evident, however the evaluative meanings are clear through both the use of individual words such as *sick, cripple, fun,* as well as whole clauses, e.g., *I did do cripple, I am still for fun.*

Organisation of the text

Numerous devices exist in language that organise discourse, including cohesive devices, chronological continuity, and logical relations. However, evaluation is another important one that maintains the "point" of the story. It contributes greatly to overall textual coherence, serving to link elements of the story that highlight the perspective of the speaker in regard to salient and often emotive information. Again, this links with the function of engaging the listener in such as way as not only to maintain informational coherence but also to convey personal stance to the listener, including the overall point of the narrative.

In linking sections of the text, evaluative language provides scaffolding throughout. Labov notes that evaluation can occur at multiple points in the text, i.e. beginning, middle, or end. For example, CP's use of evaluation as an organising device throughout the text is evident. At the outset of the story she oriented the listener to the fearful experience she was describing:

Well I was scared when I had my surgery and when I had my stroke
I was scared because I didn't know what had happened to me

(CP)

At the end of the text, CP used a coda, judging her own reactions as being normal under the circumstances:

But ain't nobody ain't nobody gon be brave going through nothing like that
I was scared
I sho was

(CP)

However, evaluative language can also be used to punctuate the discourse so that the speaker can provide reflections on specific events in order to highlight them—separate them from the rest of the text. It represents a suspension of the actual chain of events in the physical realm, while the narrator elaborates on particular feelings occurring to her at the time. Labov (1972) suggests that this interruption to the "action" occurs so that the speaker can talk directly to the listener and engage the listener further in the discourse. Consider the following example:

> *And we and they took me down to the city*
> *And the doctor said I done had one in my right hand*
> *It really tried to scare me because I couldn't write*
> **And that was one time I was really scared**
> *And I was scared then to first when they told me I had to have my heart surgery And that really scared me*
> *I said I don't know if I am gon take it or not*
> *And then I said I got to*
>
> (CP)

Then later in the same text:

> *They were all there*
> *My granddaughter and all*
> **And that was the scariest time**
> **It really is you know going through something like that**
> **And I was scared**
> **But I just put it in the Lords hands**
> **Because I know I had to do it and just do it**
>
> (CP)

In these two examples, the speaker highlights her feelings at particular points—in the first example to emphasise a particular part of the story, and in the second to conclude the story and state its significance.

DISCUSSION

This preliminary exploration suggests that it is possible for mildly to moderately aphasic individuals to make use of evaluative language to convey their attitudes and feelings, and to use it in a way that helps to organise their discourse coherently. The fact that evaluation could be ascertained from incomplete utterances is consistent with the idea that aphasic individuals do not have to have intact syntax and semantics in order to convey meaning. It is important to note that the aphasic speakers did not use different devices from non-brain-damaged speakers, but simplified their language, as noted in their pattern of repetition and their restricted range of evaluative words. Hence, a continuum appears to exist ranging from aphasic to non-brain-damaged discourse (as noted with other discourse features, e.g., Ulatowska, North, & Macaluso-Haynes, 1980, 1981). However, further studies may well uncover differences between various levels of impairment.

The role of evaluative language in organising the discourse adds another dimension to the already explored aspects of organisation of text, for example, macrostructure, syntax, semantics. It provides the speaker with another resource for creating coherence, and it provides the listener with a framework for better understanding/interpreting the meanings being conveyed despite the disruptions produced by aphasia. In addition, such evaluative devices as reported speech and repetition may function as compensatory techniques to complement lexical and syntactic problems.

Evaluative language is obviously related to personal style and occurs on a continuum in non-brain-damaged speakers. Hence, a continuum is also very likely in the aphasic population. Data collected thus far in our larger study suggest wide variability that must be taken into account in any study of evaluative language that is concerned with clinical application. For example there is clearly no "normal" benchmark for evaluative language usage. Factors such as gender, education, ethnicity, and linguistic sophistication all contribute to this variability. Males and females have different ways of telling stories (Tannen, 1994) as do different ethnic groups (Labov, 1972; Labov & Augur, 1993; Ulatowska et al., 2000). Hence one should proceed with caution when looking for straightforward clinical applications.

Clinical implications

A potential focus on evaluative language gives an added dimension to aphasia assessment and treatment by extending beyond functional tasks previously focused upon, e.g., using the telephone, buying goods. It complements our current knowledge of the abilities of people with aphasia to convey factual information, describe events, and produce procedural discourse. It also provides a way of addressing the interpersonal impact of language difficulties. As evaluative language involves expressing our perspectives on life, who we are, how we want to be seen by other people—all important identity issues for individuals with aphasia—it is clearly involved in bonding and maintaining interpersonal relationships

In light of recent research suggesting that emotive topics may facilitate better language use (Borod et al., 2000), opportunity to use evaluative language may well provide a rich and meaningful environment for aphasia therapy. Emotional motivation to share experiences provides an immediately natural context for conversation, and from our clinical experience thus far, aphasic clients of varying severities are willing to participate in emotive discourse, despite lexical and syntactic difficulties.

Addressing emotional topics in a treatment paradigm brings in new kinds of language that can be worked on in therapy, e.g., adjectives, intensifiers, repetition, metaphor etc. Some of the evaluative devices can be seen from two perspectives—one from the perspective of conveying emotional content, and another from the perspective that they can also be used as strategies to overcome language difficulties. For example, the person with aphasia may attempt reported speech when word-finding or syntactic difficulties prevent more complex explanations (Berko-Gleason et al., 1980). Repetition could also be a delaying strategy in order to delay word finding. The clinician would have to carefully investigate the function of the devices before embarking on any "therapeutic intervention".

In addition, the stroke story provides a promising way for the clinician and person with aphasia to approach important identity and social issues. In gaining a better understanding of the aphasic experience, families, health professionals, and society in general can better appreciate and deal with the notion of aphasia and what it means to live with aphasia (an increasing focus in such approaches to treatment as the Life Participation Approach; Chapey et al., 2000). Using general experiences and stories related to being aphasic as facilitators for social connection in group treatment settings has been discussed previously (Marshall, 1999; Pound, Parr, Lindsay, & Woolf, 2000). However, it would appear that the stroke story specifically may have therapeutic value in these settings, as well as individual and family sessions. As demonstrated by the participants in this study, aphasic individuals can also produce evaluative language in different modalities (i.e., written vs spoken). Hence, diaries may well be an avenue of exploration for treatment potential in regard to this kind of language.

Of course, the use of emotional topics in clinical situations can also present potential difficulties for clinicians. While counselling occurs regularly in the clinical speech pathology setting, actual linguistic intervention usually focuses primarily on emotionally neutral stimuli, e.g., Cookie Theft, WAB type of pictures. Even when stimuli are used that involve problematic situations such as a car breaking down, there is little emotion involved. Hence, using emotive topics as the focus of treatment may well involve less of a separation between language/communication treatment and dealing with emotional issues of the client than has previously been the case. While Pound et al. (2000) have suggested the use of personal portfolios as the basis of "treatment" exploring social issues related to aphasia, such media could also be used with specific linguistic goals in mind. The clinician, of course, would have to be very mindful that linguistic goals did not constrain the content of the discussion, and that evaluative language was facilitated.

Future directions

As noted above, numerous variables may influence the use of evaluative language by individuals with aphasia. In order to explore this area further, the effects of severity and type of aphasia, age, gender, ethnicity, personal style, education level, all need to be addressed.

In addition, it will be of interest to see the extent to which a speaker's story changes over time. Potential changes in stories may relate to recovery of linguistic skills, and/or may relate to the stage that the speaker is at in terms of attitude to the stroke and aphasia at particular times post onset. For example, Frank (1995) proposes that illness/trauma narratives can be divided into different stages (chaos, restitution, and quest) that reflect different psychological attitudes to illness. These stages, when described in narratives, may require a variety of linguistic/cognitive resources to convey them and so would be of interest to explore. However from our preliminary studies, chaos narratives describing the initial confusion and distress constitute the most frequent type irrespective of the time post onset, presumably attesting to the salience of trauma.

In terms of treatment implications, both working on stimulating specific evaluative linguistic devices and using emotive topics to explore the aphasia experience from a counselling perspective may be future therapeutic directions. Future studies should inform us further of these potential clinical directions.

The nature of evaluative language is clearly complex. However, the inclusion of this dimension of language in aphasiology research is an important step in increasing awareness of the impact of aphasia on interpersonal communication.

REFERENCES

Alaszewski, A. (2006). Diaries as a source of suffering narratives: A critical commentary. *Health, Risk, & Society*, *8*(1), 43–58.

Armstrong, E. (2005). Expressing opinions and feelings in aphasia: Linguistic options. *Aphasiology*, *19*(3/5), 285–296.

Armstrong, E. M. (2001). Connecting lexical patterns of verb usage with discourse meanings in aphasia. *Aphasiology*, *15*, 1029–1046.

Berko-Gleason, J., Goodglass, H., Obler, L., Green, E., Hyde, M. R., & Weintraub, B. (1980). Narrative strategies of aphasic and normal-speaking subjects. *Journal of Speech and Hearing Research*, *30*, 370–382.

Borod, J., Rorie, K. D., Haywood, C. S., Andelman, F., Obler, L. K., Welkowitz, J. et al. (1996). Hemispheric specialization for discourse reports of emotional experiences: Relationships to demographic, neurological, and perceptual variables. *Neurospychologia*, *34*(5), 351–359.

Borod, J. C., Pick, L. H., Andelman, F., Obler, L. K., Welkowitz, J., & Rorie, K. D. et al. (2000). Verbal pragmatics following unilateral stroke: Emotional content and valence. *Neuropsychology*, *14*(1), 112–124.

Chapey, R., Duchan, J. F., Elman, R. J., Garcia, L. J., Kagan, A., Lyon, J. et al. (2000). Life participation approach to aphasia: A statement of values for the future. *ASHA Leader, 15, 5*(3), 4–6.

Faircloth, C. A., Boylstein, C., Rittman, M., Young, M. E., & Gubrium, J. (2004). Sudden illness and biographical flow in narratives of stroke recovery. *Sociology of Health & Illness*, *26*, 242–261.

Frank, A. (1995). *The wounded storyteller*. Chicago: University of Chicago Press.

Hunston, S., & Thompson, G. (2003). Evaluation: An introduction. In S. Hunston & G. Thompson (Eds.), *Evaluation in text: Authorial stance and the construction of discourse* (pp. 1–27). Oxford, UK: Oxford University Press.

Kagan, A., & Duchan, J. F. (2004). Consumers' views of what makes therapy worthwhile. In J. F. Duchan & S. Byng (Eds.), *Challenging aphasia therapies: Broadening the discourse and extending the boundaries* (pp. 158–172). Hove, UK: Psychology Press.

Kovecses, Z. (2000). *Metaphor and emotion*. Cambridge, UK: Cambridge University Press.

Labov, W. (1972). *Language in the inner city*. Philadelphia: University of Pennsylvania.

Labov, W., & Augur, J. (1993). The effect of normal aging on discourse: A sociolinguistic approach. In H. Brownell & Y. Joanette (Eds.), *Discourse in neurologically impaired and normal aging adults* (pp. 115–133). San Diego, CA: Singular.

LaPointe, L. L. (2001). Darley and the psychosocial side. *Aphasiology*, *15*(3), 249–260.

Marshall, R. C. (1999). A problem-focused group treatment program for clients with mild aphasia. In R. J. Elman (Ed.), *Group treatment of neurogenic communication disorders: The expert clinician's approach* (pp. 57–66). Boston: Butterworth Heinemann.

Martin, J. R. (1995). Interpersonal meaning, persuasion, and public discourse: Packing semiotic punch. *Australian Journal of Linguistics*, *15*, 3–67.

Martin, J. R. (2003). Beyond exchange: APPRAISAL systems in English. In S. Hunston & G. Thompson (Eds.), *Evaluation in text: Authorial stance and the construction of discourse* (pp. 142–175). Oxford, UK: Oxford University Press.

McCabe, A., & Peterson, C. (Eds.). (1991). *Developing narrative structure*. Hillsdale, NJ: Lawrence Erlbaum Associates, Inc.

Moss, B., Parr, S., Byng, S., & Petheram, B. (2004). "Pick me up and not a down down, up up": How are the identities of people with aphasia represented in aphasia, stroke, and disability websites? *Disability & Society*, *19*, 753–769.

Ochs, E., & Capps, L. (2001). *Living narrative: Creating lives in everyday storytelling*. Cambridge, MA: Harvard University Press.

Parr, S., Byng, S., Gilpin, S., & Ireland, C. (1997). *Talking about aphasia: Living with loss of language after stroke*. Buckingham, UK: Open University Press.

Pound, C., Parr, S., Lindsay, J., & Woolf, C. (2000). *Beyond aphasia: Therapies for living with communication disability*. Bicester, UK: Speechmark.

Shadden, B. (2005). Aphasia as identity theft: Theory and practice. *Aphasiology*, *19*, 211–223.

Stubbs, M. (1986). A matter of prolonged fieldwork: Towards a modal grammar of English. *Applied Linguistics*, *7*(1), 1–25.

Tannen, D. (1989). *Talking voice: Dialogue, repetition, and imagery in conversational discourse*. Cambridge, UK: Cambridge University Press.

Tannen, D. (1994). *Gender and discourse*. Oxford, UK: Oxford University Press.

Taylor, G. (1986). The development of style in children's fictional narrative (pp. 215–233). In A. Wilkinson (Ed.), *The writing of writing*. Milton Keynes, UK: Open University Press.

Ulatowska, H. K., North, A., & Macaluso-Haynes, S. (1980). Production of discourse and communicative competence in aphasia. In R. H. Brookshire (Ed.), *Clinical Aphasiology: Conference Proceedings*. Minneapolis, MN: BRK Publishers.

Ulatowska, H. K., North, A. J., & Macaluso-Haynes, S. (1981). Production of narrative and procedural discourse in aphasia. *Brain and Language, 13*, 345–371.

Ulatowska, H. K., & Olness, G. S. (2001). Dialectal variants of verbs in narratives of African Americans with aphasia: Some methodological considerations. *Journal of Neurolinguistics, 14*, 93–110.

Ulatowska, H. K., & Olness, G. S. (2003). On the nature of direct speech in narratives of African Americans with aphasia. *Brain and Language, 87*, 69–70.

Ulatowska, H. K., Olness, G. S., Hill, C. L., Roberts, J., & Keebler, M. W. (2000). Repetition in the narratives of African Americans: The effects of aphasia. *Discourse Processes, 30*, 265–283.

Ulatowska, H. K., Olness, G. S., Samson, A. M., Keebler, M. W., & Goins, K. E. (2004). On the nature of personal narratives of high quality. *Advances in Speech Language Pathology, 6*(1), 3–14.

Van Dijk, T. E. (1988). *News as discourse*. Hillsdale, NJ: Lawrence Erlbaum Associates, Inc.

APHASIOLOGY, 2007, 21 (6/7/8), 775–790

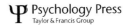

Comparing connected language elicitation procedures in persons with aphasia: Concurrent validation of the Story Retell Procedure

Malcolm R. McNeil, Jee Eun Sung, Dorothy Yang, Sheila R. Pratt, Tepanta R. D. Fossett and Patrick J. Doyle

VA Pittsburgh Healthcare System and University of Pittsburgh, PA, USA

Stacey Pavelko

University of Pittsburgh, PA, USA

Background: The Story Retell Procedure (SRP) (Doyle et al., 1998) is a well-described method for eliciting connected language samples in persons with aphasia (PWA). However, the stimuli and task demands of the SRP are fundamentally different from commonly employed picture description, narrative, and procedural description tasks reported in the aphasia literature. As such, the extent to which measures of linguistic performance derived from the SRP may be associated with those obtained from picture description, narrative, and procedural description tasks is unknown.

Aims: To assess the concurrent validity of linguistic performance measures obtained from the SRP with those obtained from picture description, narrative, and procedural description tasks by examining the correlations and the magnitude differences across the linguistic variables among the elicitation tasks. Secondarily, we examined the relationship of the percentage of information units per minute (%IU/Min) to other linguistic variables within the SRP and across the other elicitation tasks.

Methods and Procedures: This study compared the SRP to six different, frequently used sampling procedures (three sets of picture descriptions, one fairytale generation, one set of narratives, and one set of procedural description tasks) from which the same five verbal productivity, four information content, two grammatical, and two verbal disruption measures were computed. Language samples were elicited from 20 PWA, spanning the aphasia comprehension severity range. Tests of association and difference were calculated for each measure between the SRP and the other sampling methods.

Outcomes & Results: Significant and strong associations were obtained between the SRP and the other elicitation tasks for most linguistic measures. The SRP produced either no significant or significantly greater instances of the dependent variable except for the type–token ratio, which yielded a significantly lower value than the other sampling procedures.

Address correspondence to: Malcolm R. McNeil PhD, Distinguished Service Professor and Chair of Department of Communication Science and Disorders, University of Pittsburgh, 4033 Forbes Tower, Pittsburgh, PA 15260, USA. E-mail: mcneil@pitt.edu

This research was supported by VA Rehabilitation Research and Development Merit Review Project C3159R "Cognitive and linguistic mechanisms of language performance in aphasia" and the Geriatric Research, Education, and Clinical Center of the VA Pittsburgh Healthcare System. The authors gratefully acknowledge the generous participation of the volunteers for this study and the laboratory assistance of Jennifer Golovin and MaryBeth Ventura.

http://www.psypress.com/aphasiology   DOI: 10.1080/02687030701189980

Conclusions: The findings are interpreted as support for the concurrent validity of the SRP and as evidence that a single form of the SRP will yield a language sample that is generally equivalent in distribution to other sampling procedures, and one that is generally greater in quantity to those typically used to assess connected spoken language in PWA. Additionally, it was found that the %IU/Min metric predicted highly the information content linguistic measures on the SRP as well as on the other elicitation procedures. However, it did not predict well measures of verbal productivity, grammaticality, or verbal disruptions.

Among the elicited and observed procedures used to describe, classify, diagnose, measure change, quantify severity, and plan intervention for persons with aphasia (PWA), the measurement of connected spoken language has become a stable and valued procedure for many of these purposes. While being recognised as an important component in the assessment process, the most valid, reliable, and efficient methods for sampling connected spoken language have received relatively little experimental attention from clinical and experimental aphasiologists. Among the various methods used to elicit connected spoken language (e.g., picture description, story generation, personal or procedural narratives, video narration, etc.), the recently developed SRP derived from the stimuli used in the Discourse Comprehension Test (DCT) (Brookshire & Nicholas, 1997) has proven valid, reliable, and experimentally useful. Because the DCT was composed of 10 stories (plus 2 practice stories) that were equated on a number of important discourse-level linguistic variables—number of words, number of sentences, mean sentence length, number of subordinate clauses, number of T-units, ratio of clauses to T-units, listening difficulty, number of unfamiliar words, number of stated main ideas (propositions), number of implied main ideas (propositions), number of stated details, and the number of implied details—it has been used as a stimulus to elicit connected spoken language samples from non-impaired individuals and from PWA. In the SRP task, participants listen to each of the three predetermined stories constituting one of four story forms derived from the DCT stories. Participants are then instructed to retell each story in their own words, without picture support, immediately following its presentation. Participants' productions are subjected to various forms of linguistic description and quantification.

To date, research on the SRP has validated four equivalent forms (three stories each) based on linguistic variables (Doyle et al., 2000); investigated the value of picture-supported comprehension and retelling (Doyle et al., 1998); established the validity and reliability of the *information unit* scoring convention (McNeil, Doyle, Fossett, Park, & Goda, 2001); evaluated the scoring sensitivity of the percent information unit per minute efficiency measure (McNeil, Doyle, Park, Fossett, & Brodsky, 2002); investigated the inter-rater reliability of the SRP (Hula, McNeil, Doyle, Rubinsky, & Fossett, 2003); and investigated its auditory memory requirements (Brodsky et al., 2003). The SRP has the measurement advantage of having more specific predetermined targets for the retold stories than those in the other elicitation procedures, thus increasing the accuracy of the connected sample measurement. However, SRP performance reflects both comprehension and production processing and may be conditioned by the verbal memory demands of the task.

While the above-outlined psychometric properties of the test and of the scoring methods for the SRP have been investigated, concurrent validation of this procedure with other established connected spoken language sampling procedures that do not rely on comprehension or memorial factors has not. This study sought to compare several aspects of the language generated from the SRP with other published procedures for eliciting spoken language that do not rely on comprehension and memory in PWA. These were composed of two frequently used picture descriptions from published aphasia tests—the BDAE *Cookie Theft* picture (Goodglass, Kaplan, & Barresi, 2001) and the WAB *Picnic* picture (Kertesz, 1982)—two story-like picture descriptions (*Cat in Tree* and *Birthday Party*), and two sequenced picture descriptions (*The Argument* and *Directions*). PWA described "what was happening" in each picture with the pictures presented throughout the description. Two procedural description tasks (*Tell me how you would go about doing dishes by hand* and *Tell me how you would go about writing and sending a letter*), two personal narratives (*Tell me what you do on Sundays* and *Tell me where you live*), and the Cinderella Story (Berndt, Wayland, Rochon, Saffran, & Schwartz, 2000) were compared with the SRP.

The specific aims of the current study are: (a) to establish the equivalency of the SRP and other elicitation tasks by analysing the correlations among the elicitation tasks for each linguistic measure and differences in magnitude for the linguistic measures among the tasks (see Appendix for linguistic measures); (b) to establish the degree of association between the percent information units per minute (%IU/Min) as a single overall SRP metric and the other linguistic measures; and (c) to establish the associations between the %IU/Min from the SRP and the other linguistic measures from the other elicitation tasks.

METHOD AND PROCEDURES

Selection criteria

A total of 20 pre-morbidly right-handed PWA met the following selection criteria: pure tone hearing screening at 35 dB HL in at least one ear at 0.5, 1, 2, and 3 KHz; 20/40 or better visual acuity (with correction if necessary) measured with the reduced Snellen chart; performance > 8.35 (greater than 1%ile) on the 55-item Revised Token Test (RTT) (McNeil & Prescott, 1978); performance that yielded a ratio (the delayed recall/immediate recall × 100) greater than .70 on the delayed retell compared to the initial retell on the Story Retelling Test of the Arizona Battery for Communication Disorders in Dementia (ABCD) (Bayles & Tomoeda, 1993); and performance at or above 7.83 (which equates to the 20th percentile on the 180-item PICA) for individuals with left hemisphere damage on the "Two-Item" Shortened Porch Index of Communicative Ability (SPICA) (DiSimoni, Keith, & Darley, 1980).

Participants

The participants were 8 male and 12 female native speakers of English with demonstrated language performance consistent with the McNeil and Pratt (2001) definition of aphasia as determined by their performance on the selection measures. The participants had a mean age of 63 years and ranged from 43 to 82 years old (*SD* = 10), a mean of 14 years of education with a range from 11 to 23 years (*SD* = 3), and were an average of 7 months post onset with a range from 3 to 312 months (*SD* = 78). The mean RTT overall percentile score was 56 and ranged from 2 to 94 ($SD = 26$ with two participants performing within the 1st decile; one at the 2nd and 3rd deciles; three at the 4th, 5th, 6th, and 7th deciles and two at the 8th, 9th, and 10th deciles). The mean SPICA overall percentile score (estimated from the norms from the full 180-item PICA; Porch, 1981) was 78 and ranged from 52 to 92 ($SD = 11$). The mean ABCD immediate and delayed story retell ratio score was 1.02 and ranged from .75 to 1.33 ($SD = 0.14$). Descriptive information for each participant is summarised in Table 1.

Sampling methods

Connected language samples were elicited from the PWA using the six experimental tasks described above and the SRP: one of the four forms of the SRP, the Cinderella Story (Berndt et al., 2000), and the five different elicitation procedures (with two samples of each) published by Nicholas and Brookshire (1993). SRP stories were presented without picture support during presentation and retell. Participants were instructed to listen to each of the three preselected stories that make up one form of the SRP and then retell each story in their own words, as completely as possible, immediately following its presentation. The Cinderella Story was presented from its published booklet containing pictures from the "Cinderella" fairytale. After the

TABLE 1
Participant biographical data and descriptive performance measures

Participant	Gender	Age	Education Level (Yrs.)	[a]MPO	[b]RTT Percentile	[c]Estimated PICA OA Percentile	[d]ABCD Ratio
1	F	52	18	74	68	80	1.00
2	F	66	11	63	3	52	1.33
3	F	75	12	61	22	58	1.00
4	F	63	12	73	45	81	1.13
5	F	49	14	30	50	69	.75
6	F	49	17	121	63	86	.82
7	M	82	13	312	40	85	1.11
8	M	43	14	66	51	85	1.00
9	M	55	16	96	82	88	1.00
10	F	72	14	24	50	89	1.00
11	M	61	14	30	77	79	.92
12	F	60	12	91	2	76	1.00
13	M	73	14	3	39	64	1.00
14	M	61	23	27	86	66	1.00
15	F	65	12	16	91	92	1.07
16	F	75	12	17	46	83	.86
17	M	65	12	191	72	81	1.00
18	F	72	16	20	63	88	1.33
19	M	64	12	192	94	91	1.00
20	F	61	14	8	67	72	1.00
Mean	(12F;8M)	63.15	14.10	75.75	55.55	78.25	1.01
SD		10.07	2.90	77.81	26.20	11.31	.14

[a]MPO = Months Post Onset; [b]RTT = *Revised Token Test* (McNeil & Prescott, 1978); [c]PICA = *Porch Index of Communicative Ability* (Porch, 1981); [d]ABCD Ratio = *Arizona Battery for Communication Disorders of Dementia* (Bayles & Tomoeda, 1993), determined by number of delayed recall items/number of immediate recall items × 100.

participant had finished looking at the pictures, and after the pictures were removed from view, they were instructed to tell the story of Cinderella in their own words. The Nicholas and Brookshire tasks are described above and involved picture descriptions and two narrative tasks. Thus, sampling tasks were conducted according to their respective published instructions, were administered in random order across participants, and were audio-recorded for subsequent orthographic transcription and analysis.

Dependent measures

Five measures of verbal productivity (*number of utterances, number of words, number of words per minute, mean length of utterance*, and *type–token ratio*), four measures of information content (*percent of story propositions, number of correct information units, percent of correct information units, number of correct information units per minute*; and *percent of information units per minute* for the SRP only), two measures of grammaticality (*number of conjunctions* and *percent of grammatically well-formed sentences*), and two measures of verbal disruptions (*percent of mazes* and *number of abandoned sentences*) were computed for each elicitation procedure. The %IU/Min for the SRP task was calculated because that efficiency measure has been found to be more sensitive for detecting pathology than information units alone (McNeil et al., 2002).

Three speech-language pathology students trained in both language transcription and SALT (Miller & Chapman, 1998) analysis transcribed, coded, and analysed the recorded samples. Of the samples, 10% (data from two randomly selected PWA) were re-transcribed by two of the three transcribers. From this, inter- and intra-transcriber agreement was calculated for each of the language-sampling tasks and each of the dependent measures. Both within-rater and between-rater scores exceeded 90% point-to-point agreement for all dependent measures on each of the elicitation procedures.

Each of the different sampling tasks (one form from the SRP, the Cinderella Story, and the two samples from each of the five Nicholas and Brookshire elicitation tasks) were analysed separately. An SRP form is composed of three individual stories, and data from these stories were combined to compose the SRP form data. Similarly, data from both samples of each of the five different Nicholas and Brookshire elicitation procedures were combined. That is, the data were combined from each of the two aphasia test pictures (the BDAE *Cookie Theft* picture and the WAB *Picnic* picture), two sequenced picture descriptions (*Argument* and *Directions*), two story-like picture descriptions (*Cat in Tree* and *Birthday Party*), two procedural descriptions (*Doing dishes by hand* and *Writing and Sending a Letter*), and two personal narratives (*What you do on Sundays* and *Where you live*), in order to compare across task demands and to increase the corpus size for each procedure to a level more comparable to the three-story SRP task.

Because Nicholas and Brookshire (1993) suggested that a stable and representative language sample might be derived by using a single task from each of the five elicitation procedures (aphasia test picture description, story-like and sequenced picture description, procedural descriptions, and personal narrative), the same dependent measures were calculated with the data combined into two sets (Sets A and B) of five stimuli each. Set A consisted of the BDAE *Cookie Theft, Birthday Party, Argument, What you do on Sundays*, and *Doing dishes by hand* tasks. Set B consisted of the WAB *Picnic, Cat in Tree, Directions, Where you live*, and *Writing and Sending a Letter* tasks. These data, from sets A and B, and A + B combined, were then compared to the SRP, and the Cinderella Story.

Because the primary goal of the study was to establish the concurrent validity of the SRP, it was compared to each of the other sampling procedures across each of the linguistic measures. In order to determine the degree of association, Pearson Product Moment correlation coefficients were calculated for each dependent measure across each of the designated sampling procedures. In order to determine if the magnitude of any differences that exist among sampling procedures could be attributed to chance, a one-way repeated ANOVA, with Bonferroni adjustment for post-hoc comparisons, was likewise calculated. The predetermined alpha level of $p \leqslant .05$ was adjusted for multiple comparisons and set at $p \leqslant .01$ for all statistical comparisons, and a criterion of .70 was established as a substantive and statistically significant correlation between variables.

The linguistic variables of number of utterances, number of words, number of conjunctions, and number of abandoned utterances were summed for both samples (e.g. "what you do on Sundays" and "where you live") from each of the five Nicholas and Brookshire tasks, and for the three SRP stories and the single Cinderella Story. The remaining linguistic variables were averaged for each of the Nicholas and Brookshire elicitation tasks, the SRP, and for the single production of the Cinderella Story.

RESULTS

Correlations across linguistic variables between the SRP, Cinderella Story, and each of the five Nicholas and Brookshire tasks

Correlation coefficients between the SRP and each of the other elicitation procedures, for each of the 13 linguistic measures are summarised in Table 2. The SRP was correlated positively (with one exception) and significantly with the other procedures across the majority (80%; 61/77) of the 13 linguistic measures. Of these correlation coefficients, 53% (41/77) reached the criterion of .70, accounting for approximately 50% of the variance between the two variables. The great majority (85%; 40/47) of the correlations across the measures and elicitation procedures reached or exceeded the .70 criterion for the number of words per minute (6 of 6 correlations), mean length utterance (6/6), percent story propositions (3/5; story propositions were not calculated for the personal narratives), percent correct information units (5/6), number of correct information units per minute (5/6), percent grammatically well-formed sentences (5/6), percent mazes (5/6), and number of aborted sentences (5/6). Consistently lower correlation coefficients, with many non-significant, and few (7%; 2/30) reaching the .70 criterion, were derived across the elicitation procedures for the number of utterances (0/6), number of words (0/6), type–token-ratio (0/6), number of correct information units (1/6), and number of conjunctions (1/6).

While the great majority of the correlation coefficients between the SRP and the other elicitation procedures were significant ($p \leqslant .05$) across the 13 linguistic variables, the greatest number to reach the .70 criterion was found between the SRP productions and those of the Cinderella Story and the story-like pictures (69% each). The numbers of these correlations that reached criterion decreased from that of the aphasia test picture descriptions (54%), to the sequenced picture descriptions (46%), to the personal narratives (42%), and finally to the procedural descriptions (39%).

TABLE 2
Correlation coefficients (r) between the SRP and the other elicitation tasks across
all linguistic measures

Linguistic Measures	CIND	BDAE/WAB PICT.	SEQ. PICT.	NOVEL PICT.	PROCED	PERSONAL
Number of Utterances	.30	.56*	.19	.43	.25	.42
Number of Words	.47*	.46*	.38	.62*	.51*	.62*
Number of Words per Minute	.76*	.82*	.83*	.80*	.87*	.85*
Mean Length Utterance	.70*	.81*	.69*	.80*	.80*	.86*
Type-Token Ratio	.35	.33	.31	.41	.23	.37
Percent of Story Propositions	.71*	.69*	.81*	.82*	.64*	N/A
Number of Correct Information Unit	.62*	.58*	.59*	.71*	.54*	.44
Percent of Correct Information Unit	.86*	.88*	.75*	.83*	.75*	.41
Number of Correct Information Unit per Minute	.81*	.91*	.69*	.83*	.82*	.75*
Number of Conjunctions	.70*	−.11	.63*	.05	.52*	.45*
Percent of Grammatical Wellformedness	.76*	.89*	.84*	.86*	.68*	.70*
Percent of Mazes	.87*	.93*	.88*	.89*	.90*	.58*
Number of Abandoned Utterances	.81*	.78*	.78*	.70*	.47*	.82*

Note. Correlation coefficients with an asterisk are statistically significant, $p \le .05$. Shaded correlation coefficients in bold font meet or exceed the predetermined .70 criteria for a substantively high correlation coefficient.

Correlations across linguistic variables between SRP and aggregated Nicholas and Brookshire tasks

Values from each linguistic variable for the SRP and those same summed linguistic values from the five single tasks (one from each of the distinct procedures) derived from the Nicholas and Brookshire procedures, were also correlated. As described above, this yielded two forms of the procedure (Set A and B), as well as a combination of the two. These correlation coefficients are summarised in Table 3. In general, it can be seen that the same linguistic variables (number of utterances, number of words, and number of correct information units) that did not meet the .70 correlation criterion for the tasks separated by unique elicitation task demands (Figure 1) also did not meet this criterion when the tasks were combined. However, correlation coefficients for the type–token-ratio and number of conjunctions were substantively increased by this aggregation of tasks. The average correlation coefficients for those variables that did meet the criterion were .86 for the aphasia test picture descriptions, .81 for the sequenced picture descriptions, .80 for the story-like picture descriptions, .82 for the procedural descriptions, .79 for the personal narratives, 79 for set A, .81 for set B, and .80 for set A + B.

Correlations of the SRP %IU/Min metric with the SRP and the six other elicitation procedures across linguistic variables

It can be seen from Table 4 that the number of words per minute, percent story propositions, number correct information units, percent correct information units,

TABLE 3
Correlation coefficients (r) between the SRP and all linguistic measures across elicitation
Sets A, B, and A+B

Linguistic Measures	Set A	Set B	Set A+B
Number of Utterances	.30	.57*	.46*
Number of Words	.53*	.59*	.57*
Number of Words per Minute	.73*	.83*	.81*
Mean Length Utterance	.84*	.75*	.78*
Type -Token Ratio	.75*	.85*	.87*
Percent of Story Propositions	.87*	.80*	.78*
Number of Correct Information Unit	.63*	.69*	.67*
Percent of Correct Information Unit	.83*	.81*	.83*
Number of Correct Information Unit per Minute	.84*	.92*	.90*
Number of Conjunctions	.76*	.72*	.77*
Percent of Grammatical Wellformedness	.71*	.74*	.72*
Percent of Mazes	.74*	.84*	.80*
Number of Abandoned Utterances	.79*	.79*	.79*

Note. Correlation coefficients with an asterisk are statistically significant, $p \leq .05$. Shaded correlation coefficients in bold font meet or exceed the predetermined .70 criteria for a substantively high correlation coefficient.

and number correct information units per minute correlated positively, significantly, and at criterion levels with the SRP %IU/Min metric. None of the other correlation coefficients was statistically significant for the SRP. The correlation coefficients for the number of words per minute also reached criterion for the aphasia test picture

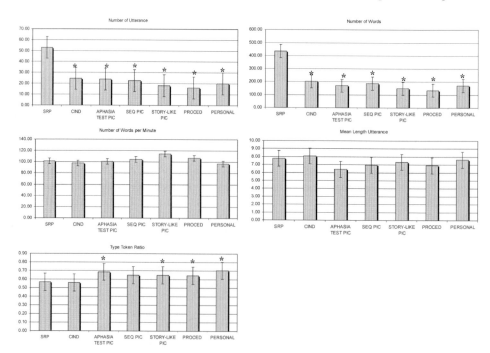

Figure 1. Verbal productivity measures across elicitation procedures. *Significant mean differences between the Story Retell Procedure (SRP) and the elicitation procedure.

TABLE 4
Correlation coefficients (r) between the SRP %IU's/Min and all linguistic measures across all elicitation tasks

Linguistic Measures	SRP	CIND	BDAE/WAB PICT.	SEQ. PICT.	NOVEL PICT.	PROCED	PERSONAL
Number of Utterances	.13	−.39	−.23	−.09	−.37	−.13	−.36
Number of Words	15	−.15	.20	.21	−.06	.14	−.13
Number of Words per Minute	.81*	.60*	.72*	.61*	.69*	.73*	.73*
Mean Length Utterance	.42	.40	.70*	67*	.65*	.60*	.46*
Type-Token Ratio	.15	.18	.33	.09	.14	.04	−.08
Percent of Story Propositions	.72*	.43	.61*	.61*	.51*	.65*	N/A
Number of Correct Information Unit	.73*	.39	.60*	.49*	.53*	.32	.22
Percent of Correct Information Unit	.70*	.70*	.76*	.55*	.71*	.56*	.50*
Number of Correct Information Unit per Minute	.93*	.76*	.87*	.67*	.78*	.72*	.63*
Number of Conjunctions	.28	.06	.40	.42	.22	.49*	.04
Percent of Grammatical Wellformedness	.42	.42	.53*	.48*	.48*	.65*	.24
Percent of Mazes	−.39	−.54*	−.53*	−.48*	−.41	−.50*	−.49*
Number of Abandoned Utterances	−.43	−.55*	−.27	−.30	−.31	−.46*	−.41

Note. Correlation coefficients with an asterisk are statistically significant, $p \leq .05$. Shaded correlation coefficients in bold font meet or exceed the predetermined .70 criteria for a substantively high correlation coefficient.

descriptions, the procedural descriptions, and the personal narratives. Likewise, the mean length of utterance reached correlation criterion for the aphasia test picture descriptions. The percent correct information units and number of correct information units per minute also reached correlation criterion for the Cinderella Story, the aphasia test picture descriptions, and the story-like picture descriptions. The number of correct information units per minute also reached criterion for the procedural description tasks. Of the correlations from the grammatical category only one was significant for the number of conjunctions and none reached criterion, while several were significant but none reached criterion for the percent grammatically well-formed sentences. Half of the correlations were statistically significant, but none of them reached criterion for verbal disruptions.

The correlations between the SRP %IU/Min and Brookshire and Nicholas' sets A, B, and A+B for each linguistic variable, shown in Table 5, generally paralleled those where the procedures were subdivided. Only the measures of number of words per minute, percent correct information units, and number correct information units per minute reached correlation criterion. The pattern of correlation coefficients among elicitation tasks was not systematic.

Magnitude of differences

The five panels of bar graphs in Figure 1 summarise data from each of the verbal productivity linguistic measures for each sampling procedures. From left to right and top to bottom, the figures represent the total number of utterances, total number of words, total number words per minute, mean length of utterance, and type–token-ratio for each elicitation procedure. The asterisk above the frequency bars indicates that the value derived from the SRP was significantly different from the value for that elicitation procedure with the multiple comparison adjusted alpha ($p \leqslant .01$). It can be

TABLE 5
Correlations (r) between the SRP %IU's/Min and all linguistic measures across elicitation Set A, Set B, Set A+B

Linguistic Measures	Set A	Set B	Set A+B
Number of Utterances	−.45*	37	−.43
Number of Words	−.02	.14	.06
Number of Words per Minute	.65*	.81*	.77*
Mean Length Utterance	.61*	.60*	.49*
Type -Token Ratio	.24	.25	.20
Percent of Story Propositions	.67*	.62*	.53*
Number of Correct Information Unit	.38	.43	.41
Percent of Correct Information Unit	.74*	.63*	.69*
Number of Correct Information Unit per Minute	.81*	.88*	.86*
Number of Conjunctions	.24	.19	.19
Percent of Grammatical Wellformedness	.52*	.58*	.55*
Percent of Mazes	−.49*	−.49*	−.49*
Number of Abandoned Utterances	−.35	−.38	−.37

Note. Correlation coefficients with an asterisk are statistically significant, p ≤ .05. Shaded correlation coefficients in bold font meet or exceed the predetermined .70 criteria for a substantively high correlation coefficient

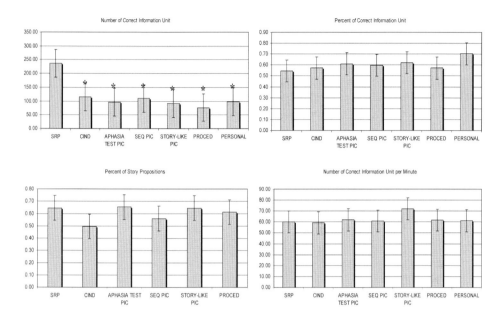

Figure 2. Information content measures across elicitation procedures. *Significant mean differences between the Story Retell Procedure (SRP) and the elicitation procedure.

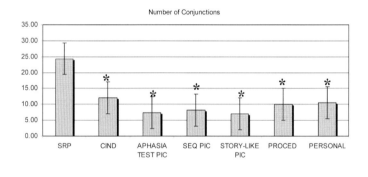

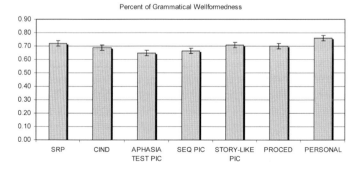

Figure 3. Grammaticality measures across elicitation procedures. *Significant mean differences between the Story Retell Procedure (SRP) and the elicitation procedure.

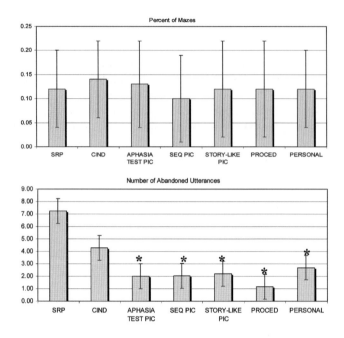

Figure 4. Verbal disruption measures across elicitation procedures. *Significant mean differences between the Story Retell Procedure (SRP) and the elicitation procedure.

seen that the SRP produced a significantly larger number of utterances ($p \leqslant .01$) and words ($p \leqslant .01$). No significant difference in magnitude of performance was evident for the number of words per minute ($p > .01$) or the mean length of utterance ($p > .01$). The SRP generated a significantly smaller type–token ratio than the other elicitation procedures ($p \leqslant .01$), except the Cinderella Story and the story-like picture descriptions, which were non-significantly different from the SRP ($p > .01$).

Figure 2 summarises the data for the information content measures composed of the total number of correct information units, percent correct information units, percent of story propositions, and number of correct information units per minute. As indicated by the asterisks, the SRP produced significantly ($p \leqslant .01$) more correct information units than each of the other elicitation procedures. No significant differences were found for any of the other information content measures for any of the elicitation procedures (all $p \geqslant .01$).

Figure 3 summarises the data for the two grammaticality measures. It can be seen in the first panel that the SRP generated significantly ($p \leqslant .01$) more conjunctions that created a compound sentence than each of the other elicitation procedures. No significant difference ($p \geqslant .01$) in the number of grammatically well-formed sentences was observed between the SRP and any of the other elicitation procedures.

Figure 4 summarises the data for the two measures selected to quantify verbal disruptions. While there was no significant difference between the percentage of mazes produced between the SRP and the other elicitation procedures ($p > .01$), the SRP did yield significantly more abandoned utterances than all other elicitation procedures (all $p \leqslant .01$) except the Cinderella Story, which was not significantly different from the SRP ($p > .01$).

DISCUSSION

A primary concern with the interpretation of the SRP and other retelling tasks as elicited, connected, spoken language sampling procedures is the fact that they require the individual to comprehend and remember the stimulus for later retelling. As such, the quality and/or the quantity of the sample could be influenced by what is comprehended and remembered, making it a procedure that is limited in its ability to provide an optimal or perhaps even valid estimate of connected spoken language. These potential limitations are minimised with connected spoken language elicitation procedures that require picture descriptions, fairytale generations, and personal narratives or procedural descriptions such as those with which the SRP was compared in this study. As such, the degree to which the SRP correlates with those elicitation procedures that do not tax the comprehension and memory systems would support its validity. This would be especially true if the magnitude of the behaviours were equivalent or greater for the SRP compared to the elicitation procedures whose comprehension and memory demands are minimised. The data derived from the SRP across the majority of the linguistic variables calculated in this investigation provide support for the concurrent validity of this retell procedure as one yielding language samples whose values are predicted from one elicitation procedure to the other. That the values derived from the SRP correlated positively and significantly across all elicitation procedures—Cinderella Story (85%), aphasia test picture descriptions (92%), sequenced picture descriptions (85%), story-like picture descriptions (77%), procedural descriptions (85%), and personal narratives (85%)—is interpreted as support for this contention. Support is also strengthened by the fact that the majority of the correlation coefficients derived across the measures reached or exceeded the .70 criterion for the Cinderella Story (69%), the story-like picture descriptions (69%), and the aphasia test picture descriptions (53%). These relationships were found for the majority (62%) of the linguistic measures and included those for the verbal productivity, information content, grammaticality, and verbal disruption domains of linguistic description generated from the SRP. To the degree that these relationships that cross elicitation procedures and linguistic measures provide a valid and reliable index of the connected spoken language of PWA, the SRP has established reasonable comparability and concurrent validity.

The average correlation coefficients for those variables that did meet the criterion were largely unchanged between the separated procedures (average correlation coefficients equalled .84 for the aphasia test picture descriptions, .78 for the sequenced picture descriptions, .82 for the story-like picture descriptions, .74 for the procedural descriptions, and .65 for the personal narratives) and those same procedures when they were aggregated (.79 for set A, .81 for set B, and .80 for sets A + B). No substantive changes in the average correlation coefficients that reached criterion were found by aggregating all ten tasks beyond those yielded by the five.

The linguistic variables that also correlated positively, significantly, and highly between the SRP and the other elicitation procedures when they were aggregated (sets A, B, and A + B) were generally the same variables that also correlated at similar levels when they were separated. The type–token ratio was the only linguistic variable in which the correlation coefficients increased substantively when the SRP was correlated with the aggregated elicitation tasks compared to when it was correlated with the individual procedures (with two samples each). This was likely due to the sensitivity of the type–token ratio to sample size (Wachal & Spreen, 1973; Wright, Silverman & Newhoff, 2003).

The SRP generated a language sample that was greater or equal in quantity to the other elicitation procedures investigated in this study for the great majority of the linguistic variables computed. That is, the SRP yielded a significantly larger number of behaviours for the number of utterances. Obtaining a larger number of behaviours may present an advantage for the purposes of analysis due to additional measurement stability/reliability. A larger number of behaviours provides the examiner more opportunities to observe linguistic complexity (e.g., morphosyntactic and discourse) as well as more and different types of errors. Non-significant differences between the SRP and the other elicitation procedures were found for words per minute, mean length of utterances, percent correct information units, number of correct information units per minute, percent story propositions, percent of grammatically well-formed sentences, and percent mazes. Therefore, together with the high correlation coefficients across most of the independent and dependent variables, we interpret the non-significant differences across elicitation procedures and the significantly larger number of behaviours for all other variables as evidence that the SRP is equivalent or superior, in terms of more opportunity to observe both positive and negative relevant behaviours, compared to the other sampling procedures as they are typically employed, and using these linguistic variables. If sample sizes are equivalent or larger, as when elicitation tasks are aggregated such as those derived in Forms A and B of the Nicholas and Brookshire tasks, this superiority may not be apparent.

It is interesting to note that when there were no significant differences across the language-sampling procedures for a particular linguistic variable (e.g., percent correct information units), the behaviours elicited on the SRP correlated highly across those procedures, with the overall average correlations across procedures and measures achieving .84 for those that reached the .70 criterion. Conversely, when the SRP yielded significantly greater linguistic behaviours compared to the other elicitation tasks, the correlations tended to fall below the criterion.

Derived from a series of studies, the %IU/Min has been advocated as a single metric for the quantification of the SRP (Brodsky et al., 2003; Hula et al., 2003; McNeil et al., 2001, 2002). As a secondary question, correlation coefficients were calculated between the %IU/Min measure and the other linguistic measures for the SRP only in order to assess the degree to which it predicts these other behaviours. The results confirmed that the measures of information content are particularly well predicted by this single metric for the SRP. The interpretation of this is that the single %IU/Min metric does not predict other relevant linguistic behaviours in PWA. Thus, linguistic measures in addition to the %IU/Min appear to be necessary in order to accurately assess the range of linguistic behaviours typically evaluated in PWA.

In summary, the data from this study support the concurrent validity of the SRP as a spoken language elicitation procedure. The high correlation coefficients among language elicitation procedures across several linguistic variables is consistent with the interpretation that the comprehension and memorial demands of the SRP, compared to the other connected spoken language sampling procedures used in this study, do not restrict the quantity or the nature of language derived from it. In addition, the well-established psychometric properties of the SRP, along with its four equivalent forms and pre-specified production targets, appear to offer a sufficient advantage to the accuracy and efficiency of transcribing and scoring the language sample to warrant its consideration over other language elicitation procedures. Finally, while the %IU/Min metric predicts information content measures on the SRP, it does not appear to be robust or general enough to predict measures of verbal productivity, grammaticality, or verbal disruptions.

REFERENCES

Bayles, K., & Tomoeda, C. (1993). *Arizona Battery for Communication Disorders of Dementia.* Tucson, AZ: Canyonlands Publishing.

Berndt, R. S., Wayland, S., Rochon, E., Saffran, E., & Schwartz, M. (2000). *Quantitative production analysis (QPA).* Philadelphia, PA: Psychology Press.

Brodsky, M. B., McNeil, M. R., Doyle, P. J., Fossett, T. R. D., Timm, N. H., & Park, G. H. (2003). Auditory serial position effects in story retelling for normal adult subjects and person with aphasia. *Journal of Speech-Language-Hearing Research, 46*(5), 1124–1137.

Brookshire, R. H., & Nicholas, L. E. (1997). *Discourse Comprehension Test.* Minneapolis, MN: BRK Publishers.

DiSimoni, F. G., Keith, R. L., & Darley, F. L. (1980). Prediction of PICA overall score by short versions of the test. *Journal of Speech and Hearing Research, 23,* 511–516.

Doyle, P. J., McNeil, M. R., Park, G., Goda, A., Rubenstein, E., & Spencer, K. A. et al. (2000). Linguistic validation of four parallel forms of a story retelling procedure. *Aphasiology, 14*(5/6), 537–549.

Doyle, P. J., McNeil, M. R., Spencer, K. A., Goda, A. J., Cottrell, K., & Lustig, A. P. (1998). The effects of concurrent picture presentations on retelling of orally presented stories by adults with aphasia. *Aphasiology, 12,* 561–574.

Goodglass, H., Kaplan, E., & Barresi, B. (2001). *Boston Diagnostic Aphasia Examination.* (3rd ed.). Philadelphia, PA: Lippincott Williams & Wilkins.

Hula, W. D., McNeil, M. R., Doyle, P. J., Rubinsky, H. J., & Fossett, T. R. D. (2003). The inter-rater reliability of the Story Retell Procedure. *Aphasiology, 17,* 523–528.

Kertesz, A. (1982). *Western Aphasia Battery.* New York: The Psychological Corporation, Harcourt Brace Jovanovich, Inc.

McNeil, M. R., Doyle, P. J., Fossett, T. R. D., Park, G. H., & Goda, A. J. (2001). Reliability and concurrent validity of the information unit scoring metric for the story retelling procedure. *Aphasiology, 15*(10/11), 991–1006.

McNeil, M. R., Doyle, P. J., Park, G. H., Fossett, T. R. D., & Brodsky, M. B. (2002). Increasing the sensitivity of the Story Retell Procedure for the discrimination of normal elderly subjects from persons with aphasia. *Aphasiology, 16,* 815–822.

McNeil, M. R., & Pratt, S. R. (2001). A standard definition of aphasia: Toward a general theory of aphasia. *Aphasiology, 15*(10/11), 901–911.

McNeil, M. R., & Prescott, T. E. (1978). *The Revised Token Test.* Austin, TX: Pro-Ed.

Miller, J., & Chapman, R. (1998). *SALT: Systematic analysis of language transcripts.* [Windows versions 1.0–5.0]. Madison, WI: Language Analysis Laboratory, Waisman Center, University of Wisconsin.

Nicholas, L. E., & Brookshire, R. H. (1993). A system for quantifying the informativeness and efficiency of the connected speech of adults with aphasia. *Journal of Speech and Hearing Research, 36,* 338–350.

Porch, B. E. (1981). *Porch Index of Communicative Ability.* Palo Alto, CA: Consulting Psychologists Press.

Wachal, R. S., & Spreen, O. (1973). Some measures of lexical diversity in aphasic and normal language performance. *Language and Speech, 16,* 169–181.

Wright, H. H., Silverman, S. W., & Newhoff, M. (2003). Measures of lexical diversity in aphasia. *Aphasiology, 17,* 443–452.

APPENDIX: DEFINITIONS OF LINGUISTIC MEASURES

Verbal productivity

- Number of utterances: Total number of speaker attempts – included all utterances.
- Number of words: Total number of completed words (main body and mazes).
- Number of words per minute: Total completed words/elapsed time in minutes (main body and mazes).
- Mean length of utterance: Mean length of utterance in words—each word counts as one word for this calculation regardless of how many bound morphemes it may contain. Words found in mazes and omitted words are not included.
- Type–token ratio: Different words/total words.

Information content

- Percent of story propositions: Story propositions accurately and completely contain all "essential" information. Information is considered essential as long as the general meaning of the story is preserved.
- Number of Correct Information Units: Total number of words that are intelligible in context and accurately convey information relevant to the eliciting stimulus.
- Percent of Correct Information Units: The total number of Correct Information Units/the total number of words.
- Number per minute of Correct Information Units: The total number of Correct Information Units/elapsed time in minutes.
- Percent Information Units per minute: Percent of Correct Information Units/ elapsed time in minutes.

Grammatical well-formedness and syntactic complexity

- Number of conjunctions: Any of the following words (AFTER, AND, AS, BECAUSE, BUT, IF, OR, SINCE, SO, THEN, UNTIL, WHILE) is considered a conjunction if used in an utterance in some meaningful way (i.e., to connect two conjoining sentences). The preceding words, however, are not considered conjunctions if they serve no functional purpose in a sentence (i.e., in cases where the speaker uses them as a filler).
- Percent of grammatically well-formed sentences: The number of accurate and complete clauses (including independent clauses, dependent clauses, and prepositional phrases)/the total number of clauses and phrases.

Verbal disruptions

- Percent of mazes: Percent of total words that are in mazes (filled pauses, false starts, repetitions, and reformulations in an utterance).
- Number of abandoned sentences: Total number of sentences where the speaker voluntarily stops before completing it.

APHASIOLOGY, 2007, 21 (6/7/8), 791–801

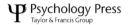

Development of a procedure to evaluate the contributions of persons with aphasia and their spouses in an interview situation

Claire Croteau, Guylaine Le Dorze, and Geneviève Baril

Université de Montréal, Canada

Background: Although there has been increasing interest in the study of conversations between people with aphasia and their partners, the participation of persons with aphasia in conversation with their spouses in the presence of a third party has not been extensively investigated. Nevertheless, opportunities for such situations are frequent, and therefore provide an interesting opportunity to examine how couples collaborate.
Aims: (1) To develop a procedure to analyse conversations that would specifically address the contributions of persons with aphasia and their spouses in an interview situation. (2) To describe spousal contributions in an interview situation, including what preceded and followed these contributions, in a group of couples with a member with aphasia. (3) To verify the inter-judge reliability of the procedure.
Methods & Procedures: Videos of three couples with aphasia in an interview situation were analysed. Contributions of the spouse when the participant with aphasia was clearly speaking with the interviewer, contexts in which spouses contributed, reactions of persons with aphasia, and their participation following contributions were described. Definitions were created, operationalised, tested, and refined on 11 other similar couples in the same interactive situation. Eight other couples were then videotaped and studied.
Outcomes & Results: Results revealed that half the contributions produced by the spouse were "repairs" and the other half were "speaking for" behaviours. Most often, contributions were unsolicited. Generally, the person with aphasia approved the spouse's contribution and continued afterwards to take an active part in the conversation. Inter-judge reliability coefficients varied between 89% and 97%.
Conclusions: The procedure employed is representative of situations encountered by couples affected by aphasia. The data collection and analysis methods could be applicable to clinical situations. It is important to consider spousal contributions and their impact on the person with aphasia in conversations when helping couples adjust to the consequences of aphasia.

There has been increasing interest in the study of conversations between people with aphasia and their partners, aiming to understand the impact of aphasia on

Address correspondence to: Claire Croteau PhD, École d'orthophonie et d'audiologie, Université de Montréal, C.P. 6128, succursale Centre-Ville Montréal, Québec H3C 3J7, Canada. E-mail: claire.croteau@umontreal.ca

This research was supported by grants from Social Sciences and Humanities Research Council of Canada and Les Fonds de la Recherche en Santé du Québec. The participants are gratefully acknowledged. We would like to also thank Christiane Malaborza, Claudia Morin, Ève Nadeau, the speech-language pathologists, and the associations of people with aphasia who referred many participants to us. We also extend our gratitude to Nina Simmons-Mackie for helpful comments.

http://www.psypress.com/aphasiology   DOI: 10.1080/02687030701192398

conversation and to describe the types and patterns of collaboration in dyads (e.g., Ferguson, 1998; Laakso & Klippi, 1999; Milroy & Perkins, 1992; Oelschlaeger & Damico, 1998, 2000; Simmons-Mackie, Kingston, & Schultz, 2004). To date, few studies have investigated how a couple in which one member has aphasia participates in interactions involving a third party. Yet, as mentioned in Croteau, Vychytil, Larfeuil, and Le Dorze (2004), such an aphasic–non-aphasic dyad might frequently converse with another speaker such as a neighbour, an acquaintance, a stranger, a professional, or a service provider. To provide a more comprehensive evaluation of the participation of persons with aphasia and their partners, these social contexts should be studied. The aim of the present project was to develop a procedure to analyse conversations that would specifically address the contributions of the non-aphasic spouses as well as the participation of the partner with aphasia when the couple is in an interview situation.

COUPLES IN AN INTERVIEW SITUATION

Manzo, Blonder, and Burns (1995), Croteau et al. (2004), and Croteau and Le Dorze (2006) studied a specific context involving three speakers, including a couple and an interviewer. In this context, some spouses spoke for the person with aphasia, a behaviour that was not always favourable to the person with aphasia as it lessened his/her participation (Croteau & Le Dorze, 2006; Croteau et al., 2004). Manzo et al. (1995) reported that spouses of men who had suffered strokes contributed significantly and substantially to the conversation without explicit invitation. They differed from spouses of men with non-stroke-related diseases (e.g., arthritis), who participated only when solicited. Furthermore, spouses oriented husbands who had had a stroke by asking them questions to help them respond. These spouses also engaged in "competitive" storytelling, i.e., they completed, corrected, or contradicted what their partner who had had a stroke had stated. Moreover, they answered questions that were directly addressed to the person who had had a stroke.

Even though these studies provide information about how spouses of stroke victims participate in an interview, additional information is needed about couples with a member with aphasia in that context. On the one hand, Manzo et al. (1995) did not report the communication impairments of their participants with stroke. On the other hand, as they focused on "speaking for" behaviours, Croteau et al. (2004) and Croteau and Le Dorze (2006) did not describe all the behaviours that a spouse may use to help the person with aphasia. For example, it is likely that spouses participate in the repair process when the partner with aphasia has communication problems. These repair behaviours have not been studied in an interview situation, although they have been described in natural conversations as discussed below.

REPAIRS IN CONVERSATION

The repair process has been generally described in terms of initiation (self-initiated or other-initiated), repair process per se (self-repair, other-repair), and resolution (Schegloff, Jefferson, & Sacks, 1977). Repair sequences are more frequent (Ferguson, 1992), longer, and more complex in conversations with a partner with aphasia than in conversations without a speaker with aphasia (Laakso & Klippi, 1999). Other-repair sequences are of interest in conversations with a person with aphasia because of the frequency with which they occur. Repair sequences often require the collaboration of both speakers (Ferguson, 1994; Laakso & Klippi, 1999; Lindsay & Wilkinson, 1999; Milroy & Perkins, 1992; Oelschlaeger & Damico, 1998; Perkins, Crisp, & Walshaw, 1999), and are often structured according to a "hint and guess" sequence (Lubinski, Duchan, & Weitzner-Lin, 1980; Laakso & Klippi, 1999). Oelschlaeger & Damico (1998) described what is accomplished through the repair process, in that spouses collaborate with the person with aphasia to find a missing word, complete a turn, and add information. Studies have also described how people with aphasia requested partner assistance in the initiation of the repair process (Laakso & Klippi, 1999; Oelschlaeger, 1999; Oelschlaeger & Damico, 1998). In terms of resolution, the reactions of the person with aphasia following his/her partner's repair have also been studied (Ferguson, 1992; Oelschlaeger & Damico, 1998, 2000).

These studies allow us to observe that the repair process is complex and includes a sequence of important elements. Additional information is needed to understand the complete repair process—i.e., from initiation to resolution—in a number of couples in which one person had aphasia. Specifically, new studies could focus on the range of contributions of spouses in conversation, the context in which they occur, and the impact these contributions have on the member with aphasia's participation in the conversation. Such studies could further our understanding of how the spouse's contribution helps the flow of conversation in different types of situations, such as interviews.

METHODOLOGICAL CONSIDERATIONS

Several studies have employed Conversational Analysis (CA) to study conversation (e.g., Ferguson, 1994; Lindsay & Wilkinson, 1999; Oelschlaeger & Damico, 1998, 2000; Sacks, Schegloff, & Jefferson, 1974; Wilkinson, 1999; Wilkinson et al., 1998). This rigorous qualitative method of analysis offers many advantages for the study of interactions. It is based on the study of natural interactions, which ensures the ecological validity of the observations. Judgements on the success of interactions are based on participant responses. Moreover, this method considers sequences of behaviours in contexts where speaker turns are linked to one another. For example, it allows one to analyse how a spouse responds to the word-finding difficulties of the partner with aphasia, to consider whether the assistance was solicited, and whether this assistance helps the partner with aphasia to continue to participate in conversation, which is essential information to orient therapy (Wilkinson et al., 1998).

However, qualitative analysis may present some disadvantages because it does not readily lend itself to quantification as does, for example, the means developed by Ramsberger and Rende (2002), which evaluates transactional success in semi-structured conversation. Thus, both qualitative and quantitative methods have both advantages and disadvantages for measuring progress and outcomes. Therefore, a combination of both qualitative and quantitative methods holds promise for both orienting and measuring therapy (Crockford & Lesser, 1994; Perkins et al., 1999).

In order to describe how spouses of a person with aphasia contribute to conversations, the present study developed a new means of analysis that was based on qualitative data and which allowed quantification. The aims were:

1. To develop a procedure to describe spousal contributions in an interview situation, as well as what preceded and followed these contributions.

2. To describe spousal contributions in an interview situation, as well as what preceded and followed these contributions, in a new group of couples with a member with aphasia.
3. To verify the reliability of the procedure.

DEVELOPMENT OF THE PROCEDURE

Part one

A preliminary qualitative study was conducted on videos of three couples with a member with aphasia in an interview situation (see description of the interview situation below). Each conversation was transcribed and analysed qualitatively with Conversation Analysis (CA, Sacks et al., 1974). The analyses aimed to characterise the contributions of the spouse when the person with aphasia was speaking with the interviewer, the context in which spouses contributed, the reactions of the persons with aphasia, and their participation following contributions. The results included a variety of spousal behaviours and reactions of persons with aphasia.

Part two

In order to eventually quantify behaviours, descriptions collected in the preliminary study were grouped and definitions of behaviours of interest were developed. In a second preliminary study, these definitions were operationalised and tested on 11 new couples with a member with aphasia involved in the same interview situation. Definitions were then refined until trained graduate students in speech and language pathology, who served as judges, were satisfied and in agreement. The results included a description of an analysis procedure, which is detailed in the Appendix.

DESCRIPTIVE STUDY METHOD

The next section focuses on a quantitative study of eight couples with aphasia using the analysis procedure developed.

Participants

Eight French-speaking couples with one member suffering from aphasia participated in the study, as presented in Table 1.

Interview situation

The interview was conducted at the University of Montreal. Participants were asked for their opinion on six various issues (e.g., divorce, technology, poverty in third-world countries, health care system, today's youth. First, one participant picked a card containing a question about one of the issues. The interviewer, an experienced speech and language pathologist, asked the participant to answer the question. When the interviewer had judged that she understood the participant's response, she asked the other member of the couple to respond to the same question. Once the second participant had responded, she/he picked another card on which another question was written. The interviewer then asked him/her to respond until she understood the

TABLE 1
Characteristics of the couples

Couples								Spouses		
Length of relationship (years)	Age	Sex	Education (years)	Type of aphasia[a]	Severity[b]	Years post CVA		Age	Sex	Education (years)
1	63	83	F	11	Broca	2	2.6	86	M	20
2	40	63	M	20	Mixed	4	3.9	58	F	13
3	29	63	F	18	Mixed	2	1.11	62	M	9
4	37	62	M	11	Broca	4	1.2	62	F	10
5	34	57	M	11	Broca	1	0.8	56	F	11
6	46	67	M	7	Broca	3	5.5	65	F	7
7	43	63	M	11	Broca	2	7.6	64	F	16
8	40	83	M	5	Subcortical	4	1.11	66	F	12

[a]Based on the responses on the Protocole Montréal-Toulouse Examen linguistique de l'Aphasie (M1B). (Nespoulous et al., 1986). [b]Based on the subjective scale of the Boston Diagnostic Aphasia Evaluation (Goodglass & Kaplan, 1983).

response. She then gave the floor over to the other spouse. Questions were asked until approximately 1 hour of material was videotaped. The first 5 minutes of recording were excluded and the next 15-minute samples were used for analysis.

Analysis

First, sections of the interview were identified in which the general questions were addressed to the person with aphasia. Next, the contributions of the spouse within these sections were analysed to identify type (repair, "speaking for", or support) and subtype (six repair subtypes and three support subtypes). Contributions were determined to be solicited or unsolicited by the participant with aphasia. The events following the contributions of the spouse were then analysed to consider the reaction of the person with aphasia and the impact of spousal contributions on his/her participation in the conversation. See Figure 1 for an illustration of the procedure, as well as the definitions in the Appendix. Here is an example of an instance where the spouse (S) produced an unsolicited repair labelled as a correction (see # 10). This repair is followed by an explicit approval (see # 11) and a major participation in the conversation by the person with aphasia (Pa) (see #11, #16 and #19 for the contributive turns).

1 I: Hum, hum. Hum, hum. (#) So, do you think there's a way to, ah, prevent these, these divorces then?
2 Pa: (# long) Me, I think, ah (# long), you'll tell me, ah, maybe that, ah (#) I...that I'm old-fashioned, ah (# long) to bring (#) God into it. (#) Period.
3 I: Yeah   [Yeah.]
4 Pa: Me, I did that (# long), but it worked.
5 I: Hum.
6 Pa: The proof.
7 I: Hum. The proof being... You've been married since, ah...
8 Pa: [Well, yeah. Thirty-one years.]
9 I: Thirty-one years.

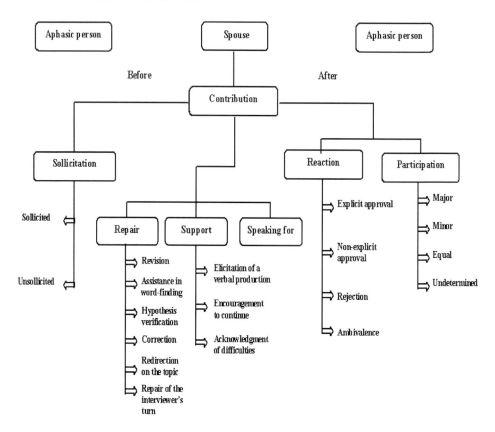

Figure 1. Parameters of the analysis procedure.

10 S: [Hey, no, no. ((laughs)) It's thirty-six years now.]
11 Pa: [Ah... ah] (pronounced intonation)
12 I: Thirty-six years!
13 Pa: [ah: m]
14 S: It'll be thirty-seven in May.
15 Pa: [(999)]
16 Pa: Ah: m (# long) The main, the basic value, (# long) it's not there. That's it.
17 I: [Of...]
18 I: Ok.
19 Pa: Hang on... (#) but I would say... I would even say (#), from where I went, I
     didn't, ah (#) I went there (# long), If I did...If I did... If I didn't hold that
     value, I wouldn't still be here (#) today.

Reliability

Reliability was established by comparing the results of a trained independent speech language pathologist with those of the third author for two of the eight conversations, which accounted for 32% of total contributions. Point-by-point reliability was 89% for the identification of contributions. Other reliability scores varied between 90% and 97%.

RESULTS

The results presented in this section concern the mean frequency of occurrence of repair and "speaking for" contributions in the 15-minute samples. The results for support and the different repair subtypes are not presented because of their low frequency of occurrence (support, $n = 1$). In general, standard deviations were high, indicating individual variation.

Contributions of spouses and persons with aphasia

Table 2 shows that spouses produced a mean of 15.13 contributions within the 15-minute samples. Half were "speaking for" contributions (Mean = 7.75) and the other half were repair contributions (Mean = 7.38). The most frequent contributions were unsolicited "speaking for" (Mean = 7.12) and unsolicited repair (Mean = 5.13). However, repair contributions were more frequently solicited (Mean = 2.25) than "speaking for" contributions (Mean = 0.63).

Following the spouse's contribution, persons with aphasia either explicitly approved the contribution half the time (Mean = 7.5) or non-explicitly (Mean = 4.75). In other words, it was uncommon for the person with aphasia to either reject a contribution (Mean = 1.63) or exhibit an ambivalent reaction (Mean = 1.25) following the spouse's contribution.

Following a contribution by the spouse, the partner with aphasia generally continued to actively participate in the conversation (Mean = 12.25). However, in a few instances the person with aphasia decreased his/her participation in the conversation. On average, minor participation in the conversation occurred 2.0 times and an equal participation in the conversation occurred 0.75 times. For minor participation, it appears that many of these instances occurred after an unsolicited "speaking for" behaviour on the part of the spouse (Mean = 1.5).

TABLE 2
Types of participation

| | | Speaking for 7.75 (5.0) | | Repairs 7.30 (6.4) | | |
		Unsolicited 7.12 (4.5)	Solicited 0.63 (0.9)	Unsolicited 5.13 (4.9)	Solicited 2.25 (2.3)	Total 15.3 (7.8)
Reaction	Explicit approvals	3.37 (2.4)	0.13 (0.4)	2.62 (2.7)	1.38 (1.7)	7.50 (4.9)
	Non-explicit approvals	2.87 (2.2)	0.13 (0.4)	1.38 (1.3)	0.37 (0.7)	4.75 (3.2)
	Rejects	0.50 (0.8)	0.25 (0.5)	0.50 (1.1)	0.38 (0.5)	1.63 (1.8)
	Ambivalent reactions	0.38 (1.1)	0.12 (0.4)	0.63 (1.4)	0.12 (0.4)	1.25 (1.8)
Participation	Major	5.12 (3.3)	0.38 (0.7)	4.62 (4.9)	2.13 (2.4)	12.25 (7.7)
	Minor	1.50 (1.1)	0.25 (0.5)	0.13 (0.4)	0.12 (0.4)	2.00 (1.3)
	Equal	0.50 (1.1)	___	0.25 (0.5)	___	0.75 (1.0)
	Undetermined	___	___	0.13 (0.4)	___	0.13 (0.4)

Means and standard deviations for the different reactions and types of participation of people with aphasia following solicited or unsolicited "speaking for" behaviours and "repairs" produced by their spouses ($N = 8$).

DISCUSSION

This study incorporated qualitative and quantitative methods in an attempt to simplify the evaluation of complex conversational behaviours in context and to consider both aphasic and non-aphasic spouses. The procedure employed is representative of situations experienced by couples affected by aphasia, i.e., visiting a professional or entertaining a guest at home. Moreover, the data collection and analysis methods could be applicable to clinical situations. In addition, by analysing sequential behaviours, a central notion of Conversation Analysis (CA), the risk of misrepresenting the observations is diminished. The procedure presented could eventually also be useful for measuring differences between couples and for testing therapeutic efficacy. In order to do so, studies of different couples including persons with a variety of types and severity of aphasia should be performed in order to better judge the frequency of behaviours in an individual couple. For example, if "speaking for" behaviours seem to be too frequent and seem to induce little or no participation on the part of the person with aphasia, this behaviour could be targeted and reduced in therapy. Moreover, the satisfactory inter-judge reliability scores obtained suggest that the procedure could be used by trained clinicians. However, a complete analysis of reliability should be performed.

Overall, our results indicate that spouses are active contributors to the interview situation when the person with aphasia has the floor. They contribute on average once a minute in a manner that appears beneficial to the flow of conversation. In general, persons with aphasia approve what their spouse has contributed and frequently continue to participate fully in the conversation after their spouse's contribution. These results indicate that the assistance provided by the spouse was beneficial to the pursuit of the conversation. This is valuable information for empowering couples in therapy.

Almost half the spouses' contributions were "speaking for" behaviours. This argues for the frequency of this type of contribution, yet it has not been the focus of much research to date. Notably, unsolicited "speaking for" contributions were the only behaviours on the part of the spouse that were followed by a decrease in conversational participation by the person with aphasia. This result emphasises the need to pursue studies of this particular conversational behaviour.

Although we observed and described different types of support and repair behaviours in the analysis procedure (see Appendix), they were of insufficient number to report in the present study. However, it may be of interest to note that most frequently spouses offer assistance in word finding and make revisions of the person with aphasia's conversational turns. Further studies with more participants will allow us to confirm this preliminary observation.

Although it is essential to study the person with aphasia in a variety of social situations, it is evident that face-to-face conversations between couples should be investigated, as well as group discussions. The procedure presented here, designed to study the contribution of spouses in an interview, could be adapted to such contexts. Moreover, the partners' individual perceptions of their contributions and participation in conversation should be considered.

In conclusion, the results of this study suggest that an understanding of aphasia and its management requires investigations focusing not just on the person with aphasia but also on his or her partner(s). Because it appears that the partner's assistance influences the person with aphasia's participation in a conversation, the clinical evaluation process should include looking at both partners. Therapy based on this kind of evaluation could help spouses provide the best assistance to their partners with aphasia and better enable both members of the couple to regain or maintain social participation.

REFERENCES

Crockford, C., & Lesser, R. (1994). Assessing functional communication in aphasia: Clinical utility and time demands of three methods. *European Journal of Disorders of Communication, 29,* 55–72.

Croteau, C., & Le Dorze, G. (2006). Overprotection, "speaking for" and conversational participation: A study of couples with aphasia. *Aphasiology, 20,* 327–336.

Croteau, C., Vychytil, A-M., Larfeuil, C., & Le Dorze, G. (2004). "Speaking for" behaviours in spouses of people with aphasia: A descriptive study of six couples in an interview situation. *Aphasiology, 18,* 291–312.

Ferguson, A. (1992). Conversation repair of word-finding difficulty. *Clinical Aphasiology, 21,* 299–310.

Ferguson, A. (1994). The influence of aphasia, familiarity and activity on conversational repair. *Aphasiology, 8,* 143–157.

Ferguson, A. (1998). Conversational turn-taking and repair in fluent aphasia. *Aphasiology, 12,* 1007–1031.

Goodglass, H., & Kaplan, E. (1983) *The assessment of aphasia and related disorders* (2nd ed.). Philadelphia, PA: Lea & Febiger.

Laakso, M., & Klippi, A. (1999). A closer look at "hint and guess" sequences in aphasic conversation. *Aphasiology, 13,* 345–363.

Lindsay, J., & Wilkinson, R. (1999). Repair sequences in aphasic talk: A comparison of aphasic–speech and language therapist and aphasic–spouse conversations. *Aphasiology, 13,* 305–325.

Lubinski, R., Duchan, J., & Weitzner-Lin, B. (1980). Analysis of breakdowns and repairs in aphasic adult communication. In R. Brookshire (Ed.), *Clinical Aphasiology Proceedings* (pp. 111–116). Minneapolis, MN: BRK Publishers.

Manzo, J. F., Blonder, L. X., & Burns, A. F. (1995). The social-interactional organization of narrative and narrating among stroke patients and their spouses. *Sociology of Health and Illness, 17,* 307–327.

Milroy, L., & Perkins, L. (1992). Repair strategies in aphasic discourse: Towards a collaborative model. *Clinical Linguistics & Phonetics, 6,* 27–40.

Nespoulous, J. L., Lecours, A. R., Lafond, D., Lemay, A., Puel, M., Joanette, Y. et al. (1986). *Protocole Montréal-Toulouse: Examen linguistique de l'aphasie (M1 Beta).* Montréal, Québec: Université de Montréal.

Oelschlaeger, M. L. (1999). Participation of a conversation partner in the word searches of a person with aphasia. *American Journal of Speech-Language Pathology, 8,* 62–71.

Oelschlaeger, M. L., & Damico, J. S. (1998). Joint productions as a conversational strategy in aphasia. *Clinical Linguistics and Phonetics, 12,* 459–480.

Oelschlaeger, M. L., & Damico, J. S. (2000). Partnership in conversation: A study of word search strategies. *Journal of Communication Disorders, 33,* 205–225.

Perkins, L., Crisp, J., & Walshaw, D. (1999). Exploring conversation analysis as an assessment tool for aphasia: The issue of reliability. *Aphasiology, 13,* 259–281.

Ramsberger, G., & Rende, B. (2002). Measuring transactional success in the conversation of people with aphasia. *Aphasiology, 16,* 337–353.

Sacks, H., Schegloff, E. A., & Jefferson, G. (1974). A simplest systematics for the organisation of turn-taking in conversation. *Language, 50,* 696–735.

Schegloff, E. A., Jefferson, G., & Sacks, H. (1977). The preference for self-correction in the organisation of repair in conversation. *Language, 53,* 31–382.

Simmons-Mackie, N., Kingston, D., & Schultz, M. (2004). Speaking for another: The management of participant frames in aphasia. *American Journal of Speech-Language Pathology, 13,* 114–128.

Wilkinson, R. (1999). Introduction. *Aphasiology, 13,* 251–258.

Wilkinson, R., Karen, B., Lock, S., Bayley, K., Maxim, J., Bruce, C. et al. (1998). Therapy using conversation analysis: Helping couples adapt to aphasia in conversation. *International Journal of Language & Communication Disorders, 33*(supplement), 144–149.

APPENDIX: ANALYSIS PROCEDURE AND DEFINITIONS

Contributions

In the sections of the interview where a major question was asked to the person with aphasia, and while watching the videos, we identified spousal contributions, defined as a conversational turn of the spouse that occurs when the person with aphasia is clearly speaking to the interviewer. Contributions were classified into three types: "speaking for", repair, and support. Other behaviours that helped maintain the topic of conversation (e.g., approbation) or signalled trouble (e.g., "Pardon me?", "What?") were not considered.

"Speaking for"

Turns where the non-aphasic spouse expresses an opinion or when he/she adds information to the conversation when the person with aphasia has the floor.

Repair behaviours

Efforts made to repair conversational trouble were divided into six subtypes, as follows:

- *Revision.* The spouse reformulates the person with aphasia's verbal or non-verbal turn.
- *Assistance in word finding.* The spouse offers assistance when a word-finding problem occurs. This can take the form of a suggested word or words, phonemic or sentence cueing.
- *Hypothesis verification.* The spouse verifies whether he/she has a good comprehension of what the person with aphasia means by proposing an idea in the form of a question (e.g., "You mean she's taking the files?").
- *Correction.* The spouse corrects what he/she believes is incorrect information.
- *Redirecting to the topic.* The spouse redirects the aphasic person to the topic being discussed.
- *Repair of the interviewer's turn.* The spouse corrects or revises the interviewer's turn.

Support

Assistance to support the person with aphasia to speak, advice on how the person with aphasia should proceed to speak, or reflection on what the person with aphasia is experiencing. Support behaviours were divided into three subtypes:

- *Elicitation of verbal production.* The spouse contributes with a hint, prompt, or question aimed at helping the person with aphasia speak, so that the latter can offer an opinion or qualify his/her statement.
- *Support to continue.* Advice from the spouse on how the person with aphasia should proceed to speak (e.g., "Talk slower.").
- *Acknowledgment of difficulties.* Verbalisations of the spouse as to what the person with aphasia is experiencing (e.g., "She has trouble expressing herself.").

Solicitation

The spouse's contributions were qualified as either previously solicited or not (verbally or non-verbally) by the person with aphasia.

Reaction

The reaction of the person with aphasia to the contribution of his/her spouse in terms of whether or not an explicit physical or verbal response is involved and whether or not the contribution allows the person with aphasia to maintain the topic. Four sub-types of reactions were identified:

- *Explicit approval*. The person with aphasia approves or repeats the spouse's contribution or part of it. Laughing by the aphasic person was considered an explicit approval.
- *Non-explicit approval*. The person with aphasia does not react explicitly to the spouse's contribution. The topic is either maintained or appropriately changed.
- *Rejection*. The person with aphasia overrules the spouse's contribution or makes a comment expressing discomfort (e.g., "Wait a minute!"). An abrupt or inappropriate change in the topic of conversation may occur.
- *Ambivalent reaction*. There is no clear reaction on the part of the person with aphasia and the topic is maintained. The person with aphasia appears ambivalent, the response is insufficient, or she/he appears more or less in agreement with the contribution.

Participation

The participation of the person with aphasia following the spouse's contribution was qualified in comparison to the spouse's participation (major, minor, equal, and undetermined) in the nine turns following the contribution. Contributive turns were calculated to qualify the participation. A turn was contributive if it added information to the outgoing conversation or if it allowed the conversation to be maintained with special emphasis (e.g., pronounced intonation or a strong reaction).

- *Major*. The number of contributive turns by the person with aphasia exceeds the number produced by the spouse.
- *Minor*. The number of contributive turns by the partner with aphasia is fewer than the number produced by the spouse.
- *Equal*. The number of contributive turns by the person with aphasia is equal to the number produced by the spouse.
- *Undetermined*. The number of contributive turns cannot be determined due to a change in conversational topic initiated by the interviewer, or because the interviewer redirects the conversation to the non-aphasic spouse.

APHASIOLOGY, 2007, 21 (6/7/8), 802–813

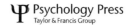

Processing distinct linguistic information types in working memory in aphasia

Heather Harris Wright

Arizona State University, Tempe, AZ, USA

Ryan A. Downey, Michelle Gravier, Tracy Love and Lewis P. Shapiro

San Diego State University, San Diego, CA, USA

Background: Recent investigations have suggested that adults with aphasia present with a working memory deficit that may contribute to their language-processing difficulties. Working memory capacity has been conceptualised as a single "resource" pool for attentional, linguistic, and other executive processing—alternatively, it has been suggested that there may be separate working memory abilities for different types of linguistic information. A challenge in this line of research is developing an appropriate measure of working memory ability in adults with aphasia. One candidate measure of working memory ability that may be appropriate for this population is the *n*-back task. By manipulating stimulus type, the *n*-back task may be appropriate for tapping linguistic-specific working memory abilities.

Aims: The purposes of this study were (a) to measure working memory ability in adults with aphasia for processing specific types of linguistic information, and (b) to examine whether a relationship exists between participants' performance on working memory and auditory comprehension measures.

Method & Procedures: Nine adults with aphasia participated in the study. Participants completed three *n*-back tasks, each tapping different types of linguistic information. They included the *PhonoBack* (phonological level), *SemBack* (semantic level), and *SynBack* (syntactic level). For all tasks, two *n*-back levels were administered: a 1-back and 2-back. Each level contained 20 target items; accuracy was recorded by stimulus presentation software. The *Subject-relative, Object-relative, Active, Passive Test of Syntactic Complexity* (SOAP) was the syntactic sentence comprehension task administered to all participants.

Outcomes & Results: Participants' performance declined as *n*-back task difficulty increased. Overall, participants performed better on the *SemBack* than *PhonoBack* and *SynBack* tasks, but the differences were not statistically significant. Finally, participants who performed poorly on the *SynBack* also had more difficulty comprehending syntactically complex sentence structures (i.e., passive & object-relative sentences).

Conclusions: Results indicate that working memory ability for different types of linguistic information can be measured in adults with aphasia. Further, our results add to the growing literature that favours separate working memory abilities for different types of linguistic information view.

Address correspondence to: Heather Harris Wright PhD, Department of Speech and Hearing Science, Arizona State University, P. O. Box 870102, Tempe, AZ 85287-0102, USA.
E-mail: Heather.Wright.1@asu.edu

© 2007 Psychology Press, an imprint of the Taylor & Francis Group, an informa business
http://www.psypress.com/aphasiology
DOI: 10.1080/02687030701192414

Recent investigations have suggested that adults with aphasia present with a working memory deficit (e.g., Caspari, Parkinson, LaPointe, & Katz, 1998; Downey et al., 2004; Friedmann & Gvion, 2003; Yasuda & Nakamura, 2000), and this deficit may contribute to the language-processing difficulties found in these individuals (Caspari et al., 1998; Friedman & Gvion, 2003; Wright & Shisler, 2005). Working memory capacity has been conceptualised as a single "resource" pool for attentional, linguistic, and other executive processing (e.g., Just & Carpenter, 1992). It has also been suggested that there may be separate working memory abilities for different types of linguistic information (e.g., Caplan & Waters, 1999; Friedmann & Gvion, 2003, 2006). Moreover, individuals with aphasia may exhibit differential difficulty in processing distinct types of linguistic information, such as phonological, semantic, and syntactic (Angrilli, Elbert, Cusumano, Stegagno, & Rockstroh, 2003; Martin, Wu, Freedman, Jackson, & Lesch, 2003; Vallar, Corno, & Basso, 1992; Waters & Caplan, 1996, 1999), which may contribute to their overall difficulties with language. Friedmann and Gvion (2003) suggested that the effect of a verbal working memory deficit on sentence comprehension is dependent on the type of processing (i.e., semantic, syntactic, phonological) required in the sentence.

A challenge in investigating working memory in aphasia is developing an appropriate measure. This has met with mixed success. Historically, adaptations of Daneman and Carpenter's Reading Span test (1980) have been administered to individuals with aphasia in an effort to measure working memory capacity. Such tasks require participants to process multiple types of information (i.e., phonological, semantic, syntactic) simultaneously, while also remembering sentence-final words for later recall or recognition. Not surprisingly, many individuals perform poorly on such tasks (Caspari et al., 1998; Tompkins, Bloise, Timko, & Baumgaertner, 1994; Wright, Newhoff, Downey, & Austermann, 2003). Yet, due to the conflation of distinct linguistic information types involved in such a task, it is impossible to determine where breakdowns occur.

One candidate measure of working memory ability that may be appropriate for this population is the n-back task (the task is described in detail in the Method section). Downey et al. (2004) suggested that an n-back task might be useful in differentiating individuals with aphasia based on working memory ability. To perform the n-back task different cognitive processes are required, including storing n information in working memory and continuously updating contents of working memory by dropping the old, unnecessary information and adding the newly presented information (Jonides, Lauber, Awh, Satoshi, & Koeppe, 1997). This task is commonly used to measure working memory ability in functional neuroimaging studies for several reasons. The task does not require an overt verbal response; participants can respond with a button press. Task difficulty can be increased parametrically by increasing the n back, thus increasing memory load and taxing the participant's working memory system. Also, by including several levels of the n-back (i.e., 0-back, 1-back, 2-back), a baseline task is not needed; rather, comparisons can be made between the different task levels. Finally, by manipulating stimulus type, the n-back task may be appropriate for tapping linguistic-specific working memory abilities. For these reasons, the n-back task may be an appropriate measure of working memory ability in adults with aphasia and differentiating individuals based on linguistic-specific working memory ability.

The present study is a follow-up to the study by Downey and colleagues (2004). In the initial study, we determined if the *n*-back task, using semantically related stimuli, was appropriate to use with adults with aphasia and if a relationship existed between performance on the working memory measure and performance on a syntactic, auditory comprehension measure. Participants' performance declined as *n*-back task difficulty increased, but no relationship was found between performance on the *n*-back and comprehension measures. However, the two tasks tapped different types of linguistic information (i.e., semantic and syntactic). Friedmann and Gvion (2003) hypothesised that to measure the effect of a working memory limitation on sentence comprehension, the type of reactivation required, the memory load, and the working memory limitation all need to be the same (i.e., phonological, syntactic, etc.), and they demonstrated this with adults with conduction aphasia. That is, the participants with conduction aphasia presented with a phonological working memory deficit and struggled when comprehending sentences that required phonological reactivation. Continuing to investigate this tripartite relationship in adults with aphasia by tapping different types of linguistic information is a logical next step to further unravel the relationship between sentence comprehension and working memory. The purposes of the current study, then, were (a) to measure working memory ability in adults with aphasia for processing specific types of linguistic information, and (b) to examine whether a relationship exists between participants' performance on working memory and auditory comprehension measures.

METHOD

Participants

Nine adults with aphasia participated in the study. Participants included one female and nine males, ages 44 to 80 (Mean = 57.3; *SD* = 13.1). Years of education completed ranged from 8 to 20+ (Mean = 14.9, *SD* = 2.2). All participants presented with unilateral left hemisphere damage subsequent to cerebrovascular accident (CVA). Clinical criteria for participation included (a) no more than one stroke located in the left hemisphere, (b) at least 6 months post onset of the stroke, (c) pre-morbid right-handedness, and (d) no history of dementia or other neurological illness. In addition to the previously mentioned inclusion criteria, all participants also met the following criteria: (a) aided or unaided hearing acuity within normal limits; (b) normal or corrected visual acuity; and (c) sufficient dexterity control to make responses using a computer keyboard or button-box. All participants presented with aphasia as confirmed by clinical diagnosis and performance on the *Western Aphasia Battery* (WAB; Kertesz, 1982). Aphasia quotients (AQ) were obtained for each participant who received the WAB. Participants included two adults classified with Broca's aphasia, one with transcortical motor aphasia, one with conduction aphasia, and five with anomic aphasia. Although a more homogeneous group of participants in terms of behavioural presentation and severity of impairment would be preferred, participants were included in the study because they presented with damage in left anterior brain regions. Some also presented with damage extending to posterior regions. Table 1 presents group demographic and clinical description data.

TABLE 1
Clinical and demographic data for participants

Pt[1]	Age	Educ[2]	Sex	m/p CVA[3]	WAB AQ[4]	Aphasia type	Lesion information
1	51	16	M	51	58	Broca's	Left middle cerebral artery (MCA) infarct; upper left temporal & parietal lobes & left basal ganglia
2	62	20+	M	31	81.7	Conduction	Left temporal & frontal lobes; insular region
3	44	17	M	17	68.1	Transcortical-motor	Left basal ganglia & contiguous portions of the subinsular cortex; portions of left frontal & temporoparietal lobes
4	76	12	M	152	48.1	Broca's	Left frontotemporal cerebral infarct
5	47	16	F	104	91.1	Anomic	No data available
6	55	20	M	27	88.6	Anomic	Left MCA
7	45	17	M	56	72.3	Anomic	Left MCA infarct with small intracerebral acute haematoma
8	56	14	M	88	91.9	Anomic	Left frontal cortical region; left basal ganglia
9	80	12	M	62	84.7	Anomic	Superior aspect of left perisylvian region extending to frontoparietal convexity
Mean	57.3	14.9		43	76.1		

[1]patient; [2]years of education completed; [3]months post cerebrovascular accident; [4]Western Aphasia Battery Aphasia Quotient.

Stimuli and tasks

N-*back tasks.* We developed three *n*-back tasks, each tapping different types of linguistic information. They included the *PhonoBack*, which tapped the phonological level, *SemBack*, tapping the semantic level, and *SynBack*, which tapped the syntactic level. For all tasks, two *n*-back levels were administered: a 1-back and 2-back, each containing 20 target items used for determining performance. All 1-back tasks comprised four blocks: one practice block of 10 items containing 2 targets; a second practice block of 12 items, with 3 targets; a third block of 32 items with 10 targets; and a fourth block of 33 items with 10 targets. All 2-back tasks similarly consisted of four blocks: 10 practice with 2 targets; 15 practice with 3 targets; 37 experimental with 10 targets; and 39 experimental with 10 targets. Thus, the percentages of tokens that were targets in the 1-back and 2-back were 31% and 27%, respectively. These percentages were selected to be consistent with *n*-back tasks in the literature while also falling within the ability level of the participants, to keep the tasks from being frustratingly long. The 1-back level required a response when the current token was the same as the one immediately preceding it (e.g., apple…peach…*peach*…). For the 2-back level, participants responded to any token that was identical to the item appearing two tokens prior (e.g., plum…apple…*plum*…).

The *PhonoBack* stimuli consisted of 25 CVC words, five ending in each of five frames: -at, -it, -in, -ill, and -ig. The *SemBack* stimuli consisted of five words from each of five different semantic categories: fruits, tools, furniture, animals, and clothing. Stimuli were controlled across categories for length and frequency of occurrence. The *SynBack* stimuli included five-word sentences with either active ("The doctor kissed the banker") or passive ("The banker was kissed by the doctor") sentence structures. Ten nouns and ten verbs were used; length, frequency of occurrence, and role (object/subject) were controlled. See Table 2 for stimuli used in the different *n*-back tasks.

Each *n*-back task also consisted of two levels of processing—identity and depth. For identity versions, targets were identical to prime items presented *n* back. For all tasks, instructions were as follows: "*Push the button when the word (sentence) you just heard is the same as the one [n] back.*" Only depth versions of the *PhonoBack* and *SemBack* were administered. We anticipated that the depth version of the *SynBack* would be too challenging for this population, thus it was not administered. For the *PhonoBack* depth, participants responded when target items rhymed with the prime presented *n* back (e.g., cat – rat). For the *SemBack* depth, participants responded when target items matched the category of the prime presented *n* back (e.g., grapes – lime).

SOAP. Love and Oster (2002) developed the *Subject-relative, Object-relative, Active, Passive Test of Syntactic Complexity* (SOAP), and have demonstrated its validity and sensitivity for certain comprehension abilities in brain-damaged populations, as well as its ability to differentiate between subgroups of aphasia. Briefly, the SOAP requires participants to listen to a sentence produced by the experimenter and then point to the one picture, among two foils, that corresponds to the sentence. The test sentences conform to the following syntactic structures and are processed with differential success, depending on each aphasic individual's comprehension deficits: subject-relative, object-relative, active, and passive. Because it contains 10 trial sentences from each of the four syntactic structures, the SOAP provides a sensitive and selective profile of an individual's comprehension ability across a range of processing difficulty.

Experimental procedures

Assessment was completed prior to the experimental sessions. During the assessment phase, informed consent was obtained, the WAB was administered, and vision and hearing screenings were conducted. For the experimental study, each participant attended three sessions in a sound-insulated room. All participants received all 11 *n*-back conditions and the SOAP. The *PhonoBack* and *SemBack* identity versions were

TABLE 2
Stimuli for *PhonBack*, *SemBack*, and *SynBack* tasks

***PhonoBack* words**		
-at: bat, hat, rat, pat, mat[1]	-in: pin, fin, bin, tin, kin	-ill: till, hill, pill, sill, gill
-ap: tap, cap, map, nap, sap	-ig: wig, rig, jig, pig, fig	
***SemBack* words**		
Animals: wolf, cat, snake, bird, rabbit		Tools: hammer, drill, pliers, hatchet, axe
Furniture: chair, desk, dresser, couch, stool		Fruit: apple, orange, lemon, grape, lime[2]
Clothes: shirt, hat, jacket, blouse, pants		
***SynBack* words**		
Verbs: pushed, called, punched, kicked, thanked, blamed, teased, kissed chased, hugged[3]		
Noun phrases: actor, golfer, doctor, banker, singer, teacher, lawyer, baker, jogger, mayor[4]		

[1]only words used in *PhonoBack* Identity tasks; [2]only words used in *SemBack* Identity tasks; [3]all verbs used in passive and active tenses; [4]all noun phrases used as subjects and objects.

completed in the first session and the depth versions completed in the second session. Presentation order for the *PhonoBack* and *SemBack* was counterbalanced across participants and sessions. During the third session, the *SynBack* and SOAP were administered; presentation order was counterbalanced across participants. Participants were given ample time to respond during the SOAP; the *n*-back tasks were internally time-driven by a 4000-ms stimulus onset asynchrony (SOA) regardless of stimulus length.

Practice items for the *n*-back tasks were administered to ensure that participants understood the instructions and were comfortable performing the tasks. Participants completed practice items on the computer identical to the experimental *n*-back tasks. To reduce any chance of task perseveration from one condition to the next, task training and practice preceded each condition. The participant was instructed to press a button on a button response box when the item heard matched the item *n* items back.

Stimuli were played through computer speakers or headphones at a volume comfortable for each participant. Accuracy and response times (RT) were recorded by stimulus presentation software with millisecond precision. Because participants were not specifically instructed to respond with any rapidity—only "quickly, as another item will be coming up soon"—RTs are not viewed here as an index of processing time and were not subjected to further analysis. Administration and scoring of the SOAP were performed according to the procedures developed and standardised by Love and Oster (2002).

RESULTS

N-back

To compare accuracy performance across levels of processing for the different *n*-back tasks, the *SynBack* data were not included because participants did not complete *SynBack* depth tasks. A repeated measures analysis of variance (ANOVA) of information type (phonological, semantic) by level of processing (Identity, Depth) by *n*-back level (1-back, 2-back) was performed. The main effect for information type was significant, $F(1, 8) = 5.40$, $p < .05$, as were the main effects for level of processing, $F(1, 8) = 12.89$, $p < .01$, and *n*-back level, $F(1, 8) = 75.57$, $p < .0001$. Participants were more accurate on the *SemBack* task compared to the *PhonoBack*. Participants also were more accurate at the identity level than depth level and on the 1-back compared to the 2-back. The interactions were not significant. To compare participants' accuracy performance across the different *n*-back tasks a repeated measures ANOVA of information type (phonological, semantic, syntactic) by *n*-back level was performed. Significant main effects were found for information type, $F(2, 16) = 13.54$, $p < .001$, and *n*-back level, $F(1, 8) = 30.00$, $p < .001$. Planned comparisons were performed. Although participants' accuracy scores were better during *SemBack* tasks compared to *PhonoBack* and *SynBack* tasks, no significant findings emerged when controlling for family-wise error using an adjusted *p* of .0167 (.05/3).

Finally, we inspected individual participant's performances on the *n*-back tasks to determine if individual patterns were consistent with that of the group. Generally, all participants performed better on the 1-back tasks when compared to the corresponding 2-back tasks. When inspecting individual data within and among the different linguistic information versions some inconsistencies with group performance were found. For the *PhonoBack*, two participants performed appreciably better on the depth version compared to the identity version (i.e., P7 for 2-back, P8 for 1-back). When comparing across the tasks, one participant performed worse on the *SemBack* compared to the *PhonoBack* (i.e., P7 for depth tasks). In all other instances, individual patterns were comparable to that of the group. See Figures 1–3 for participants' accuracy performance on the *n*-back tasks.

SOAP

The SOAP was administered to assess participants' auditory comprehension for four syntactic structures. Participants' performance on the SOAP was grouped according to sentence canonicity and then subjected to statistical analysis. Using a paired sample *t*-test, participants comprehended the canonical sentences (i.e., active, subject-relative) significantly better than the non-canonical sentences (i.e., passive, object-relative), $t(9) = 2.90$, $p < .05$ (see Figure 4).

Relationship between working memory and language comprehension

Friedmann and Gvion (2003) hypothesised that a verbal working memory deficit affects sentence comprehension when the type of processing required is the same for both. The sentence comprehension task (i.e., SOAP) required processing syntactic information, thus it would be expected that participants who performed poorly on the *SynBack* would also perform poorly on the more complex sentence forms (i.e., non-canonical sentences) of the SOAP. Kendall's Tau correlation, corrected for ties, was computed to determine the probability that participants' performance on the

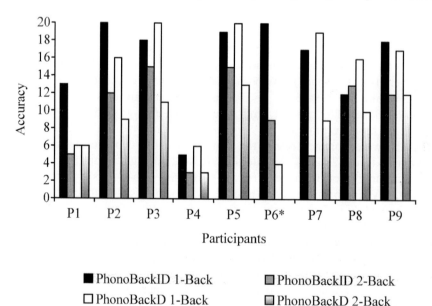

*P6 completed PhonoBackD 2-Back but missed all targets during the task

Figure 1. Participants' accuracy on the *PhonoBack* tasks.

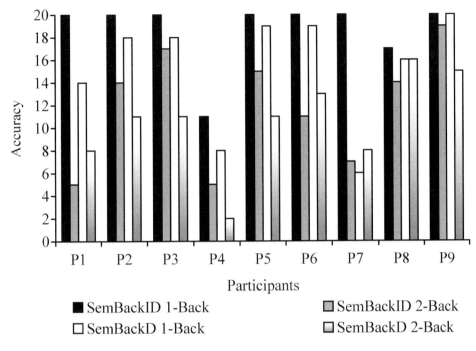

Figure 2. Participants' accuracy on the *SemBack* tasks.

SynBack 2-back identity task was similar to their performance on the SOAP non-canonical sentence forms. The non-parametric statistical analysis was performed because homogeneity of variance could not be assumed. Results indicated a significant relationship between participants' performances on the *SynBack* 2-back and the SOAP non-canonical sentences, tau = .67, $p < .05$.

We also inspected individual patterns. Four participants (P1, P2, P4, P6) missed more than 50% of the targets on the *SynBack* 2-back task. These participants also evinced lower scores on the non-canonical sentences compared to the canonical sentences. Other participants (P3, P5, P8, P9), who differed by less than 10% in accuracy between canonical and non-canonical sentences on the SOAP and performed well on the SOAP, yielded higher hit rates on the *SynBack* task. One participant did not fit either grouping; P7 performed poorly on the *SynBack* but demonstrated a stable performance across all sentence forms on the SOAP (see Figures 3 and 4).

DISCUSSION

The primary goals of this study were to measure working memory ability for processing specific types of linguistic information and to identify whether a relationship existed between working memory ability and auditory comprehension of different syntactic structures in adults with aphasia. Participants' performance declined as *n*-back task difficulty increased. Further, participants performed more poorly on the depth versions of the *PhonoBack* and *SemBack* compared to the identity versions. Although participants overall performed better on the *SemBack* than *PhonoBack* and *SynBack* tasks, the differences were not statistically significant.

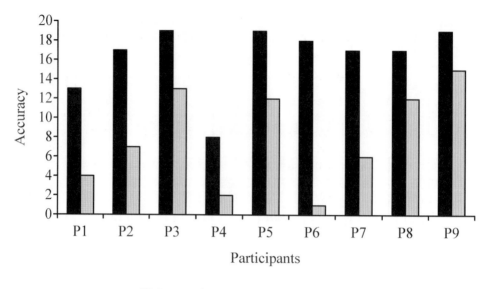

Figure 3. Participants' accuracy on the *SynBack* tasks.

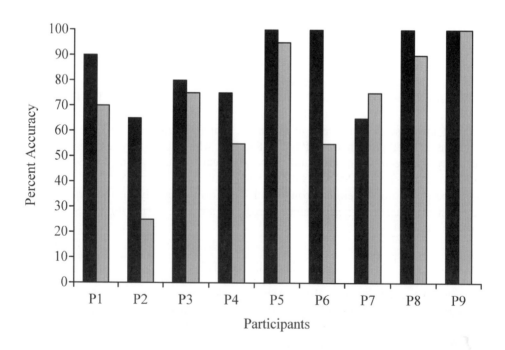

Figure 4. Participants' percent accuracy on the Subject-relative, Object-relative, Active, Passive Test of Syntactic Complexity (SOAP; Love & Oster, 2002).

Finally, participants' performance on the *SynBack* 2-back task significantly correlated with their performance on the SOAP non-canonical sentence forms.

Working memory performance

The participants were able to perform the working memory tasks, supporting our previous work (Downey et al., 2004) that the tasks are appropriate for measuring working memory ability in adults with aphasia. As expected, the participants with aphasia performed similarly to participants without neurological impairment (Jonides et al., 1997; Yoo, Paralkar, & Panych, 2004), with traumatic brain injury (Levin et al., 2004), and with schizophrenia (Callicott et al., 2000) in previous studies using an *n*-back task; that is, participants' accuracy declined as the *n*-back increased.

   Previous *n*-back studies have manipulated stimulus type to tap different types of working memory, such as spatial, visual, auditory, and verbal (e.g., Hinkin et al., 2002; Kubat-Silman, Dagenbach, & Absher, 2002; McEvoy, Smith, & Gevins, 1998). No known study to date has manipulated *n*-back stimuli to tap different types of linguistic information as we did. Many of the participants' performances differed across the *n*-back tasks. For example, some participants (P1, P2, P4, P6) had better hit rates on the *SemBack* tasks compared to the *PhonoBack* and *SynBack* tasks, suggesting that these individuals with aphasia demonstrate differential difficulty in processing distinct types of linguistic information. That is, they had more difficulty processing phonological and syntactic information versus lexico-semantic. Belleville, Caza, and Peretz (2003) found that individuals with anterior lesions present with structural (i.e., phonological, syntactic) deficits and a relative strength in processing lexico-semantic information. Although our participants who demonstrated this differential performance did present with anterior damage at the cortical and/or subcortical level, other participants who performed similarly across the three *n*-back tasks also presented with anterior damage. Further, many of the participants presented with damage in both anterior and posterior brain regions. At this point, our results do not support any hypotheses regarding the relationship between lesion location and processing of different types of linguistic information.

Sentence comprehension and WM

Our results add to previous findings indicating that individuals with aphasia may exhibit differential difficulty in processing distinct types of linguistic information, such as phonological, semantic, and syntactic (Angrilli et al., 2003; Martin et al., 2003; Vallar et al., 1992; Waters & Caplan, 1996, 1999), which may contribute to their overall difficulties with language. Friedmann and Gvion (2003, 2006) demonstrated that individuals with conduction aphasia presenting with a phonological working memory deficit struggle when comprehending sentences that require phonological reactivation, yet have minimal difficulty comprehending syntactically complex sentences. Thus, demonstrating that a linguistic-specific working memory deficit does affect sentence comprehension when that specific type of processing (i.e., semantic, syntactic, phonological) is required. We found similar results with a different type of linguistic process—syntactic. The participants who demonstrated a syntactic working memory deficit had the most difficulty comprehending syntactically complex sentences.

Although all participants demonstrated a decline in accuracy as the *n*-back task increased in difficulty, four participants' working memory for syntactic information was severely stressed as the *SynBack* level increased. These participants' performance on the sentence comprehension task also deteriorated as task difficulty increased; that is, comprehending non-canonical sentence forms compared to canonical sentence forms. Further, those participants who performed better on the *SynBack* overall and had a smaller decline in performance from the 1-back to 2-back on the *SynBack* did not have any trouble comprehending the more syntactically complex sentences. The one exception, P7, demonstrated poor performance on all 2-back tasks as well as both *SemBack* Depth tasks (i.e., 1-back and 2-back) suggesting that he may have a more "overarching" working memory deficit.

Conclusions and future directions

Results of this preliminary study investigating working memory ability and its relationship with sentence comprehension ability in aphasia are promising. First, we demonstrated that working memory ability for different types of linguistic information can be measured in adults with aphasia. Further, it had been hypothesised that a syntactic working memory deficit may contribute to the syntactic comprehension deficit found in some individuals with aphasia. However, prior to this study this hypothesis had not been tested and no measure of working memory ability for syntactic information had been proposed. Although these results are preliminary they add to the growing literature that favours the separate working memory abilities for different types of linguistic information view. To further evaluate the relationship between working memory and language comprehension, the next step in this line of research is to include sentence comprehension tasks that require different types of processing as well as working memory tasks for different types of linguistic information, and to include adults with aphasia with distinct lesion sites (i.e., anterior vs posterior).

REFERENCES

Angrilli, A., Elbert, T., Cusumano, S., Stegagno, L., & Rockstroh, B. (2003). Temporal dynamics of linguistic processes are reorganised in aphasics' cortex: An EEG mapping study. *Neuroimage, 20,* 657–666.

Belleville, S., Caza, N., & Peretz, I. (2003). A neuropsychological argument for a processing view of memory. *Journal of Memory and Language, 48,* 686–703.

Callicott, J., Bertolino, A., Mattay, V., Langheim, F. J. P., Duyn, J., & Coppola, R. et al. (2000). Physiological dysfunction of the dorsolateral prefrontal cortex in schizophrenia revisited. *Cerebral Cortex, 10,* 1078–1092.

Caplan, D., & Waters, G. (1999). Verbal working memory capacity and language comprehension. *Behavioral Brain Sciences, 22,* 114–126.

Caspari, I., Parkinson, S., LaPointe, L., & Katz, R. (1998). Working memory and aphasia. *Brain and Cognition, 37,* 205–223.

Daneman, M., & Carpenter, P. A. (1980). Individual differences in working memory and reading. *Journal of Verbal Learning and Verbal Behavior, 19,* 450–466.

Downey, R. A., Wright, H. H., Schwartz, R. G., Newhoff, M., Love, T., & Shapiro, L. P. (2004). *Toward a measure of working memory in aphasia.* Poster presented at Clinical Aphasiology Conference, Park City, UT, USA.

Friedmann, N., & Gvion, A. (2003). Sentence comprehension and working memory limitation in aphasia: A dissociation between semantic-syntactic and phonological reactivation. *Brain and Language, 86*, 23–39.

Friedmann, N., & Gvion, A. (2006). *Is there a relationship between working memory limitation and sentence comprehension? A study of conduction and agrammatic aphasia.* Technical session presented at Clinical Aphasiology Conference, Ghent, Belgium.

Hinkin, C. H., Hardy, D. J., Mason, K. I., Castellon, S. A., Lam, M. N., & Stefaniak, M. et al. (2002). Verbal and spatial working memory performance among HIV-infected adults. *Journal of the International Neuropsychological Society, 8*, 532–538.

Jonides, J., Lauber, E. J., Awh, E., Satoshi, M., & Koeppe, R. A. (1997). Verbal working memory load affects regional brain activation as measured by PET. *Journal of Cognitive Neuroscience, 9*(4), 462–475.

Just, M. A., & Carpenter, P. A. (1992). A capacity theory of comprehension: Individual differences in working. *Psychological Review, 99*, 122–149.

Kertesz, A. (1982). *Western Aphasia Battery*. New York: Grune & Stratton.

Kubat-Silman, A. K., Dagenbach, D., & Absher, J. R. (2002). Patterns of impaired verbal, spatial, and object working memory after thalamic lesions. *Brain and Cognition, 50*, 178–193.

Levin, H. S., Hanten, G., Zhang, L., Swank, P. R., Ewing, C. L., & Dennis, M. et al. (2004). Changes in working memory after traumatic brain injury in children. *Neuropsychology, 18*, 240–247.

Love, T., & Oster, E. (2002). On the categorization of Aphasic typologies: The S.O.A.P, a test of syntactic complexity. *Journal of Psycholinguistic Research, 31*, 503–529.

Martin, R. C., Wu, D., Freedman, M., Jackson, E. F., & Lesch, M. (2003). An event-related fMRI investigation of phonological versus semantic short-term memory. *Journal of Neurolinguistics, 16*(4–5), 341–360.

McEvoy, L., Smith, M., & Gevins, A. (1998). Dynamic cortical networks of verbal and spatial working memory: Effects of memory load and task practice. *Cerebral Cortex, 8*, 563–574.

Tompkins, C. A., Bloise, C. G. R., Timko, M. L., & Baumagaertner, A. (1994). Working memory and inference revision in brain-damaged and normally aging adults. *Journal of Speech and Hearing Research, 37*, 896–912.

Vallar, G., Corno, M., & Basso, A. (1992). Auditory and visual verbal short-term memory in aphasia. *Cortex, 28*, 383–389.

Waters, G., & Caplan, D. (1996). The measurement of verbal working memory capacity and its relation to reading comprehension. *The Quarterly Journal of Experimental Psychology, 49*A(1), 51–79.

Waters, G., & Caplan, D. (1999). Verbal working memory capacity and on-line sentence processing efficiency in the elderly. In S. Kepmer & R. Kliegle (Eds.), *Constraints on language: Aging, grammar and memory* (pp. 107–136). Boston, MA: Kluwer.

Wright, H. H., Newhoff, M., Downey, R., & Austermann, S. (2003). Additional data on working memory in aphasia. *Journal of International Neuropsychological Society, 9*(2), 302.

Wright, H. H., & Shisler, R. (2005). Working memory in aphasia: Theory, measures, and clinical implications. *American Journal of Speech-Language Pathology, 14*, 107–118.

Yasuda, K., & Nakamura, T. (2000). Comprehension and storage of four serially presented radio news stories by mild aphasic subjects. *Brain and Language, 75*, 399–415.

Yoo, S-S., Paralkar, G., & Panych, L. P. (2004). Neural substrates associated with the concurrent performance of dual working memory tasks. *International Journal of Neuroscience, 114*, 613–631.

APHASIOLOGY, 2007, 21 (6/7/8), 814–828

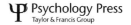

Executive dysfunction as an explanatory basis for conversation symptoms of aphasia: A pilot study

Tali Frankel, Claire Penn, and Digby Ormond-Brown

University of the Witwatersrand, Johannesburg, South Africa

Background: Lack of communicative success for people with aphasia is no longer seen as purely a linguistic deficit. Instead, the integrity of the executive functions (EF) is thought to be at least partly responsible for successful communication, particularly during conversation. In order to inform clinicians regarding both conversation and EF, a merging of two paradigms—conversational and neuropsychological approaches—is proposed.

Aims: First, we explore the relevance of both neuropsychological and conversational approaches to the assessment of aphasia. Second, we present the executive battery that was designed and administered to a single participant (MS) to assess various aspects of EF. The results of a Conversation Analysis (CA) undertaken on an excerpt of MS's conversation are given. Results of the EF analysis are presented with the CA in order to highlight proposed relationships that may impact on conversational strengths and difficulties.

Methods and Procedures: The executive battery was designed to assess the following constructs: attention, verbal and nonverbal working memory, memory, planning, generation, and concept formation. The participant was video-recorded in conversation with a familiar interlocutor. Transcriptions were derived and subjected to Conversation Analysis. A discussion of conversational features is presented in conjunction with results from the executive battery.

Outcomes and Results: Several areas including simple sustained attention, interference control, memory, and planning appeared to be preserved. This profile occurred together with the ability to maintain concentration and track meaning during interactions with one interlocutor. Memory for previously stated information was preserved as well as the ability to think and plan ahead. These strengths also co-occurred with intact turn taking and topic management. However MS's performance also indicated difficulty with shifting attention, verbal and nonverbal working memory, generation, and concept formation. The latter two especially appeared to be mediated by the effects of perseveration, which resulted from a reduced ability to shift focus. In terms of conversation, MS reported difficulty in multi-party settings. In addition, conversational repair was affected by poor generation and selection of strategies as well as an inability to shift away from current ineffectual forms of expression to more effective, flexible, and potentially successful forms of communication.

Conclusions: The notion of merging two distinct and historically separate paradigms presents unique and valuable opportunities for creative and effective treatment of individuals with aphasia who have reached plateaus or who, as in this case, present with relatively intact linguistic skills on formal testing but experience daily frustration during conversation.

Address correspondence to: Tali Frankel, School of Human and Community Development, University of the Witwatersrand, Private Bag 3, Wits 2050, Johannesburg, South Africa.
E-mail: tdfranky@absamail.co.za

This paper was presented at the Clinical Aphasiology Conference, Ghent, Belgium, May 2006.

---

http://www.psypress.com/aphasiology   DOI: 10.1080/02687030701192448

In this paper we explore the notion that communicative success for people with aphasia depends, at least in part, on the integrity of the executive functions (EF). This is achieved with reference to a case study by examining the conversation of MS, a person with aphasia, in relation to her executive profile as derived from a battery designed to test relevant EF.

This preliminary study proposes the merging of two paradigms to aphasia that up to now have been largely distant in terms of theory and application. The first paradigm—a conversational one—has been largely seen as focusing on the strengths of the individual, and approaches to therapy are geared towards building these strengths and enhancing social interaction. The other paradigm that originates from a neuropsychological approach is based on revealing the nature and extent of deficit through formal testing and assessing the explanatory basis of symptoms.

EXECUTIVE FUNCTIONS

Executive functions (EF) have been described as a collection of high-level, interconnected control processes that allow us to generate, choose, organise, and regulate goal-directed, adaptive, and non-automatic behaviours. They include "working memory, self-monitoring and self-regulating, inhibiting irrelevant stimuli, shifting between concepts or actions, generation and application of strategies, temporal integration and integrating multimodal inputs from throughout the brain" (Keil & Kaszniak, 2002, p. 306).

Primarily, EF is thought to rely on neural activity in the frontal and prefrontal cortex (PFC) and its connections to the sub-cortex. In addition to the important anatomical connections thought to support EF, the PFC shares a variety of neurotransmitter substances, associations that are also important for cortical transactions related to motor functions. These associations are additionally suggestive of the PFC's role in higher integrative functions subserving the organisation of behaviour (Fuster, 1989).

Deficits of executive function have been proposed as all or part of the underlying mechanisms of language impairment in at least some types of aphasia. A body of recent research suggests for example that deficits in attentional capacity, working memory, divided attention, cognitive effort, or intention may be implicated as potential contributors to the communication problems in aphasia (Coelho, 2005; Crosson et al., 2005; McNeil et al., 2004).

The link between deficient executive function and difficulty with social communication was found in Purdy's (2002) study of 15 individuals with aphasia. Her research demonstrated that despite an ability to learn communicative techniques, patients switched techniques only 41% of the time after their initial communication attempt failed. Those who switched were successful 67% of the time. Her participants often persisted in using verbal means, without recognising that nonverbal means provided a better opportunity for communication. She hypothesised that individuals with aphasia "lack the ability to initiate, plan, monitor and correct their communicative performance and thus are unable to use their available verbal and nonverbal abilities to achieve their goals" (Purdy, 2002, p. 5).

Miyake, Emerson, and Friedman (2000) similarly found that aphasic individuals who had been rated as good communicators coped well with dual task demands without showing performance decrement, whereas people who had been rated as poor communicators showed marked deterioration on dual task performance. This observation was apparent despite comparable results on formal language tests for both groups. Miyake et al. (2000) concluded that differences in aphasic patients' communicative success may be related to their abilities to perform certain tasks designed to capture aspects of executive functioning.

CONVERSATION

The above findings suggest the need for more ecologically valid forms of communicative assessment. A common phenomenon especially in mild aphasia is that formal language test results often belie the extent of the difficulty experienced in conversational settings. There is a strong possibility that linguistic tasks used in current research may not sufficiently stress skills to a degree that they produce changes in function. As Oelschlaeger and Damico (2003) suggest, "we need to employ other assumptions about language and conversation and we need to use more authentic research stances if we are to understand the pragmatic life of brain-damaged patients" (p. 211). We propose that deficits in EF can account for some of these conversational difficulties because conversation represents a complex integration of processes such as planning, sequencing, organisation, and monitoring during novel activity. These functions, along with generating, selecting, and applying strategies, have been classified as executive in nature and are frequently disrupted in individuals with frontal lobe damage (Rende, 2000). Further, the availability of such organisational, planning, and learning processes has been shown to be associated with faster recovery (Bailey, Powell, & Clark, 1981). The ultimate goal of any speech-language intervention is to harness these learning processes to improve communication in everyday settings, where unpredictable demands and fluctuating conditions require goal-oriented behaviour and flexible problem solving (Helm-Estabrooks, 2002).

A further benefit of studying conversation is that certain grammatical behaviours that have previously been interpreted as direct symptoms of an underlying linguistic deficit may actually arise from the interactional context in which they are produced (Beeke, Wilkinson, & Maxim, 2003). Grammatical structures allow the listener to anticipate pragmatic, structural, and linguistic sequences. The ability to analyse the communicative environment to which the aphasic individual needs to adapt through conversation, allows an in-depth assessment of the structure of the interaction, providing insight into the individual's conversational flexibility in real-time and real-life settings—essentially a reflection of novel and complex adaptive behaviours—the domain of executive functioning (Penn, 2000). The goal of the present study is thus to explore the interface between conversational performance and executive functioning in a single individual.

CASE STUDY

Case description

MS is a 58-year-old woman, a qualified teacher of Art and English with additional degrees in business management and counselling, who suffered a stroke 5 years ago. Both CT and MRI scans confirmed an infarct of the left fronto-parietal lobe corresponding to the distribution of the left middle cerebral artery territory. No other associated intracerebral or subarachnoid components were identified. Administration of the Western Aphasia Battery (WAB) (Kertesz, 1982) yielded an aphasia quotient of 93.4 and a cognitive quotient of 90.25.

Conversational characteristics

MS was video-recorded during conversation with the first author as well as with a friend (A). Data collection complied with guidelines stipulated by Conversation Analysis practice (Ten Have, 1999). Recordings were each 30 minutes long, and extracts of 10 minutes taken from the middle portion of the interactions were used for transcription and analysis. Appendix A provides the key for the transcription symbols. Turn taking, topic management, and repair sequences were assessed as these have been acknowledged to form the basic tenets of conversational ability and are likely to set the context for more micro-level behaviours (Lesser & Milroy, 1993). Characteristics of MS's conversation revealed the presence of a mild non-fluent aphasia with agrammatism and significant word-finding difficulty. Specific examples of MS's turn-taking, topic management, and repair skills are demonstrated later in the text.

Turn taking. Analysis revealed that MS and her interlocutors, A and T, experienced even turn distribution. Furthermore, MS's turns were often of equal length and content to that of her interlocutors', although some of her turns were much longer to accommodate self-repairs, revisions, and multiple attempts at a single utterance. Finally, MS managed the split-second handovers whereby one speaker finishes a turn and either selects the next speaker or the next speaker self-selects for the next turn at talk. MS was able to respond to being selected as well as being able to self-select when appropriate.

Topic management. MS's skills were intact in terms of topic initiation, maintenance, shift, and bias. In the interchange with interlocutor A, two main topics were raised, the first relating to whether or not MS should entertain a friend at tea time without A (MS initiated this topic), and the second topic relating extensively to a minor procedure A was undergoing the following day (which A initiated). MS showed considerable skill in terms of maintaining the second topic for the majority of the conversation, while contributing successfully to topic shift by asking a variety of questions and making comments related to the main topic.

Repair. The repair of conversational breakdown afforded the main area of difficulty for MS. The two transcripts captured eight instances of repair. Only one of these was other initiated (i.e., initiated by A), while the others were all initiated by MS herself as an attempt to revise her own messages. This may indicate the effectiveness of her communication in most instances despite the fact that she expresses frustration with her lack of ability to speak fluently. She frequently engaged in self-initiated self-repair whereby she interrupted her own utterance within the same turn by cutting off a word or phrase and attempting to correct herself. She was also able to respond to other-initiated self-repair (where she repaired a trouble spot, to which attention was drawn by her interlocutor A).

Executive functions

A battery of tests was used to test MS's executive functions. The design of this battery took into account the particular challenges involved in assessing EF due to her aphasia. These include the fact that many EF tests have verbal and other language requirements, which may be inaccessible unless suitably modified. EF tests also place non-routine demands on the person taking the test. In order to increase test sensitivity it is necessary to administer more complex tasks to highlight deficits that are not apparent when testing simpler cognitive functions. However, this makes it increasingly difficult to differentiate cognitive processes and speaks for the need to administer control tasks to rule out confounding variables, such as neglect (Keil & Kaszniak, 2002). A range of cognitive, sensory, motoric, perceptual, and demographic variables that may influence test performance and tasks that require drawing or writing may have to be adapted, particularly for individuals who will have to use their non-dominant hand to comply (Riepe, Riss, Bittner, & Huber, 2004). Finally EF tests rely heavily on the amount of time taken to complete, and accommodations may need to be made for individuals with slowed processing or motor output.

In this particular study, tasks were chosen for their specificity in terms of their ability to measure a particular construct. In addition, tasks were chosen for their lack of reliance on complicated verbal explanations in favour of those whose requirements could be simply explained and demonstrated. Comprehension of the test requirements was further ensured by having MS repeat the instructions before testing.

Her performance on the constructional and visuospatial components of the WAB served as control tasks. In addition, MS was able to repeat digits, read individual letters, numbers, and words, and recognise and name colours, as well as show good performance on the reading and comprehension sub-tests of the WAB. MS was assessed over two testing sessions, a week apart. Her profile will be discussed with reference to each specific function and how proposed deficits or strengths linked to conversational performance as characterised by CA. The constructs assessed, tests used for assessment, adaptations made, and MS's results are presented in Appendix B.

Identifying parallels in EF and conversational assessments

Preserved areas of EF and cognition and conversation parallels

MS showed preserved functions for sustained attention, suppression (interference control), memory, and planning—incorporating scheduling/strategy use/rule adherence. This co-occurred with preserved topic management and turn-taking skills in the one to setting.

Simple sustained attention. Previous research has identified deficits in sustained attention in individuals with aphasia resulting from left-hemisphere lesions. Furthermore, problems with sustained attention have been hypothesised to account for auditory comprehension deficits (Helm-Estabrooks, Tabor-Connor, & Albert, 2000). As is evident from her scores, MS did not suffer from simple attention difficulties. However, she reported difficulty with group interactions, during which she found it difficult to track and comprehend interactions. Group interactions draw on different attentional skills, including divided and shifting attention (Schapiro & Sacchetti, 1993) as well as verbal working memory skills, and will be discussed below. Her ability to keep track of conversation with a single interlocutor is depicted in Example 1. MS frequently makes use of back channel responses such as "OK" in turn 2 and "Oh ok" in turn 7, indicating that she is following the conversation and is providing evidence of this. She also repeats A's phrases (turn 9) and makes meaningful contributions (turn 13) indicating that she has remained attentive to what A has been saying.

Example 1
1.   A: The sister came in this morning
2.   MS: OK
3.   (2)
4.   A: and (.) she had a look at the pamphlet
5.   MS: What pamphlet? Oh! (.) the pamphlet
6.   A: Ja and (.) no (.) solids the whole day
7.   MS: Oh ok
8.   A: No solids only (1) liquids and only clear liquids
9.   MS: Only clear liquids?
10.   A: Only clear liquids
11.   MS: So you-
12.   A: (.) Nothing solid
13.   MS: So you might have fruit juices
14.   (2)
15.   A: I might I can have plain fruit juice like apple juice

Complex attention (suppression/interference control). Although poor scores on the Stroop Colour Word Test are generally indicative of brain damage and slowed rate of information processing, the interference score itself is of the most interest as this indicates the integrity of the ability to ward off distractions. MS's scores would seem to further corroborate good sustained attention scores, with the ability to resist distraction while simultaneously pointing to other complex attention deficits, based on her generally slow response times (Golden, 1978). During conversation, sustained attention and resistance to distractions (interference control) have been associated with the ability to be generally attentive, comprehend on-line discourse, and maintain topics during conversation (Frankel & Penn, in press). Analysis of MS's conversational skills confirms her ability in all these areas in a one-to-one speaking situation. In Example 2, MS promptly takes her turn and handles the split-second timing of handovers promptly and efficiently without delays (turns 104, 106, and 110). The distribution of turns is equal, and there is no evidence of overlap or interruption, suggesting that at this point MS is able to claim and hold the floor during this conversation. She is further able to stay on topic and contributes meaningfully.

Example 2
103. A: And if I miss supper over here I've got something I've got (3) I've got
        Provita. I've got cheese
104. MS: OK
105. A: I've got
106. MS: No well if you miss supper by being over there then she is supper um not
        miss no then there is supper um I think that u- uhm nurses will get you
        supper
107.   (5)
108. MS: Um the nurses will get you SUPPER
109. A: Well I think (2) uh I'll go down (2) lunchtime and speak to Nicky and
        explain the position to her. Maybe she can do- Maybe she'll do something.
110. MS: Yes yes fantastic

Memory. Long-term memory deficits among aphasic persons for both verbal and nonverbal information have previously been identified. Amnestic conditions of differing severity may impact on conversational performance in a number of ways. An individual may simply not remember previous encounters or information presented in the past by themselves or others. This may cause them to repeat already stated information or to request clarification regarding something that their interlocutor may assume they would have remembered based on earlier encounters. Should the individual with aphasia not wish to draw attention to this forgetfulness, conversational repair may not be initiated at the expense of full participation in the current exchange.

MS's performance on the Medical College of Georgia Complex Figures Test (Spreen & Strauss, 1998) (this test requires participants to copy a complex drawing and then reproduce it from memory after a 30 minute delay) indicated that her long-term memory was intact. This was further evidenced by her ability to refer to information that had been discussed some time previously. In the previous sample, A had mentioned that he was now allowed to eat solids that day in preparation for the procedure. In Example 3, MS clearly demonstrates that she has remembered this information. In turn 72, after A had mentioned that he thought he would have something to eat that morning, MS strongly objects (turn 73), and then in turn 75 acknowledges that A did the right thing by not eating as his instructions were clearly to abstain from solid food that day.

Example 3
69.   MS: What did you have last night?
70.   A: I had cereal
71.   MS: Oh (.) yes?
72.   A: A bit of cereal that's all. This morning I had nothing. I thought I'll go down and I'll have something-
73.   MS: NO! NO!
74.   A: But I decided no
75.   MS: Yes no this is right you decided no {pointing to pamphlet, with instructions from the hospital}

Planning/scheduling/strategy use/rule adherence. "Planning" as a notion exists on a continuum from the conceptual to the motoric. In the context of executive functions, the emphasis clearly falls on the conceptual nature of planning. The challenge of applying the notion of planning to varying levels of conversational output is considerable and would have to include planning on a conceptual level in terms of more global features such as topic management to discrete aspects such as syntactic construction of sentences. Furthermore, decreased syntactic complexity may not reflect poor planning, but rather the adaptation of the aphasic speaker to the demands of the communicative environment by minimising syntactic demands in order to reduce or avoid communication breakdown.

MS's performance on a computerised version of the Tower of London task (Shallice, 1982), indicated good forward planning with successful completion of all of the problems presented. A sample of her conversation, below, suggests the presence of forward planning in terms of her message. In turn 61 A had asserted that he was not allowed to eat solid foods that day preceding the procedure. In line 62, the extensive pause (handovers usually take place with split-second timing, and MS is usually able to comply with this convention), suggests some sort of processing or thinking on her part. When she speaks again in turn 63, it is to clarify the content of A's utterance about when exactly he is allowed to eat again. Once this information is provided in turns 64 and 66, MS reiterates the information by asserting that the last time A ate was the previous evening. However, the sentence is marked with paraphasias ("soup" for "eat"; "tonight" for "last night"), interjections, and numerous pauses. The pauses in particular, and to a lesser extent the interjections, appear to serve the purpose of allowing some time to frame or plan the next phrase or utterance, which she eventually checks with the question "yes?" tagged onto the end of her turn.

Example 4
61.   A: There are no solids
62.   (2)
63.   MS: Oh (.) t- no solids the whole day from breakfast until tomorrow morning
64.   A: Until tomorrow after it's all done=
65.   MS: =until?
66.   A: Maybe lunch time tomorrow.
67.   MS: Ok until uh so you don't have to soup (.) no until uh (.3) tomorrow morning
            mm mm mm (1) mm um (1) I think that the last food you had was till tonight
            no (.6) till last night yes?
68.   A: Ja ja ja last night

Areas of deficient EF and cognition and conversation parallels

MS showed deficits in specific areas tested including shifting attention, verbal and nonverbal working memory, generation (fluency/initiation), and concept formation (abstract reasoning) tasks. The latter two appeared to be significantly mediated by deficits of response inhibition (shifting attention), which resulted in perseveration. This factor accounted for her poor performance on both the fluency tasks, the Wisconsin Card Sorting Test, and possibly Raven's Progressive Matrices. The effects of these deficits were most keenly felt during instances of self-initiated self-repair, where MS attempted to repair her own utterances, often with frustrating outcomes.

Shifting attention (response inhibition). Difficulties with divided attention have been identified in individuals with aphasia. These individuals fatigue easily, have impaired selective attention and scanning, and poor shifting of attention back and forth. Such attention deficits seem to manifest in social conversations—particularly during group interaction—where tracking meaning becomes particularly taxing (Godfrey & Shum, 2000). Shifting and dividing attention have further been associated with the ability to adapt to rapid topic shifts and speaker turns during group conversations (Frankel & Penn, in press)—a particular challenge for MS.

Complex attention tasks look at response inhibition and shifting attention among other things. MS's performance on the echopraxic tasks significantly indicated the presence of shifting difficulties. This finding was further confirmed by poor performance on Part B of the Trail Making Test. These shifting difficulties, evident when individuals have trouble inhibiting an action before it is required or after it should stop, results in behaviour that is either impulsive or perseverative. In MS, the presence of response inhibition deficits appeared to underlie perseverative behaviour, of the stuck-in-set kind. This is the inappropriate maintenance of a framework of response after introduction of a new task (Albert & Sandson, 1986). It was further evident in MS's difficulty on the Wisconsin Card Sorting Test.

There is an interesting instance of difficulty with shifting set in Example 5. The excerpt begins with a discussion of whether or not ginger beer is available at the tea garden. This line of conversation appears to be resolved in turn 24. There are five intervening turns, during which A has moved onto discussing other drinks he may be allowed, when, without warning, MS returns to the ginger beer discussion (turn 30). This sudden return to a topic previously closed, rather than the stilted expression, may in fact be at least partly responsible for the trouble spot that ensues in turn 31, with A asking "What's that?". The transcript seems to point to a difficulty with reference rather than comprehension of the sentiment expressed about "something" being unavailable. Evidence for this appears in the following lines when, immediately following resolution of the trouble spot (which MS in this instance manages well), A returns to his previous line of thought.

Example 5
17. A: Oh Gingerbeer is the one that I was thinking of. Gingerbeer might go-
18. MS: Where do you get that from?
19. A: I can get from downstairs I'm sure they must have it.
20. MS: No they don't have it
21. A: They don't have Gingerbeer?
22. MS: {Pulls a questioning face and shrugs shoulders in an "I don't know" gesture}
23. A: Right
24. MS: I doubt it=
25. A: =They have lemonade?
26. MS: Yes they have
27. A: Right they've got lemonade. They've got cream soda uh energy drink
                                               [   ]   [   ]
28. MS: OK   Oh
29. A: Black tea and coffee (1) no milk
30. MS: Oh I don't know if they got Gingerbeer if not the Gingerbeer I don't think
         they have it.
31. A: What's that?
32. MS: Gin(.)gerbeer (.) BEER
33. A: Oh Gingerbeer

Verbal and nonverbal working memory. The notion of working memory is complex, although it is clear that the integrity of working memory has far-reaching implications across multiple cognitive domains. Its definitions and relations link it to higher-order abilities as the cognitive system that permits interactions between attention, perception, and memory. Logie (1999) refers to nonverbal working memory as the capacity to hold an event in mind, across a temporal delay, in order to guide a future response by manipulating that which is held in mind and integrating it with prior knowledge in preparation for use in a range of tasks. Its role in problem-solving tasks is therefore critical, and deficits in this area have been extensively noted in brain-injured populations.

In terms of conversation, working memory deficits typically involve the inability to recall new information or maintain and manipulate current information. Patients who cannot hold recently stated information might lose the thread of social interactions in that they cannot integrate new utterances with a previously stated one (Schapiro & Sacchetti, 1993). This inability means that patients lose the facility for developing coherence, and conversations may become difficult to follow and meaningless, as they represent disembodied texts that have no prior mention or orientation. One could therefore expect impaired topic management resulting in ineffective participation in topic shift, and poor topic maintenance as a result of difficulty recalling previously stated information and how it may relate to a current discussion (Watt & Penn, 2000). These difficulties would be exacerbated during group interactions, especially when multiple speakers may engage in a number of topics and there is considerable amount of input to process.

MS had significant difficulty with the backward portion of the Digit Span test. Her difficulty with verbal working memory ability corresponds with predictions regarding the difficulty of tracking meaning during multi-party conversations in which topics and speakers change rapidly. In addition, MS's performance on the Self Ordered Pointing Test (nonverbal working memory; Spreen & Strauss, 1998) indicated difficulty with visual working and strategic memory. The fact that the test requires the person taking the test to plan, sequence, initiate, and monitor their own pointing responses provides evidence that the task captures important aspects of executive functioning. Performance on this task has a moderate correlation with activities of daily living (Spreen & Strauss, 1998, p. 212). It is therefore interesting to note that despite reduced scores on this task, MS was able to engage in some level of self-monitoring when she was realised she was having difficulty with the task. She adopted a strategy whereby she repeatedly chose the picture in the same position, as she reasoned that different pictures were unlikely to occur in the same space on consecutive pages. Perseveration was ruled out on this task, as MS actually verbalised her strategy. This skill may be reflected in her ability to utilise the tracking and integration skills needed for interactions with either one other person or a small group of people. She displayed excellent topic shift in the one-to-one setting and had no difficulty with topic management in the conversation sample recorded, as seen in the conversational samples above.

Generation/fluency/initiation. Individuals with frontal lobe deficits have been shown to have impaired strategy-generation processes. Once a person has been taught cognitive and behavioural strategies to compensate for his or her communication impairment, it is important that they generalise these strategies to real-life situations. However, patients with aphasia have been shown to have significant difficulty generalising verbal and nonverbal behaviours (Purdy, 2002). MS's performance on both the Five Point Test and the Design Fluency task yielded similarly poor results. Once again her performance was significantly hampered by repetitive and perseverative designs. MS therefore appears to present with an overriding tendency towards perseveration during tasks requiring the output of novel and generative material, resulting from difficulty with shifting attention as extrapolated from her poor scores on the echopraxic and Trails tasks, which may account for several of her conversational characteristics.

Rende's summary (2000) of this difficulty is most pertinent to MS. In aphasia the predominant problem of cognitive flexibility relates to perseveration, and therefore manifests in a lack of spontaneous flexibility and an inability or decreased ability to use flexible strategies to improve their communication. This view accurately depicts MS's difficulty in conversation during periods of frustration when, unable to communicate effectively, she is often unable to shift away from strategies that are not efficient and which do not facilitate communication to different techniques that may assist her more. In the example below, MS is attempting to engage in self-initiated self-repair, whereby she cuts off her own utterances during the same turn in order to revise a previous statement. In turn 95, MS attempts to revise her initial statement no less than five times, each time separated by the interjection "uh". However, this approach does not assist her and she finally gives an exasperated sigh "Agh!", the prolonged "MMM", and then buries her head in her hands. Finally on her sixth attempt, she conveys her intended message.

Example 6
95.   MS: W-what if m- uh uh no yes uh what if they there uh (0.6) sees you at uh five o'
           clock. What happens if Wiver fees you at Agh! M- uh- (4) MMM {buries
           head in hands}
96.   A: Relax relax slowly (3) Take a deep breath and (.) talk again
97.   MS: Um what happens if Iver fetches you at five o'clock or six o' clock?

Concept formation/abstract reasoning. Concept formation or abstraction ability refers to "the ability to shift cognitive strategies in response to changing environmental contingencies" (Lezak, 1995, p. 219). Tests like the Wisconsin Card Sorting Test are thought to measure executive function because they require strategic planning, organised searching, the ability to use environmental feedback to shift cognitive sets, goal-oriented behaviour, and the ability to modulate impulsive responding. The Progressive Matrices are designed to assess the ability to "perceive and ... identify relationships" (Raven, Raven, & Court, 1998, p. SPM 1). Essentially it is the ability to generate new, largely nonverbal (hence its usability in the aphasic population) concepts that make it possible to think clearly (Raven et al., 1998).

Thus performance on these tests could contribute substantially to an understanding of an underlying ability to perceive and conceptualise elements within any situation (in this case, the focus being communicative encounters), and the ability to respond accordingly by gathering a number of potential responses in an organised manner and then systematically choosing the most appropriate response given contextual demands. This cognitive construct is characterised by the ability to identify the gestalt and then respond in a flexible and appropriate manner.

MS achieved significantly poor scores on the Wisconsin Card Sorting Test (WCST). She was able to make only one shift (mean = 5.41, SD = 1.3), and her percentage of responses that constituted perseveration was 56.23% (mean = 15.6, SD = 11.5). This tendency towards perseveration underscores a cognitive inflexibility that does not allow the flexible cognitive shifts necessary for reformulating strategies to meet changing contextual and conversational demands. In the same vein, MS's performance on the Raven's Progressive Matrices indicated similar difficulties with concept formation.

Of all the cognitive deficits assessed, MS's consistent inability to shift set, i.e., her tendency towards perseveration, illuminates the underlying cognitive deficit that may interfere with successful strategy revision during conversation. When confronted with a trouble spot or conversational breakdown, the ability to initiate and engage in repair is undermined by MS's difficulty with changing a given strategy to a different one, even if other avenues afford a better chance of communicative success. In fact, it is possible that other strategies such as drawing or gesture may be limited by the same deficits in creative and flexible expression as her verbal attempts, and therefore do not necessarily represent solutions. MS's experience of not being able to alter or change modes of expression sufficiently to convey her meaning effectively are frequently expressed with a dismissive shrug and the statement "I can't speak." This is clearly depicted in Example 7, where MS is talking to the first author about the event of the stroke. In turns 1, 5, 15, nonverbal gestures, such as eye rolling, tongue clicking, sighing, and shrugging, evidence her impatience with her difficulty with self-expression. In turn 7 there is a long silence, followed by "MMMMM"—uttered in a loud guttural voice—and then she gives up her effort at speech with "I can't talk" in turn 15. The therapist hazards a guess as to what MS may have been trying to say, which allows the breakdown to be repaired and the conversation to continue. However, it is notable that MS appears to be unable to find an alternative means of communicating her message and instead despairs with overt displays of frustration.

Example 7
1. MS: That he couldn't see {clicks tongue, shakes head, holds hand up to indicate that she has not communicated what she wanted to}
2. T: OK
3   MS: mm-mm
4. T: That's not what you wanted to say
5. MS: Yes what I wanted to say is what he um I want to know what he couldn't see {sighs and rolls eyes}
6. T: OK
7. MS: (4.3) MMMMM:
8. T: It's difficult to get it out
9. MS: Yes it's ki-difficult to get it out uh (0.3) uh: phone
10. T: Pat phoned someone
11. MS: Yes=
12. T: =OK
13. MS: Pat phoned my brother there
14. T: Your brother (0.3) the doctor
15. MS: Yes (3) I want to tell you that he phoned my brother at the um at the u {sighs} (0.6) I can't talk {shrugs}
16. T: At the hospital

DISCUSSION

This case study supports the increasingly accepted view that EF and cognitive deficits are likely to account for numerous manifestations of communication difficulty in individuals with aphasia, particularly in conversation. In this case, MS presented with preserved turn-taking and topic management skills but demonstrated poor resolution of conversational breakdown in terms of her inability to initiate compensatory or alternative forms of expression. Despite a growing body of research asserting that people with aphasia can present with varying degrees of impairment in a number of cognitive domains, speech language pathologists have not traditionally been involved in their assessment or treatment (Helm-Estabrooks, 2002). Still, it is becoming clearer that cognitive functions are important predictors of successful treatment and rehabilitation of stroke patients (Riepe et al., 2004). Cognitive impairment is a strong predictor of poor functional outcome post stroke because it impairs the rehabilitation process. Therefore, clinicians should be able to identify the presence, nature, and severity of such deficits to be truly effective in the treatment of the range of cognitive-communicative disorders associated with aphasia. However, assessment and interpretation of tests is complex and requires comprehension of both the principles of EF in general, as well as a thorough understanding of the adaptations required for use with an aphasic population. Additional training and experience in accommodating test procedures for and interpreting test results of adults with acquired speech and language deficits is therefore necessary.

Therapeutic implications also arise from this case study. The possibility exists for fine-tuning conversational approaches to intervention. MS's programme would therefore include non-traditional therapeutic approaches including executive and metacognitive types of therapeutic intervention (Coehlo, 2005; Ylvisaker & Feeney, 1998). It could perhaps be argued that EF testing is equivalent to a type of "poor man's neuroimaging". Certainly in a context like South Africa, where access to advanced neurodiagnostic tools is limited and costly, this is a compelling argument. However, even when opportunities for such validation exist, EF testing would appear to provide not only an explanatory basis for communication symptoms in aphasia but also a facilitating framework for focusing our therapeutic endeavours.

Future research would benefit from taking a longitudinal approach, measuring executive function deficit and recovery in conjunction with conversational profiling over long periods of time. In addition, longitudinal neuroimaging would greatly inform clinicians in terms of locus of EF deficit and its impact on spontaneous communication skills. As has been suggested in this paper and others, and which would warrant further investigation, the hypothesis that we can improve conversation by encouraging EF needs to be tested. This area of research presents an exciting frontier, which needs to be approached in collaborative and novel ways. By merging conversational and neuropsychological approaches to aphasia, we may be able to present more authentic and meaningful support to those of our clients who have not benefited from working within the confines of one paradigm alone.

REFERENCES

Albert, M. L., & Sandson, J. (1986). Perseveration in Aphasia. *Cortex, 22*, 103–115.

Bailey, S., Powell, G., & Clark, E. (1981). A note on intelligence and recovery from aphasia: The relationship between Raven's Matrices Scores and change on the Schuell Aphasia Test. *British Journal of Disorders of Communication, 16*, 193–203.

Beeke, S., Wilkinson, R., & Maxim, J. (2003). Exploring aphasic grammar 2: Do language testing and conversation tell a similar story? *Clinical Linguistics and Phonetics, 17*(2), 109–134.

Coehlo, C. A. (2005). Direct attention training as a treatment for reading impairment in mild aphasia. *Aphasiology, 10*(3/4/5), 275–283.

Crosson, B., Moore, A. B., Gopinath, K., White, K. D., Wierenga, C. E., Gaiefsky, M. E. et al. (2005). Role of the right and left hemispheres in recovery of function during treatment of intention in aphasia. *Journal of Cognitive Neuroscience, 17*(3), 392–406.

Frankel, T., & Penn, C. (in press). The phenomenon of conversational perseveration in traumatic brain injury. *Aphasiology*.

Fuster, J. M. (1989). *The prefrontal cortex*. New York: Raven Press.

Godfrey, H. P. D., & Shum, D. (2000). Executive functioning and the application of social skills following traumatic brain injury. *Aphasiology, 14*(4), 433–444.

Golden, J. C. (1978). *Stroop Color and Word Test*. Illinois: Stoelting Company.

Helm-Estabrooks, N. (2002). Cognition and aphasia: A discussion and a study. *Journal of Communication Disorders, 35*, 171–186.

Helm-Estabrooks, N., Tabor Connor, L., & Albert, M. L. (2000). Treating attention to improve auditory comprehension in aphasia. *Brain and Language, 74*, 469–472.

Keil, K., & Kaszniak, A. W. (2002). Examining executive function in individuals with brain injury: A review. *Aphasiology, 16*(3), 305–336.

Kertesz, A. (1982). *Western Aphasia Battery*. New York: The Psychological Corporation.

Lesser, R., & Milroy, L. (1993). *Linguistics and aphasia: Psycholinguistics and pragmatic aspects of intervention*. Essex, UK: Longman Group Ltd.

Lezak, M. D. (1995). *Neuropsychological Assessment (3rd ed.)*. New York: Oxford University Press.

Logie, R. H. (1999). Working memory. *The Psychologist, 12*(4), 174–178.

McNeil, M. R., Doyle, P. J., Hula, W. D., Rubinksy, H. J., Fossett, T. R. D., & Matthews, C. T. (2004). Using resource allocation theory and dual-task methods to increase the sensitivity of assessment in aphasia. *Aphasiology, 18*(5–7), 521–542.

Miyake, A., Emerson, M. J., & Friedman, N. P. (2000). Assessment of executive functions in clinical settings: Problems and recommendations. *Seminars in Speech and Language, 21*(2), 169–183.

Oelschlaeger, M. L., & Damico, J. S. (2003). Word searchers in aphasia: A study of the collaborative responses of communicative partners. In C. Goodwin (Ed.), *Conversation and brain damage* (pp. 211–227). New York: Oxford University Press.

Ormond Software Enterprises (1999). *The Wisconsin Card Sorting Test*. Johannesburg: Digby Brown Enterprises.

Penn, C. (2000). Paying attention to conversation. *Brain and Language, 71*(4), 185–189.

Purdy, M. (2002). Executive function ability in persons with aphasia. *Aphasiology, 16*(4/5/6), 549–557.

Raven, J., Raven, J. C., & Court, J. H. (1998). *Standard Progressive Matrices*. Oxford, UK: Oxford Psychologists Press.

Rende, B. (2000). Cognitive flexibility: Theory assessment and treatment. *Seminars in Speech and Language, 21*(2), 121–133.

Riepe, M. W., Riss, S., Bittner, D., & Huber, R. (2004). Screening for cognitive impairment in patients with acute stroke. *Dementia and Geriatric Cognitive Disorders, 17*, 49–53.

Rourke, S. B., & Adams, K. M. (1996). The neuropsychological correlates of acute and chronic hypoxemia. In I. Grant & K. M. Adams (Eds.), *Neuropsychological assessment of neuropsychiatric disorders* (pp. 379–422). New York: Oxford University Press.

Schapiro, S. R., & Sacchetti, T. S. (1993) Neuropsychological sequelae of minor head trauma. In S. Mandel, R. T. Sataloff, & S. R. Schapiro (Eds.), *Minor head trauma: Assessment, management and rehabilitation* (pp. 86–106). New York: Springer-Verlag.

Shallice, T. (1982). Specific impairments of planning. *Philosophical Transactions of the Royal Society of London, 298*, 199–209.

Spreen, O., & Strauss, E. (1998). *A compendium of neuropsychological tests: Administration, norms and commentary (2nd ed.)*. New York: Oxford University Press.

Ten Have, P. (1999). *Doing conversation analysis*. London: Sage Publications.

Watt, N., & Penn, C. (2000). Predictors and indicators of return to work following traumatic brain injury in South Africa: Findings from a preliminary experimental database. *South African Journal of Psychology, 30*(2), 27–37.

Ylvisaker, M., & Feeney, T. J. (1998). *Collaborative brain injury intervention*. San Diego, CA: Singular Publishing Group.

APPENDIX A

Conversation analysis: Transcription symbols (Lesser & Milroy, 1993)

(0.0)	Gaps in tenths of seconds
(.)	Micropause
(hhh)	Laughter
==	Latched utterances (no pause between turns)
:	Prolonged syllable (e.g., mme for "me" and heee for "he")
?	Rising intonation contour (e.g., when asking a question)
[ ]	Overlapping utterances (speakers talk at the same time)
-	Cut off prior word or sound
CAPITALS	Relatively loud speech
underlined	Extra stress/emphasis
{...}	Nonverbal behaviours

APPENDIX B

Executive functioning battery

CONSTRUCTS	TESTS	ADAPTATIONS	SCORES
Simple Attention – Sustained attention	(a) Digit Span (forward) (Lezak, 1995) (b) Bells Cancellation Tests (Lezak, 1995).	(a) None needed. MS's performance on the repetition sub-test of the WAB indicated an ability to repeat lengthy phrases (b) No time limit imposed	(a) 6 forward (normal limits; Lezak, 1995). (b) 33/35 (norm = 32 or more; Lezak, 1995).
Complex Attention (a) Suppression (interference control) (b) Shifting (response inhibition)	(a) (i) Stroop Colour-Word Interference Test (Golden, 1978) (ii) Echopraxic Tasks (Spreen & Strauss, 1998). (b) Trail Making (Lezak, 1995).	(a) (i) The score is based on a ratio of time taken to complete the second task compared to the first. (ii) Tasks that required foot tapping of the unaffected leg were used. (b) The motoric pattern needed to complete Parts A and B was identical. Speed was measured as a ratio between the two parts.	(a) (i) Interference score = 131.95; normal limits (mean = 123.04; SD = 35.77) (Golden, 1978). (ii) Six errors in one minute (five errors in a minute indicate deficit) (Spreen & Strauss, 1998) (b) Trails B = 255 (mean = 122; SD = 62) (Rourke & Adams, 1996).
Verbal working memory and Nonverbal working memory	Digit Span (backwards) (Lezak, 1995) Self-Ordered Pointing Test (Spreen & Strauss, 1998).	None needed None needed	2 digit sequence (norm = 4 to 5 digit sequence) (Lezak, 1995). 10 errors, (mean = 4.68, SD = .53) (Spreen & Strauss, 1998)
Memory	Medical College of Georgia complex figures (Spreen & Strauss, 1998)	None needed as there was no time limit.	36 (mean = 31.19; SD = 3.68) (Spreen & Strauss, 1998).
Planning/scheduling/ strategy use/rule adherence	Tower of London (Shallice, 1982)	Tester manipulated computer mouse. Timing constraints were discarded.	MS solved all of the 12 problems independently
Generation/fluency/ initiation	(a) Five Point Test (Spreen & Strauss, 1998) (b) Design Fluency (Spreen & Strauss, 1998)	None needed	(a) 47% of total designs were perseverative, the cut-off being 15% (Spreen & Strauss, 1998). (b) 5 (mean = 11.8; SD = 4.4) (Spreen & Strauss, 1998).
Concept formation/abstract reasoning	(a) Wisconsin Card Sorting Test (Ormond Software Enterprises, 1999)	(a) The examiner manipulated the mouse	(a) 1 correct sort (mean = 5.4, SD = 1.3). 84 incorrect responses (mean = 24.9; SD = 19.4) 72 perseverative responses (mean = 15.6; SD = 11.5). (b) 10th percentile rank (Raven et al., 1998)